DATA INTERPRETATION FOR MEDICAL STUDENTS

Second Edition

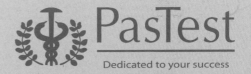

PasTest

Dedicated to your success

DATA INTERPRETATION FOR MEDICAL STUDENTS

Second Edition

Paul K Hamilton

BSc(Hons), MB BCh BAO(Hons)
MRCP(UK) MD

Consultant Physician

Belfast Health and Social Care Trust

Belfast

United Kingdom

Ian C Bickle

MB BCh BAO(Hons), FRCR

Consultant Radiologist
RIPAS Hospital
Brunei Darussalam

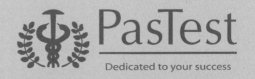

PasTest
Dedicated to your success

© 2012 PASTEST LTD
Egerton Court
Parkgate Estate
Knutsford
Cheshire
WA16 8DX

Telephone: 01565 752000

First published 2006, reprinted 2007, second edition 2012

ISBN: 190563577X

ISBN: 9781905635771

A catalogue record for this book is available from the British Library.

The information contained within this book was obtained by the authors from reliable sources. However, while every effort has been make to ensure its accuracy, no responsibility for loss, damage or injury occasioned to any person acting or refraining from action as a result of information contained herein can be accepted by the publishers or authors.

PasTest Revision Books and Intensive Courses

PasTest has been established in the field of postgraduate medical education since 1972, providing revision books and intensive study courses for doctors preparing for their professional examinations.

Books and courses are available for the following specialties:

MRCGP, MRCP Parts 1 and 2, MRCPCH Parts 1 and 2, MRCPsych, MRCS, MRCOG Parts 1 and 2, DRCOG, DCH, FRCA, PLAB Parts 1 and 2, Dental Students, Dentists and Dental Nurses.

For further details contact:

PasTest, Freepost, Knutsford, Cheshire WA16 7BR

Tel: 01565 752000 Fax: 01565 650264

www.pastest.co.uk enquires@pastest.co.uk

Illustrations by Ben Stockham
Text prepared by Carnegie Book Production, Lancaster, UK

Printed and bound in the Uk by Page Bros, Norwich

Contents

Preface to the second edition

The practice of medicine in the twenty-first century is centred on data interpretation. Never before have so many tests been available to help diagnose disease and monitor patient progress. One difficulty facing students and junior doctors is in choosing which tests to request. This is especially important in the current financial climate where ordering a range of unnecessary tests will be very costly for the health service. Once a test result is back, the investigator must be able to interpret the result confidently and accurately. We encourage investigations to be assessed in a sequential manner, with their interpretation dictating subsequent tests, rather than a 'blunder-bus' approach. This is professionally more satisfying and more educational, and encourages thoughtful medicine and sensible use of resources.

We hope that the latest edition of this book will help you as you begin interpreting all forms of data for your patients. All aspects of the book have been reviewed for the second edition. New sections have been written to incorporate latest developments, difficult concepts have been further clarified, and more example cases have been added to test your understanding. The imaging section has been extended in keeping with the increasing influence that this plays in everyday clinical medicine.

The first edition has been more successful than we could have imagined; however, after 5 years a refresher was much needed.

It is our hope that, in some small way, the care of patients will be improved from the use of this text.

Acknowledgements

We have included material that we feel represents common scenarios and that best illustrates the various investigations in medicine. All material has received intensive feedback during the production process to ensure that it is readable and usable. We both greatly value constructive criticism, and ideas to improve this text further would be very welcome. Please e-mail us on datainterpretationformedicalstudents@pastest.co.uk if you have any suggestions.

A hugely influential contributor to this book must be mentioned first. Sandy Davey is a current medical student in Queen's University Belfast. His unique qualities, limitless enthusiasm and bravery to comment have helped shape the final draft of this book. We both owe him a huge debt of gratitude.

A special mention must also be made of the contributions of Professor Patrick Bell who reviewed the book critically.

We also owe our Commissioning Editor at Pastest, Elizabeth Kerr, our sincere thanks and apologies – thanks for supporting us throughout this project and making valuable comments; apologies for having to put up with our incessant demands, impatience and peculiarities.

Thanks are extended to Joel Rankin for assisting with the ECGs, Dr Barry Kelly for providing a selection of radiographs, and Dr Ann Johnston for reviewing the neurology section.

PH would like to thank his parents and sister Kerry for their never-ending support and encouragement. He also thanks Anna for her incredible patience during the writing process.

ICB would like to thank Haiza who, despite his spending hours putting this book together, still agreed to marry him!

Like the world of medicine, our own lives has changed since the 1st edition in 2005. We have both been blessed with beautiful daughters to whom we dedicate this 2nd edition.

Chloe and Nur Ayesha, you are the sunshine in your Daddy's eyes.

Normal values

Haematology

Full blood picture

Haemoglobin (Hb)	
Males	13.5–18 g/dl
Females	11.5–16 g/dl
Mean cell volume (MCV)	76–96 fl
Packed cell volume (PCV)	
Males	0.4–0.54
Females	0.37–0.47
Red cell distribution width (RDW)	12–15%
White cell count (WCC)	$4.0–11.0 \times 10^9/l$
Neutrophils	$2.0–7.5 \times 10^9/l$
Lymphocytes	$1.5–4.0 \times 10^9/l$
Eosinophils	$0.04–0.4 \times 10^9/l$
Monocytes	$0.2–0.8 \times 10^9/l$
Basophils	$0.0–0.1 \times 10^9/l$
Platelets	$150–400 \times 10^9/l$
Reticulocytes	0.5–2.5% of red blood cells
Erythrocyte sedimentation rate (ESR)	
Males	0–15 mm/h
Females	0–22 mm/h
HbA1c (glycated haemoglobin)	3.8–6.4%

Tests of clotting

Activated partial thromboplastin time (APTT)	35–45 s
Prothrombin time (PT)	12–16 s
Fibrinogen	2–4 g/l
Bleeding time	3–9 min
D-dimer	<0.5 mg/l

Haematinics

Iron studies	
Iron	11–32 mol/l
Total iron-binding capacity (TIBC)	42–80 mol/l
Ferritin	12–200 µg/l
Folate	>2 µg/l
Vitamin B$_{12}$	>150 ng/l

Biochemistry

Urea and electrolytes (U&Es)

Sodium (Na$^+$)	135–145 mmol/l
Potassium (K$^+$)	3.5–5.0 mmol/l
Urea	2.5–6.7 mmol/l
Creatinine	79–118 µmol/l (dependent on muscle mass)
Chloride (Cl$^-$)	95–105 mmol/l
Bicarbonate (HCO$_3^-$)	24–30 mmol/l

Liver function tests

Total bilirubin	3–17 µmol/l
Aspartate aminotransferase (AST)	5–35 IU/l
Alanine aminotransferase (ALT)	5–35 IU/l
Alkaline phosphatase (ALP)	30–150 U/l
γ-Glutamyl transpeptidase (GGT)	
Male	11–58 IU/l
Female	7–33 IU/l
Albumin	35–50 g/l

Bone profile

Corrected calcium (Ca^{2+}) (total)	2.10–2.65 mmol/l
Phosphate (PO$_4^{3-}$)	0.8–1.45 mmol/l
Alkaline phosphatase (ALP)	30–150 U/l
Albumin	35–50 g/l

Poisoning

Alcohol	Nil
Carboxyhaemoglobin	<5% of total haemoglobin
Paracetamol	Nil
Salicylates	Nil

Tumour markers

α-Fetoprotein (AFP)	
<50 years	<10 kU/l
50–70 years	<15 kU/l
70–90 years	<20 kU/l
β Human chorionic gonadotrophin (β-hCG)	<5 U/l
CA-125	<35 U/ml
CA-19-9	<37 U/ml
Carcinoembryonic antigen (CEA)	<10 ng/ml

Prostate-specific antigen (PSA; males)

40–49 years	<2.5 ng/ml
50–59 years	<3.5 ng/ml
60–69 years	<4.5 ng/ml
70–79 years	<6.5 ng/ml

Arterial blood gas analysis

pH	7.35–7.45
Arterial partial pressure of oxygen breathing room air (PaO_2)	11–13 kPa
Arterial partial pressure of carbon dioxide breathing room air ($PaCO_2$)	4.7–6.0 kPa
Bicarbonate	24–30 mmol/l
Base excess (BE)	−2 to +2 mmol/l
Anion gap	12–16 mmol/l

Immunoglobulins

IgA	0.8–4.0 g/l
IgG	7.0–14.5 g/l
IgM	0.45–2.0 g/l

Other

Amylase	25–125 U/l
C-reactive protein (CRP)	<10 mg/l
Creatine kinase (CK)	
Male	25–195 IU/l
Female	25–170 IU/l
CK-MB	<25 IU/l
Globulin	18–36 g/l
Glucose	See page 152
Lactate	0.5–2.0 mmol/l
Lactate dehydrogenase (LDH)	70–250 IU/l
N-terminal pro-brain natriuretic protein (NT-proBNP)	<125 pmol/l
Osmolality (plasma)	280–300 mosmol/kg
pH	7.35–7.45
Total protein	60–80 g/l
Troponin I	<0.1 µg/l
Troponin T	<0.03 µg/l
Urate	0.15–0.50 mmol/l

Endocrinology

Cortisol
    9am   200–700 nmol/l
    10pm   50–250 nmol/l

Cortisol	
9am	200–700 nmol/l
10pm	50–250 nmol/l
Free thyroxine (T_4)	7.6–19.7 pmol/l
Thyroid-stimulating hormone (TSH)	0.4–4.5 mU/l
Total thyroxine (T_4)	70–140 nmol/l

Therapeutic drug levels

Digoxin (6 hours post-dose)	0.8–2.0 nmol/l
Lithium	0.5–1.5 mmol/l

Cerebrospinal fluid

Glucose	2.5–4.4 mmol/l (two-thirds of plasma value)
Red cell count (RCC)	0/mm^3
Total protein	<0.45 g/l
White cell count (WCC)	<5/mm^3

Urine

Creatinine clearance	
Male	85–125 ml/min
Female	75–115 ml/min
Metanephrines	<5.5 µmol/day
Osmolality	250–1250 mosmol/kg
Protein	<0.2 g/day

Sweat

Chloride	<60 mmol/l

HAEMATOLOGY

HAEMATOLOGY

One of the most frequently requested tests in medicine is the full blood picture (FBP). This contains a wealth of information about the components of blood. The typical constituent parts of the FBP are as shown in the box.

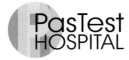

PasTest HOSPITAL

FULL BLOOD PICTURE
A typical FBP comprises the following tests:
Haemoglobin concentration (Hb)
Mean cell volume (MCV)
Mean corpuscular haemoglobin (MCH)
Packed cell volume (PCV)
Red cell distribution width (RDW)
White cell count (WCC) incorporating a differential white cell count
Platelet count
Reticulocyte count

Abnormalities with red blood cells

Anaemia

Anaemia describes a low level of haemoglobin. It is usually defined by an arbitrary cut-off haemoglobin concentration (eg 13 g/dl in men aged >15 years, 12 g/dl in non-pregnant women aged >15 years and 11 g/dl in pregnant women), below which a patient is deemed to be anaemic.

Before deciding on the particular subtype of anaemia present in a patient, it is worth looking at the other cell types described on the full blood picture. If there are problems with red cells, white cells and platelets, then the major problem is likely to be a disease of the bone marrow, and the test most likely to give the diagnosis would be a bone marrow biopsy.

If the only problem on the full blood picture is low haemoglobin, the next stage is to check the reticulocyte count. Reticulocytes are immature red blood cells, and will be found in increased amounts in patients who are bleeding and in those in whom red cells are being destroyed (haemolysis). The history should distinguish between these types. If the reticulocyte count is not elevated, the next step in diagnosis is to look at the size of the red cells (erythrocytes).

Anaemia can be split into three big groups by looking at the size of the red blood cells. In microcytic anaemia red cells are small, in normocytic anaemia they are normal size and in macrocytic anaemia they are large. The mean cell volume (MCV) provides an average measurement of red cell size.

TYPE OF ANAEMIA	SIZE OF ERYTHROCYTES
Microcytic	Small
Normocytic	Normal
Macrocytic	Large

The diagram on page 5 shows the various causes based on this classification of anaemia.

Note that the MCV provides a measure of average cell size, and this is reliable in most instances. If, however, a patient has two ongoing pathologies, such as iron deficiency and folate deficiency, the MCV can be unreliable. They may have two populations of red cells, one with a low MCV and another with a high MCV. When these measures are averaged, the MCV will be normal. For this reason, the red cell distribution width (RDW) is sometimes measured. This gives an indication of the distribution of red cell sizes. This measure will be raised if two red cell populations are present.

Fig 1.1: The various causes of the major classifications of anaemia.

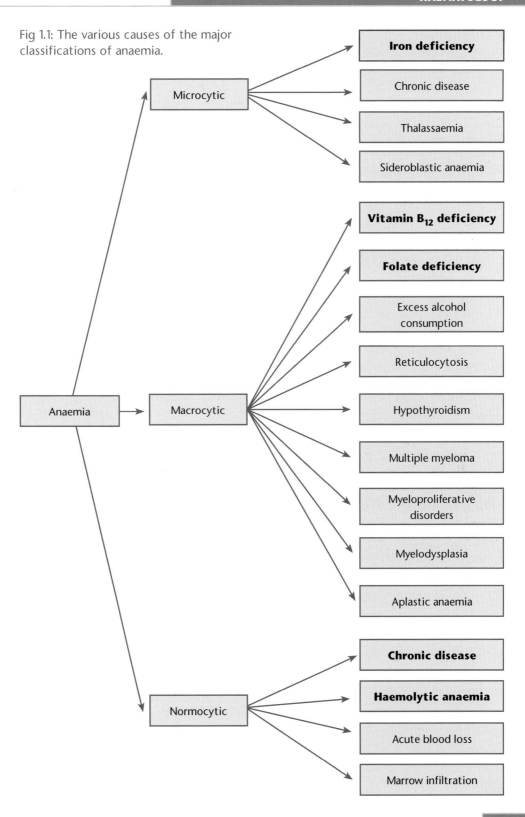

Haematinics

Deficiencies in any of three key nutrients – iron, vitamin B_{12} and folate – can result in anaemia. These nutrients are called haematinics. Iron deficiency is the most common cause of anaemia, and is commonly found in association with blood loss.

DEFICIENCY	TYPE OF ANAEMIA
Iron	Microcytic
Vitamin B_{12}	Macrocytic
Folate	Macrocytic

Finding a haematinic deficiency is only the first part of establishing the cause of anaemia. Where possible, the cause of the nutrient deficiency should also be sought. For example, iron deficiency is often due to blood loss from the gastrointestinal tract, and endoscopy is often used to search for this.

Knowledge of exactly where haematinics are absorbed from the gastrointestinal tract can sometimes help localise the pathology underlying anaemia. These sites are shown in the box below.

HAEMATINIC	ABSORBED FROM
Iron	Duodenum and jejunum
Vitamin B_{12}	Terminal ileum
Folate	Small bowel

Iron studies

A good understanding of how the body handles iron is required before iron studies can be interpreted.

Iron is best absorbed from the upper small bowel in the ferrous (Fe^{2+}) state. Iron is transported across the intestinal cell and into the plasma. Iron in the plasma is carried to developing red cells in the bone marrow by a protein called transferrin. Iron is stored in the body as ferritin and haemosiderin. Red cells have transferrin receptors (soluble transferrin receptors, sTfRs) which can be measured in plasma.

COMPONENTS OF AN IRON PROFILE

Serum iron

Serum total iron-binding capacity (serum TIBC)

Serum ferritin

Transferrin saturation

Serum soluble transferrin receptors

In iron deficiency states, iron studies are as follows:

IRON PARAMETER	RESULT
Serum iron	Reduced
Serum total iron-binding capacity	Increased – the body tries hard to bind any iron around the system
Serum ferritin	Reduced – since iron stores are low
Transferrin saturation	Reduced
Serum sTfRs	Increased – since red cells attempt to absorb any iron in the system

The serum ferritin level is the single best test for iron deficiency, with levels of below 15 µg/l being suggestive.

To make matters a little more confusing, ferritin behaves as an acute phase reactant – its level increases with active inflammation, in the same way as the erythrocyte sedimentation rate (ESR) and C-reactive protein (CRP) (see pages 17 and 74). This means that, in states of iron deficiency associated with an ongoing inflammatory process (eg an active infection), the serum ferritin level may be high. However, the sTfR will reveal the true state of affairs.

Unfortunately sTfR is not routinely available, and often clinical judgement is required in such situations. Sometimes, it can be difficult to be sure that a patient is iron deficient, and in such circumstances a trial of iron treatment may be necessary. Once the diagnosis has been established, it is imperative that a reason for the iron deficiency be sought.

In cases of diagnostic uncertainty, a bone marrow biopsy can be obtained and stained for the presence of iron. In iron deficiency states, little or no iron will be seen in the marrow.

Iron studies are also abnormal in states of iron overload. This is commonly seen in haemochromatosis and in haematological conditions that require frequent blood transfusions. In such cases, serum iron, ferritin and transferrin saturation are raised. The total iron-binding capacity (TIBC) is usually low.

In anaemia of chronic disease, iron studies are commonly as follows:

IRON PARAMETER	RESULT
Serum iron	Normal or slightly reduced
Serum total iron-binding capacity	Reduced
Serum ferritin	May be raised as acute phase reactant
Transferrin saturation	Reduced
Serum sTfR	Normal – reflecting the true state of body iron levels

Goddard AG, James MW, McIntyre AS, et al. (2011) Guidelines for the management of iron deficiency anaemia. *Gut* doi:10.1136/gut.2010.228874.

Vitamin B_{12}

Vitamin B_{12} deficiency may result from inadequate intake, but the most common reason for deficiency relates to poor absorption.

In health, vitamin B_{12} is bound to a protein called intrinsic factor secreted by gastric parietal cells. The vitamin is then absorbed from the ileum. Poor absorption generally results from the absence of intrinsic factor or disease of the ileum.

The most common disease causing vitamin B_{12} deficiency is pernicious anaemia, in which there is defective intrinsic factor production. The disease is associated with autoantibodies against gastric parietal cells and intrinsic factor (see Chapter 8).

Schilling test

The Schilling test may be used to distinguish between the various causes of vitamin B_{12} deficiency. In this test, patients are given two doses of vitamin B_{12}. One dose is radioactively labelled and given orally. The other dose is given intramuscularly with the aim of flushing absorbed radiolabelled vitamin B_{12} into the urine. The urine is collected over a period of 24 hours. Normally, a proportion of the oral vitamin B_{12} dose will be absorbed and excreted, so that more than 10% of the oral dose will be excreted in the urine. With vitamin B_{12} malabsorption, this amount will be reduced. Unfortunately, despite the eloquence of the Schilling test, it is being used with decreasing frequency, and in some areas is no longer available.

The test is repeated with an oral preparation of intrinsic factor being given at the same time as the oral dose of vitamin B_{12}. If the test results are now normal, one can assume that the patient's problem lies with inadequate intrinsic factor. If the test is still abnormal, the problem most likely lies in the ileum.

One possible cause of ileal disease is bacterial overgrowth. In order to test for this possibility, the patient can be given a course of antibiotics. If the Schilling test returns to normal after this, the diagnosis of bacterial overgrowth can be made. Alternatively, bacterial overgrowth can be diagnosed using a breath test. The most commonly used test is the hydrogen breath test. A carbohydrate load is given orally. Bacteria in the small bowel metabolise the carbohydrate, liberating hydrogen which is absorbed and detected in exhaled air.

Folate

Folate analysis is simple. Serum folate levels are measured with a deficiency identified if levels are low.

Haemolytic anaemia

There are many causes of haemolytic anaemia, but in each case there is abnormal destruction of red blood cells.

Evidence of haemolysis

When red blood cells are destroyed, haemoglobin is degraded, and bibirubin liberated. Bilirubin is conjugated in the liver and passed into the bowel in the bile. Here, it is converted into urobilinogen. Some of this is passed in the stools; some is reabsorbed, and excreted in the urine, where it can be detected using a urinalysis strip. In cases of haemolysis, the plasma unconjugated bilirubin will rise, and increased amounts of urobilinogen will be detected in the urine. The level of lactate dehydrogenase (LDH) will also rise.

When red cells are destroyed inside blood vessels, haemoglobin is released. Haptoglobins bind to free haemoglobin and escort it to the liver. However, haptoglobins can become saturated and in such circumstances haemoglobin may be passed in the urine (haemoglobinuria), or converted to haemosiderin which is then passed in the urine (haemosiderinuria). Alternatively, further reactions can occur which result in the presence of methaemalbumin in the circulation.

INTRAVASCULAR HAEMOLYSIS IS SUGGESTED BY

- low haptoglobins
- haemosiderinuria
- methaemalbumin (detected in the Schumm test)

With excessive red cell destruction, the bone marrow works hard to replace the number of circulating cells. The number of primitive red cells (reticulocytes) in the circulation therefore increases.

The causes of haemolytic anaemia are illustrated in the diagram on page 11.

Osmotic fragility test

Hereditary spherocytosis is a condition associated with an abnormal red blood cell membrane where red cells become spherical in shape. The cells are less resilient to damage in this condition. This can be assessed using an osmotic fragility test. Spherocytes have increased osmotic fragility.

Direct antiglobulin test

In autoimmune haemolytic anaemias, antibodies attack red cells and cause their destruction. The main laboratory test for autoimmune haemolytic anaemia is the direct antiglobulin test (DAT or Coombs' test). In this test, antibodies to human immunoglobulin are added to a sample of red cells from the patient. If the red cells are coated in antibodies (ie if the patient has an autoimmune haemolytic anaemia), they will agglutinate.

World Health Organization (2008). *Worldwide Prevalence of Anaemia*, 1993–2005. Geneva: WHO.

Fig 1.2: The causes of haemolytic anaemia.

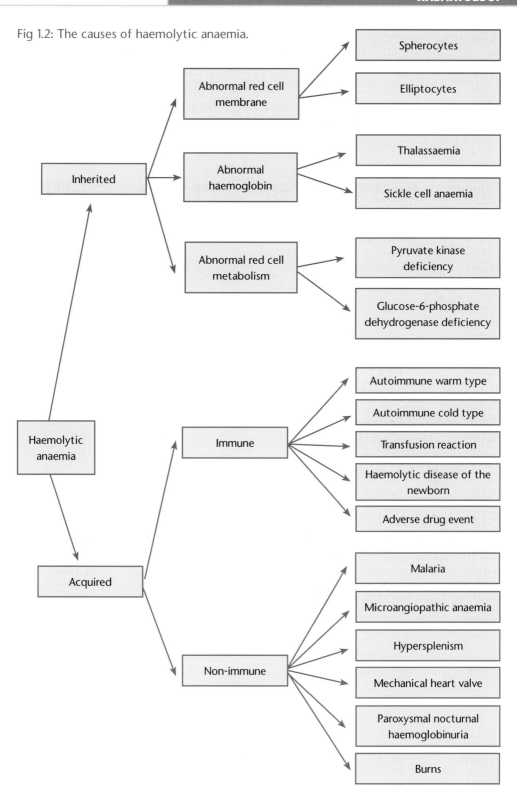

Polycythaemia

Polycythaemia is defined as a packed cell volume (PCV) greater than 0.51 in males or greater than 0.48 in females.

POLYCYTHAEMIA
Males – PCV >0.51
Females – PCV >0.48

Red cell mass

In order to distinguish between true and apparent polycythaemia, the red cell mass must be measured. In true polycythaemia, the red cell mass is raised. Apparent polycythaemia is due to a reduction in plasma volume rather than an increase in red cell mass.

Red cell mass is measured by labelling red cells with a radioactive isotope. A predicted red cell mass can be calcuated based on the patient's height and weight. True polycythaemia is diagnosed if the red cell mass is more than 25% higher than that predicted.

To distinguish between causes of true polycythaemia, further tests should be arranged. These usually include:

- arterial blood gas analysis (to look for hypoxia)
- erythropoietin level (to detect inappropriately high levels)
- an ultrasound of the abdomen (to detect structural renal or hepatic disease and to visualise the spleen)
- further investigations depending on the most likely cause.

Haemoglobinopathies

Haemoglobin electrophoresis can be used to diagnose a variety of diseases in which the structure of haemoglobin is abnormal. The most common diseases of this type are sickle cell disease and the thalassaemias. In sickle cell disease, haemoglobin electrophoresis shows the presence of HbS.

Polycythaemia can be subdivided as shown in Fig 1.3.

Fig 1.3: Causes of polycythaemia.

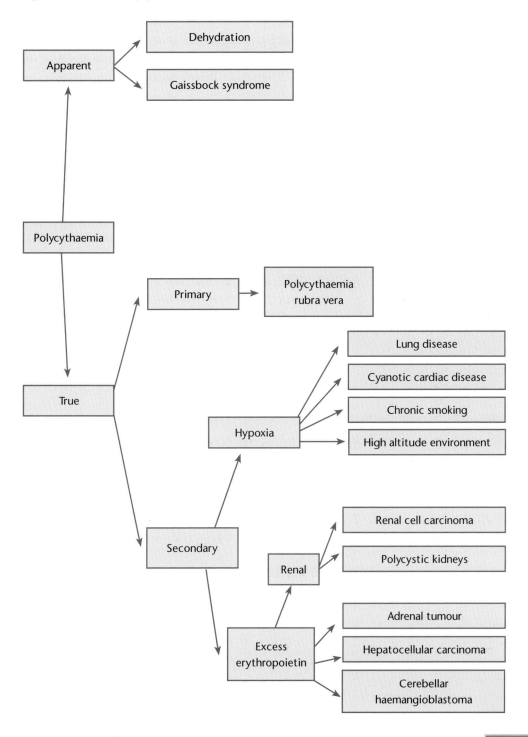

Abnormalities with white blood cells

Abnormal white cell counts

Abnormalities in white blood cell counts are common. The most frequently occurring abnormalities are listed in the boxes below with common causes.

COMMON CAUSES OF NEUTROPHILIA (NEUTROPHILS >7.5 X 10⁹/l)

Bacterial infections	Malignancy
Inflammation	Myeloproliferative disorders
Necrosis, eg after myocardial infarction	Metabolic disorders, eg renal failure
Treatment with corticosteroids	

COMMON CAUSES OF NEUTROPENIA (NEUTROPHILS <2.0 X 10⁹/l)

Post-chemotherapy
Post-radiotherapy
Adverse drug reactions, eg clozapine, carbimazole
Viral infection
Felty syndrome

COMMON CAUSES OF LYMPHOCYTOSIS (LYMPHOCYTES >3.5 X 10⁹/l)

Viral infections
Chronic infections, eg TB
Chronic lymphocytic leukaemia
Lymphomas

COMMON CAUSES OF EOSINOPHILIA (EOSINOPHILS >0.5 X 10⁹/l)

Allergic disorders	Skin diseases, eg eczema
Parasite infection	Malignancy, eg Hodgkin disease
Hypereosinophilic syndrome	Allergic bronchopulmonary aspergillosis

Abnormalities with platelets

Thrombocytosis

Thrombocytosis describes a high platelet count (>400 x 10^9/l). The common causes are shown in the box below.

COMMON CAUSES OF THROMBOCYTOSIS	
Primary haematological diseases:	**Reactive thrombocytosis secondary to:**
• Essential thrombocythaemia and other myeloproliferative disorders • Chronic myeloid leukaemia • Myelodysplasia	• Infection • Inflammation • Malignancy • Bleeding • Pregnancy • Post-splenectomy

Thrombocytopenia

Thrombocytopenia describes a low platelet count (<150 x 10^9/l). The common causes are shown in the box below.

CAUSES OF THROMBOCYTOPENIA

Reduced platelet production due to bone marrow failure:
- Infections (particularly viral, eg infectious mononucleosis)
- Drug induced, eg penicillamine
- Leukaemia
- Aplastic anaemia
- Myelofibrosis (later stages)
- Bone marrow replacement with tumour, eg myeloma or metastases
- Myelodysplasia
- Megaloblastic anaemia

Increased platelet destruction:
- Immune-mediated platelet destruction
  - Autoimmune idiopathic thrombocytopenia purpura (AITP)
  - Drug induced, particularly heparin-induced thrombocytopenia (HIT)
- Hypersplenism
- Thrombotic thrombocytopenic purpura/haemolytic uraemic syndrome
- Disseminated intravascular coagulation (DIC)
- After a massive blood transfusion

PLATELET CLUMPING

This is a relatively common cause for an apparently low platelet count. If a blood sample is sent to the laboratory in a tube containing anticoagulant, clumping will not occur and the true platelet count will be apparent. It is therefore always worth sending a 'citrated' sample for a platelet count if unexpected thrombocytopenia is found.

Pancytopenia

Pancytopenia is the term used to describe the pattern present when there are low levels of red blood cells, white blood cells and platelets in the circulation. There are a wide variety of causes, the most common of which are shown in the box.

COMMON CAUSES OF PANCYTOPENIA

- Aplastic anaemia
- Bone marrow infiltration, eg with tumour
- Hypersplenism
- Megaloblastic anaemia
- Sepsis
- Systemic lupus erythematosus (SLE)

Erythrocyte sedimentation rate

The erythrocyte sedimentation rate (ESR) measures how rapidly red blood cells form sediment when a column of blood is kept upright for 1 hour. The further the red cells sink in the hour, the higher the ESR.

The ESR is a non-specific marker of disease. In inflammatory processes, raised levels of plasma proteins result in red blood cells forming clumps called rouleaux. These clumps of cells sink more easily than single cells, and thus, in the presence of such proteins, the ESR is high.

The ESR normally rises with advancing age, but levels of more than 35 mm/h should raise the suspicion of a disease process in any age group. Causes of a raised ESR are myriad. Common examples are listed in the box below.

COMMON CAUSES OF A RAISED ESR

- Infectious disease
- Neoplastic disease (particularly multiple myeloma)
- Connective tissue disease (particularly giant cell arteritis and polymyalgia rheumatica)
- Anaemia
- Renal disease

Blood film abnormalities

Examination of a peripheral blood film can aid or clinch a diagnosis in a range of clinical scenarios. Correct identification of various cell types requires significant training, but knowledge of the different terminology used can greatly aid interpretation of blood film reports. The following abnormal cell types are among those most commonly seen.

Abnormal erythrocyte colour or shape

ABNORMALITY	MEANING	FOUND IN
Hypochromic cells	Pale red cells	Iron deficiency or defective haemoglobin synthesis
Microcytosis	Small cells	Iron deficiency or defective haemoglobin synthesis
Macrocytosis	Large cells	Megaloblastic anaemia, high alcohol intake, liver disease
Pencil cells	Pencil-shaped cells	Iron deficiency
Spherocytes	Spherical cells	Hereditary spherocytosis, haemolytic anaemia, burns
Elliptocytes	Elliptical cells	Hereditary elliptocytosis, thalassaemia major, iron deficiency
Acanthocytes	Spiky-appearing cells	Abetalipoproteinaemia, post-splenectomy, liver disease
Target cells	Target-like cells	Thalassaemia, iron deficiency, post-splenectomy, liver disease
Stomatocytes	Cells with mouth-shaped area of pallor	Hereditary stomatocytosis, high alcohol intake, liver disease
Ecchinocytes	Also known as burr cells – less spiky than acanthocytes	Post-splenectomy, liver disease, uraemia
Sickle cells	Sickle shaped	Sickle cell anaemia (homozygous HbS disease)

ABNORMALITY	MEANING	FOUND IN
Fragmented cells	Broken pieces of cell	Microangiopathic haemolytic anaemia, haemolytic uraemic syndrome, thrombotic thrombocytopenic purpura, mechanical heart valves, disseminated intravascular coagulation
Tear cells (dacryocytes)	Tear-shaped cells	Myelofibrosis and other causes of extramedullary haematopoiesis
Poikilocytosis	Abnormal shapes of red cells	Iron deficiency
Anisochromia	Varying shades of colour	Iron deficiency

Abnormalities inside erythrocytes

ABNORMALITY	FOUND IN
Heinz bodies	Unstable haemoglobin states
Howell–Jolly bodies	Hyposplenism, post-splenectomy
Pappenheimer bodies	Post-splenectomy, haemolytic anaemia, sideroblastic anaemia
Basophilic stippling	Lead poisoning, thalassaemia, myelodysplasia
Cabot rings	Myelodysplasia, megaloblastic anaemia

Abnormal white blood cells

ABNORMALITY	FOUND IN
Hypersegmented neutrophils	Megaloblastic anaemias, chronic infections
Toxic granulation of neutrophils	Bacterial infection, poisoning, burns, chemotherapy
Auer rods	Acute myeloid leukaemia
Smear cells	Chronic lymphocytic leukaemia

Leukoerythroblastic blood film

This is a term used to describe the overall appearance of a blood film in which immature red and white blood cells are seen in peripheral blood. There are several causes.

CAUSES OF A LEUKOERYTHROBLASTIC BLOOD FILM
• Bone marrow infiltration, eg with tumour • Idiopathic myelofibrosis • Severe sepsis • Haemolysis

Coagulation disorders

Haemostasis (the process of stopping bleeding) is a complex process. It involves the interplay of blood vessel walls, platelets and clotting factors. The common tests used to assess coagulation are as follows:

COMMON TESTS OF COAGULATION
• Prothrombin time (PT) • International normalised ratio (INR) • Activated partial thromboplastin time (APTT) • Bleeding time

Prothrombin time

The PT is dependent on clotting factors I, II, V, VII and X. In clinical practice, it is most commonly measured to assess the synthetic function of the liver (eg in liver failure), or to monitor the effects of warfarin therapy.

International normalised ratio

To allow comparison of coagulation results between laboratories, the PT is often converted to the INR, by applying a correction factor. This takes into account differences in laboratory methods, and means that the patient's INR should be the same regardless of the laboratory used to measure it.

The INR is the parameter most commonly used to monitor the effects of warfarin. In a patient with normal coagulation, the INR will be close to 1.0 before warfarin is commenced. As warfarin is introduced, the INR rises. The higher the INR, the less coagulable the blood becomes (ie the more difficult it will be for the blood to clot). Target INRs are set, and warfarin dosing must be adjusted to aim for these targets.

DISEASE	TARGET INR
Deep venous thrombosis (DVT)	2.5
Pulmonary embolism (PE)	2.5
Atrial fibrillation	2.5
Mechanical prosthetic heart valve	2.5
Recurrent DVT/PE in a patient with a therapeutic INR	3.5

The essence of warfarin prescribing involves increasing the dose if the INR is too low, reducing the dose if the INR is too high, and omitting it if the INR is dangerously high or the patient is bleeding. An example of a warfarin prescribing chart is shown on page 486.

Activated partial thromboplastin time

The APTT depends on all clotting factors except factor VII. In clinical practice, the APTT is used most commonly in patients receiving an infusion of heparin. The APTT is monitored frequently, and the rate of the heparin infusion adjusted to achieve the desired level of anticoagulation. With the common prescribing of low-molecular-weight heparin, in preference to unfractionated heparin, this process is now performed infrequently. A frequent cause of concern relates to elevated APTTs in patients with central venous catheters. The proximal end of such catheters are often filled with heparin to keep the lumina patent when they are not being used. A spuriously high APTT will be obtained if blood is withdrawn from one such lumen. If the APTT is tested on a sample of blood tested peripherally, the true value will be obtained.

Coagulation correction testing

In cases of deranged coagulation, laboratories will often perform a coagulation correction test. This is performed to detect problems in coagulation arising because of a low level of a particular clotting factor. Essentially, normal plasma (containing normal clotting factors) is mixed with the patient's sample. If the patient is deficient in clotting factors, a deranged coagulation profile would be expected to normalise. There will be no change, however, if an inhibitor of coagulation is present. Specialised assays for individual clotting factors are also available.

Bleeding time

Bleeding time is measured directly at the bedside. A sphygmomanometer cuff is inflated around the patient's arm to 40 mmHg. A specially designed blade is then used to make a small puncture in the arm. Blood is removed from the area at fixed time intervals (eg 15 s) using a piece of filter paper to soak it up. The time taken for bleeding to stop is recorded. Elevated bleeding times indicate defective platelet function or low platelet numbers. This test should not be performed if the patient is known to have severe thrombocytopenia.

Bear in mind that patients with abnormal numbers or deranged function of platelets may also have abnormal bleeding. Patients with von Willebrand disease may have normal coagulation profiles.

> **DON'T FORGET**
> Patients with von Willebrand disease may have normal coagulation profiles.

Disseminated intravascular coagulation

Disseminated intravascular coagulation (DIC) is a disease of two apparently conflicting problems. On the one hand, fibrin deposition in various organs results in areas of micro-infarction. On the other hand, the body's supplies of clotting factors become used up because of all the clotting, leaving the patient prone to bleeding.

DISSEMINATED INTRAVASCULAR COAGULATION

A disease in which clotting and bleeding cause problems simultaneously.

Typical laboratory findings in DIC are as follows:

Raised PT and APTT	Since clotting factors are reduced
Reduced fibrinogen	Due to widespread fibrin formation
Raised D-dimer	Due to the body's attempt to break down the excess fibrin deposits

D-dimer

D-dimer is the most commonly measured fibrinogen/fibrin degeneration product. It is detected following clot formation in the vasculature, as the body's fibrinolytic system attempts to break the clot down. D-dimer levels are often tested in cases of suspected deep venous thrombosis and pulmonary embolism, and in the majority of cases will be raised. However, D-dimer levels are also raised in many other conditions, and a raised level should always be interpreted in light of the clinical scenario.

Laboratory findings in bleeding disorders

	PT	APTT	FIBRINOGEN
Warfarin treatment	Increased	Normal (or Increased)	Normal
Heparin treatment	Normal (or increased)	Increased	Normal
Haemophilia A or B	Normal	Increased	Normal
Liver disease	Increased	Increased	Normal
DIC	Increased	Increased	Reduced

Plasma cell dyscrasias

Diseases of plasma cells are common, and their investigation is often a cause for confusion. They represent a spectrum of disorders, with multiple myeloma being the most important at the undergraduate level, and monoclonal gammopathy of unknown significance (MGUS) being the most common. The hallmark of these conditions is that plasma cells secrete M protein in excess. The effects of multiple myeloma can be far-reaching, and can lead to the following features:

- Anaemia

- Renal impairment

- Low levels of normal immunoglobulins with resultant infections

- Bone involvement, causing bony pain, hypercalcaemia, lytic lesions and problems if bones collapse

- Hyperviscosity of the blood.

The conditions should be suspected if any of the following abnormalities are present:

- Elevated ESR

- Hypercalcaemia

- Anaemia

- Renal impairment

- Abnormal M-protein detected on plasma protein electrophoresis

- Abnormal quantities of immunoglobulin light chains in the serum (with an abnormal $\kappa{:}\lambda$ ratio)

- Low levels of immunoglobulins

- Lytic lesions on X-ray of bones

- Detection of Bence Jones protein in the urine (this represents immunoglobulin light chains)

- Abnormal plasma cells seen on bone marrow biopsy

- Elevated β_2-microglobulin.

Case 1.1

A 48-year-old retired civil servant is concerned with her pale colour and feelings of faintness that have occurred over the past 4 weeks. She had felt well before this and enjoyed regular trips to southern France. Brief clinical examination reveals pallor. Her blood tests come to your attention.

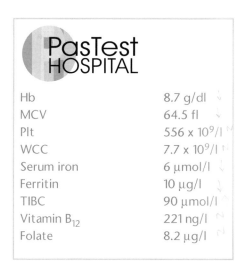

Hb	8.7 g/dl
MCV	64.5 fl
Plt	556 x 10^9/l
WCC	7.7 x 10^9/l
Serum iron	6 µmol/l
Ferritin	10 µg/l
TIBC	90 µmol/l
Vitamin B$_{12}$	221 ng/l
Folate	8.2 µg/l

1. **How would you interpret these results?**
2. **How would you proceed with investigation?**

Answer 1.1

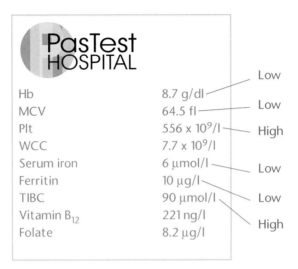

PasTest HOSPITAL

Hb	8.7 g/dl	Low
MCV	64.5 fl	Low
Plt	556 x 10⁹/l	High
WCC	7.7 x 10⁹/l	
Serum iron	6 μmol/l	Low
Ferritin	10 μg/l	
TIBC	90 μmol/l	Low
Vitamin B$_{12}$	221 ng/l	
Folate	8.2 μg/l	High

1. This patient has a microcytic anaemia. Her iron profile is in keeping with iron deficiency with a low iron, low ferritin and high TIBC. There is a mild thrombocytosis which may indicate active bleeding.

2. The most common cause for these findings in young women is menorrhagia. In an older female or male of any age, investigations should be carried out to exclude a sinister cause – in particular an occult gastrointestinal tract malignancy. Investigations should begin with a thorough history and clinical examination which should include rectal examination. The next line of investigation usually involves gastrointestinal tract endoscopy.

Case 1.2

A 57-year-old woman attends her GP complaining of tiredness. The GP knows her medical history well as she also suffers from Graves' disease. A full blood count was analysed as well as haematinics.

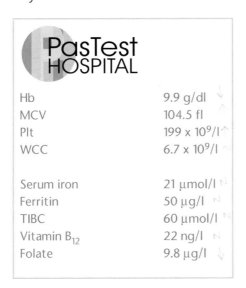

Hb	9.9 g/dl
MCV	104.5 fl
Plt	199 x 10^9/l
WCC	6.7 x 10^9/l
Serum iron	21 µmol/l
Ferritin	50 µg/l
TIBC	60 µmol/l
Vitamin B$_{12}$	22 ng/l
Folate	9.8 µg/l

1. **Interpret these blood results.**

Following these results the GP also requests another test shown below.

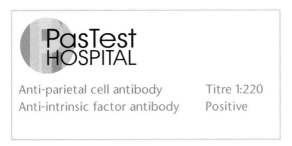

Anti-parietal cell antibody	Titre 1:220
Anti-intrinsic factor antibody	Positive

2. **What is the diagnosis?**

Answer 1.2

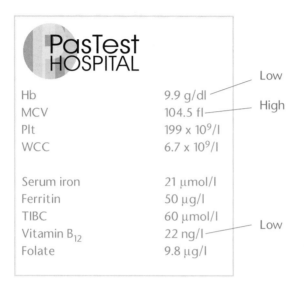

Hb	9.9 g/dl	Low
MCV	104.5 fl	High
Plt	199 x 10⁹/l	
WCC	6.7 x 10⁹/l	
Serum iron	21 μmol/l	
Ferritin	50 μg/l	
TIBC	60 μmol/l	
Vitamin B₁₂	22 ng/l	Low
Folate	9.8 μg/l	

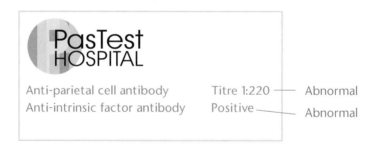

Anti-parietal cell antibody	Titre 1:220	Abnormal
Anti-intrinsic factor antibody	Positive	Abnormal

1. The haemoglobin is low with an elevated mean cell volume. This patient has a macrocytic anaemia. Haematinics show a low vitamin B_{12} level. Iron studies and folate level are within normal limits.

2. The positive antibodies to gastric parietal cells and intrinsic factor indicate that the likely underlying cause of the anaemia is pernicious anaemia. You will note that the patient was already known to have an autoimmune disease – Graves' disease. Always remember that patients with one autoimmune disease are prone to developing another.

A Schilling test would have been useful in this case. The initial test would show low levels of radiolabelled vitamin B_{12} in the urine. Once the patient was given oral intrinsic factor, urine vitamin B_{12} excretion would be expected to return to normal.

Case 1.3

A 49-year-old woman with systemic sclerosis complains of malaise and palpitations. Her disease has been quiescent for 2 years and she is not on any immunosuppressant medications. She has a balanced diet and has had no previous surgery. Her rheumatologist requests the following tests:

PasTest HOSPITAL

Hb	8.2 g/dl
MCV	109.4 fl
Plt	169 x 10^9/l
WCC	6.2 x 10^9/l
Serum iron	23 µmol/l
Ferritin	49 µg/l
TIBC	62 µmol/l
Vitamin B_{12}	31 ng/l
Folate	>10 µg/l

Anti-parietal cell antibody	Titre < 1:120
Anti-intrinsic factor antibody	Negative

Schilling test	Without oral intrinsic factor: 0.03 µg radioactive vitamin B_{12} in 24-h urine sample (3% of oral dose)
	With oral intrinsic factor: 0.03 µg radioactive vitamin B_{12} in 24-h urine sample (3% of oral dose)
Hydrogen breath test	Early peak in hydrogen excretion

---

1. **What would you infer from these results?**

2. **What is the reason for performing a hydrogen breath test?**

Answer 1.3

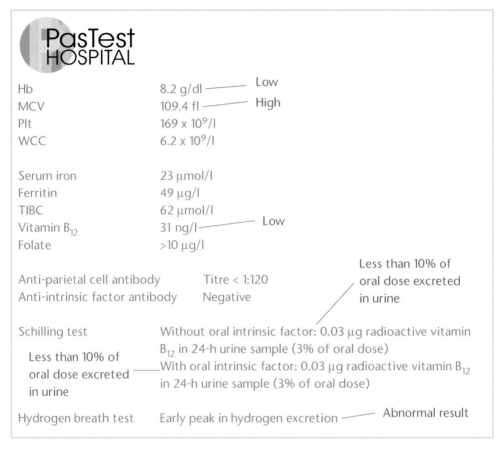

PasTest
HOSPITAL

Hb	8.2 g/dl	Low
MCV	109.4 fl	High
Plt	$169 \times 10^9/l$	
WCC	$6.2 \times 10^9/l$	

Serum iron	23 μmol/l	
Ferritin	49 μg/l	
TIBC	62 μmol/l	
Vitamin B$_{12}$	31 ng/l	Low
Folate	>10 μg/l	

Anti-parietal cell antibody   Titre < 1:120   Less than 10% of oral dose excreted in urine

Anti-intrinsic factor antibody   Negative

Schilling test   Without oral intrinsic factor: 0.03 μg radioactive vitamin B$_{12}$ in 24-h urine sample (3% of oral dose)

Less than 10% of oral dose excreted in urine   With oral intrinsic factor: 0.03 μg radioactive vitamin B$_{12}$ in 24-h urine sample (3% of oral dose)

Hydrogen breath test   Early peak in hydrogen excretion   Abnormal result

1. This patient has a macrocytic anaemia. Vitamin B$_{12}$ is the only deficient haematinic, but the autoantibodies for pernicious anaemia are negative. The history states that the diet is balanced and no surgery has taken place on the bowel to interfere with the absorption of vitamin B$_{12}$. The Schilling test is abnormal. Normally, at least 10% of the oral dose of radiolabelled vitamin B$_{12}$ is excreted in the urine. In this case, the excreted dose is low, and supplementation with intrinsic factor makes no difference. The likely pathology is therefore in the ileum.

2. The abnormal hydrogen breath test result points to the cause of anaemia – small bowel bacterial overgrowth. Patients with systemic sclerosis are prone to developing this condition. Definitive testing for bacterial overgrowth involves culturing small bowel contents. One would expect a normal Schilling test after an adequate course of appropriate antibiotics.

Case 1.4

A 34-year-old accountant with a 15-year history of Crohn's disease attends for outpatient review. He feels reasonable, although has not yet been able to hold down full employment after numerous hospital admissions and surgery over the past 10 years. His last surgery involved small bowel resection and anastomosis after further failure of medical therapy. The doctor in the clinic requests the following tests.

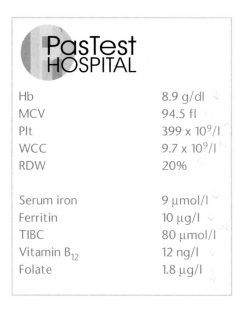

PasTest HOSPITAL

Hb	8.9 g/dl
MCV	94.5 fl
Plt	399 x 10⁹/l
WCC	9.7 x 10⁹/l
RDW	20%
Serum iron	9 µmol/l
Ferritin	10 µg/l
TIBC	80 µmol/l
Vitamin B$_{12}$	12 ng/l
Folate	1.8 µg/l

What is your interpretation of these tests?

Answer 1.4

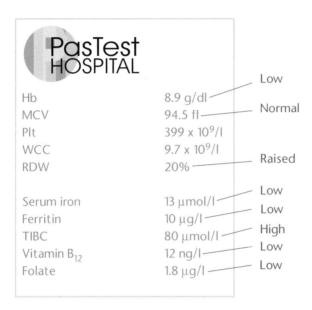

PasTest HOSPITAL

Hb	8.9 g/dl	Low
MCV	94.5 fl	Normal
Plt	399 x 10⁹/l	
WCC	9.7 x 10⁹/l	
RDW	20%	Raised
Serum iron	13 µmol/l	Low
Ferritin	10 µg/l	Low
TIBC	80 µmol/l	High
Vitamin B₁₂	12 ng/l	Low
Folate	1.8 µg/l	Low

This man has a normocytic anaemia. He is deficient in iron, vitamin B_{12} and folate. The red cell distribution width (RDW) is raised, indicating a wide variation in the size of circulating red cells. The patient is likely to have a dimorphic blood picture, with small red cells resulting from iron deficiency, and large cells resulting from deficiencies of vitamin B_{12} and folate. Crohn's disease is an inflammatory bowel disease involving the whole gastrointestinal tract so has the potential to cause deficiencies in all three haematinics. In this case, multiple operations have left him with a very short small bowel ('short gut syndrome').

Case 1.5

A 55-year-old woman with essential hypertension attends the medical clinic. Her blood pressure remains elevated despite treatment with four drugs. Her consultant commences her on methyldopa. Four weeks later she attends the accident and emergency department feeling generally unwell. The A&E doctor sends off a variety of blood tests, which are shown here.

PasTest HOSPITAL

Hb	9.2 g/dl
MCV	93.4 fl
Plt	376 x 10^9/l
WCC	7.2 x 10^9/l
Serum iron	25 μmol/l
Ferritin	154 μg/l
TIBC	65 μmol/l
Vitamin B$_{12}$	198 ng/l
Folate	6.5 μg/l
Total bilirubin	45 μmol/l
AST	25 IU/l
ALT	22 IU/l
GGT	15 IU/l
ALP	98 U/l

She is admitted to the medical unit, and several other tests are requested.

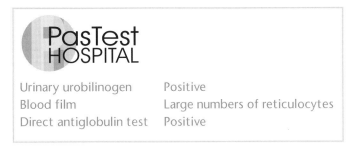

PasTest HOSPITAL

Urinary urobilinogen	Positive
Blood film	Large numbers of reticulocytes
Direct antiglobulin test	Positive

1. **Interpret the results above**

2. **What is the likely diagnosis?**

Answer 1.5

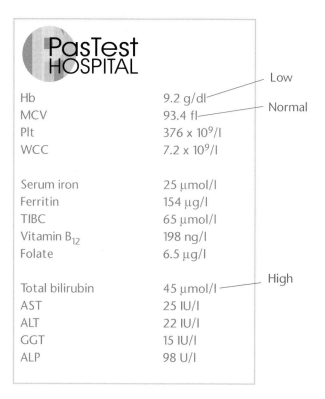

PasTest
HOSPITAL

Hb	9.2 g/dl	Low
MCV	93.4 fl	Normal
Plt	376 x 10⁹/l	
WCC	7.2 x 10⁹/l	
Serum iron	25 μmol/l	
Ferritin	154 μg/l	
TIBC	65 μmol/l	
Vitamin B₁₂	198 ng/l	
Folate	6.5 μg/l	
Total bilirubin	45 μmol/l	High
AST	25 IU/l	
ALT	22 IU/l	
GGT	15 IU/l	
ALP	98 U/l	

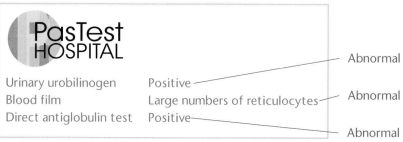

PasTest
HOSPITAL

Urinary urobilinogen	Positive	Abnormal
Blood film	Large numbers of reticulocytes	Abnormal
Direct antiglobulin test	Positive	Abnormal

1. This patient has a normocytic anaemia. Her haematinics are normal. She has a raised blood bilirubin level and urobilinogen in the urine which would be in keeping with haemoglobin breakdown. Her blood film shows a reticulocytosis indicating that the bone marrow is working hard to make new red blood cells. The direct antiglobulin test is positive indicating that the patient's red cells are coated with antibodies.

2. The patient has an autoimmune haemolytic anaemia, which is most likely to be an adverse effect of treatment with methyldopa.

Case 1.6

When on elective in Malawi, you are asked to see a patient. He is 35 years old and complains of anorexia and abdominal discomfort. Examination is unremarkable. A full blood picture is requested.

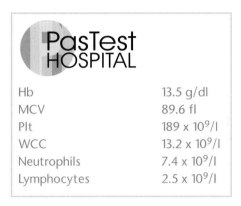

PasTest
HOSPITAL

Hb	13.5 g/dl
MCV	89.6 fl
Plt	189 x 10^9/l
WCC	13.2 x 10^9/l
Neutrophils	7.4 x 10^9/l
Lymphocytes	2.5 x 10^9/l

What is the likely diagnosis?

Answer 1.6

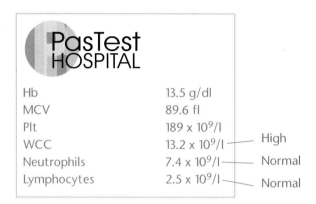

PasTest HOSPITAL		
Hb	13.5 g/dl	
MCV	89.6 fl	
Plt	189 x 10⁹/l	
WCC	13.2 x 10⁹/l	High
Neutrophils	7.4 x 10⁹/l	Normal
Lymphocytes	2.5 x 10⁹/l	Normal

This question is a little sneaky. The key to finding the answer is to remember that the total WCC is equal to the sum of the component parts of the differential white cell count.

DON'T FORGET

Total white cell count = neutrophil count + lympocyte count + eosinophil count + monocyte count + basophil count

In this case, the neutrophil count and lympocyte count together cannot account for the total white cell count ((7.4×10^9/l) + (2.5×10^9/l) <13.2×10^9/l)). There must be a further type of white blood cell in elevated numbers. It is impossible to tell for certain what this cell type might be. However, the likely diagnosis here is helminthic (worm) infection. A full differential white cell count would reveal a raised level of eosinophils.

Case 1.7

You see a 64-year-old woman in A&E. She has severe chronic obstructive pulmonary disease (COPD), and has been an inpatient on several occasions in the past year. She appears short of breath, and complains of a worsening cough productive of green sputum. This has become worse over the last 3 days. Part of her admission blood tests are shown.

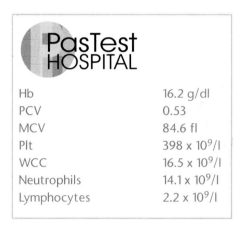

Hb	16.2 g/dl
PCV	0.53
MCV	84.6 fl
Plt	398 x 10^9/l
WCC	16.5 x 10^9/l
Neutrophils	14.1 x 10^9/l
Lymphocytes	2.2 x 10^9/l

Outline the abnormalities shown, and discuss their most likely causes.

Answer 1.7

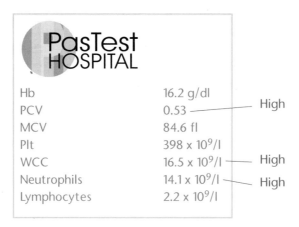

Hb	16.2 g/dl	
PCV	0.53	High
MCV	84.6 fl	
Plt	398 x 10^9/l	
WCC	16.5 x 10^9/l	High
Neutrophils	14.1 x 10^9/l	High
Lymphocytes	2.2 x 10^9/l	

The first abnormality relates to the raised packed cell volume (PCV) indicating polycythaemia. The most likely cause in this case is a true polycythaemia secondary to chronic hypoxia resulting from COPD. Useful tests to confirm this would be an estimation of red cell mass to confirm true polycythaemia, and an arterial blood gas sample to demonstrate hypoxaemia.

The second abnormality relates to the elevated white cell count. Note that the neutrophil count is markedly elevated, and that the sum of the neutrophil and lymphocyte counts almost adds up to the total white cell count. The small discrepancy is due to the presence of a small number of other white blood cells (eosinophils, monocytes and basophils) in the circulation. The most likely cause for this picture is a bacterial infection of the lower respiratory tract.

Case 1.8

A 74-year-old man presents to the A&E department after a 5 minute episode of loss of vision affecting the right eye. Further questioning revealed that the patient had a similar episode 2 days previously. On each occasion the vision was lost rapidly, 'like a curtain being drawn' over the visual field. Direct questioning revealed that he had been lethargic for several weeks, and experienced some pain in his jaw on chewing. Initial blood tests revealed the following:

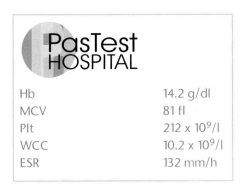

Hb	14.2 g/dl
MCV	81 fl
Plt	212 x 10^9/l
WCC	10.2 x 10^9/l
ESR	132 mm/h

1.   **What is the likely diagnosis?**

2.   **What treatment would you prescribe immediately?**

Answer 1.8

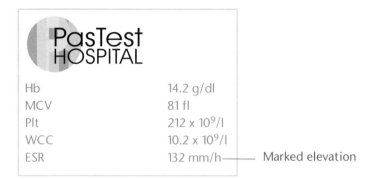

PasTest
HOSPITAL

Hb	14.2 g/dl
MCV	81 fl
Plt	212 x 10^9/l
WCC	10.2 x 10^9/l
ESR	132 mm/h —— Marked elevation

1. The episode of loss of vision is typical of amaurosis fugax. Taken together with the history of lethargy and jaw pain on eating (jaw claudication), the clinical suspicion must be of temporal arteritis. Such patients are at high risk of complications, including blindness. The extremely high ESR measured here would support this diagnosis. Temporal arteritis is one of the few causes of an ESR greater than 100 mm/h.

2. Treatment should be given rapidly, and should comprise high-dose prednisolone (eg 60–80 mg orally immediately), followed by a reducing dose regimen.

Case 1.9

You are the junior doctor on the vascular surgical unit. One of your patients, a 75-year-old man with peripheral vascular disease, is due to undergo bypass vascular surgery on his legs. You request a battery of preoperative blood tests. The following results give the nursing staff some concern.

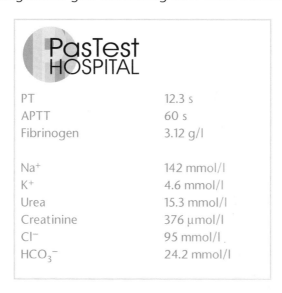

PasTest HOSPITAL

PT	12.3 s
APTT	60 s
Fibrinogen	3.12 g/l
Na$^+$	142 mmol/l
K$^+$	4.6 mmol/l
Urea	15.3 mmol/l
Creatinine	376 μmol/l
Cl$^-$	95 mmol/l
HCO$_3^-$	24.2 mmol/l

What should you do next?

Answer 1.9

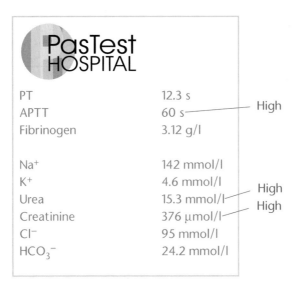

PasTest HOSPITAL

PT	12.3 s
APTT	60 s ——— High
Fibrinogen	3.12 g/l
Na$^+$	142 mmol/l
K$^+$	4.6 mmol/l
Urea	15.3 mmol/l — High
Creatinine	376 µmol/l — High
Cl$^-$	95 mmol/l
HCO$_3^-$	24.2 mmol/l

This situation is a common cause for concern. The details omitted from the history above are that the patient has chronic renal failure, and receives haemodialysis three times per week via his indwelling central venous catheter. The raised urea and creatinine are a reflection of the chronic renal failure in this case (see Chapter 2 for more information).

The cause of the deranged coagulation is most likely because blood has been drawn from the central venous catheter, which is often flushed with a heparin solution. The next step should be to repeat the coagulation profile using blood taken from a peripheral vein.

Case 1.10

A 58-year-old patient with immunodeficiency is admitted to the intensive care unit with severe pneumonia. Despite aggressive antibiotic therapy, his condition does not improve. On his third day in the unit, the nurses report that he is beginning to bleed around the sites of his indwelling venous lines. The doctor in charge requests a coagulation profile. The blood is taken from a peripheral vein.

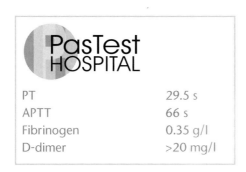

PasTest HOSPITAL	
PT	29.5 s
APTT	66 s
Fibrinogen	0.35 g/l
D-dimer	>20 mg/l

What is the likely diagnosis?

Answer 1.10

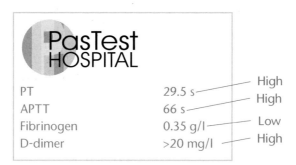

PasTest HOSPITAL		
PT	29.5 s	High
APTT	66 s	High
Fibrinogen	0.35 g/l	Low
D-dimer	>20 mg/l	High

The PT and APTT are raised suggesting a tendency to bleed. The fibrinogen level is low indicating that fibrinogen has been used up. The D-dimer level is markedly raised indicating that the body's fibrinolytic system is working hard to disperse clots.

This pattern of abnormalities is typical of DIC, a not uncommon complication in patients with critical illness. Blood product support will be required, and the advice of a haematologist would be helpful.

Case 1.11

A 24-year-old woman from the Maldives is in Ireland on honeymoon.
She attends the emergency department after falling and spraining her wrist.
The doctor is concerned about the results of her full blood picture:

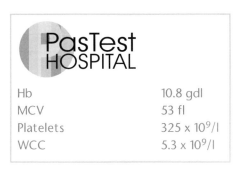

PasTest HOSPITAL	
Hb	10.8 gdl
MCV	53 fl
Platelets	325 x 10⁹/l
WCC	5.3 x 10⁹/l

What is the most likely diagnosis and what test(s) would you arrange?

Answer 1.11

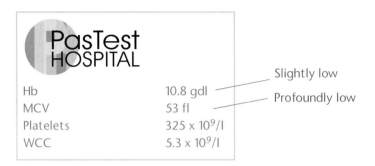

Hb	10.8 gdl	Slightly low
MCV	53 fl	Profoundly low
Platelets	325 x 10⁹/l	
WCC	5.3 x 10⁹/l	

This patient has a microcytic anaemia. The striking abnormality on her FBP is that the MCV is extremely low, whereas the haemoglobin concentration is only slightly below the reference range. She originates from the Maldives – an area where thalassaemia is common. It is probable that this woman has thalassaemia (most likely to be β-thalassaemia trait). Haemoglobin electrophoresis will confirm the diagnosis. Concomitant iron deficiency is possible, so sending blood for iron studies would also seem sensible.

Case 1.12

A 45-year-old man with a history of asthma is admitted with symptoms and signs in keeping with cardiac failure. There are no risk factors for ischaemic heart disease. The cause for the cardiac failure remains uncertain until a junior doctor reviews his FBP and suggests the correct diagnosis.

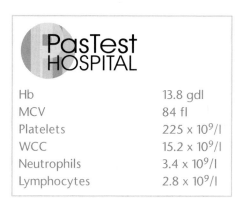

PasTest
HOSPITAL

Hb	13.8 gdl
MCV	84 fl
Platelets	225 x 10^9/l
WCC	15.2 x 10^9/l
Neutrophils	3.4 x 10^9/l
Lymphocytes	2.8 x 10^9/l

What is the rare disease that the junior doctor suspected?

Answer 1.12

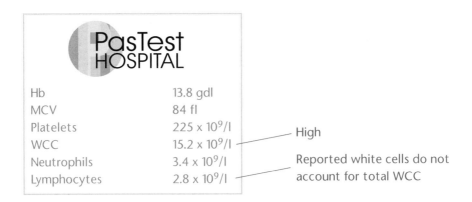

Hb	13.8 gdl
MCV	84 fl
Platelets	225 x 10^9/l
WCC	15.2 x 10^9/l — High
Neutrophils	3.4 x 10^9/l
Lymphocytes	2.8 x 10^9/l — Reported white cells do not account for total WCC

The key to even thinking about the rare disease in this case starts with the basics in interpreting the patient's FBP. The neutrophil and lymphocyte counts do not account for the elevated total WCC. The missing piece of information in the question is the eosinophil count which is highly abnormal in this case. The diagnosis here is Churg–Strauss syndrome, a rare vasculitic disease associated with a peripheral eosinophilia.

Case 1.13

An elderly patient is admitted to the rehabilitation ward 4 weeks after having surgery to repair a fractured neck of femur. Her postoperative course was complicated by pneumonia and renal failure, both of which have been treated successfully. She has not been out of bed since the operation. You review her recent full blood pictures:

PasTest
HOSPITAL

	14/06/11	28/06/11	01/07/11	15/07/11	10/07/11
Hb	11.6 gdl	12.2	11.8	12.4	12.1
MCV	80 fl	81	79	79	81
Platelets	227 x 10^9/l	264	90	32	8
WCC	5.4 x 10^9/l	4.5	4.7	4.9	4.5

What is the major problem, and name one possible drug-induced cause?

Answer 1.13

PasTest
HOSPITAL

	14/06/11	28/06/11	01/07/11	15/07/11	10/07/11
Hb	11.6 gdl	12.2	11.8	12.4	12.1
MCV	80 fl	81	79	79	81
Platelets	227 x 10^9/l	264	90	32	8
WCC	5.4 x 10^9/l	4.5	4.7	4.9	4.5

Steadily falling platelet count

On 1 July, the patient developed thrombocytopenia. This has worsened steadily and significantly since. An extremely rare adverse drug reaction, 'heparin-induced thrombocytopenia (HIT)', can occur in patients receiving unfractionated or low-molecular-weight heparin. It is likely that this patient was receiving low-molecular-weight heparin in an attempt to prevent thromboembolic disease.

Case 1.14

A patient attends the emergency department because of a swollen leg on the right side. He has a history of dementia, and is unsure for how long the leg has been swollen. On inspection, the right calf is 0.3 cm larger than the left, there is no erythema and the calf is non-tender. You order a blood test to help with management.

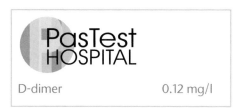

D-dimer	0.12 mg/l

How would you proceed?

Answer 1.14

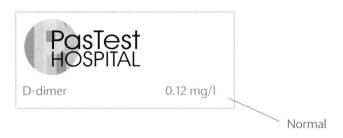

PasTest
HOSPITAL

D-dimer   0.12 mg/l

                                                              Normal

This patient gives an unconvincing history for deep venous thrombosis (DVT), and there is very little clinical evidence for it. A normal D-dimer in this situation, when the pre-test probability for the condition is low, is helpful in making DVT extremely unlikely in this man. The patient can be reassured that it is extremely unlikely that he has a clot in his leg.

Case 1.15

A 62-year-old woman is admitted with septic arthritis of the knee. A D-dimer blood test is sent in error, but comes back as follows:

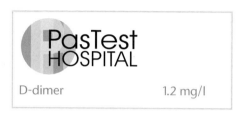

D-dimer   1.2 mg/l

Would you arrange investigations to test for thromboembolic disease?

Answer 1.15

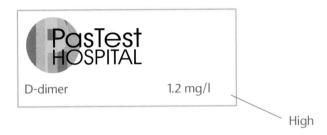

PasTest
HOSPITAL

D-dimer   1.2 mg/l

High

D-dimer is an extremely helpful blood test when sent in the correct
circumstances. In a patient with a reasonable chance of having a blood clot, an
elevated D-dimer would support the diagnosis. All too often, however, D-dimer
is measured in patients with no clinical suggestion of thromboembolic disease.
There are many causes for a raised D-dimer other than clot (eg commonly
found in acutely unwell patients malignancy, and following surgery or
trauma), so, unless the patient has signs or symptoms in keeping with
thromboembolism, the test should generally not be ordered. No investigations
for thromboembolic disease are required in this woman in whom we are given
no reason to suspect a blood clot.

BIOCHEMISTRY

2

BIOCHEMISTRY

Urea and electrolyte profile

A urea and electrolyte (U&E) profile is the most commonly requested biochemical blood test. U&Es, in combination with a full blood picture (FBP), are performed for virtually all new hospital admissions. The U&E profile incorporate measures of electrolytes (sodium and potassium), along with renal function (urea and creatinine). U&Es are often used as a screening test in unwell patients, and frequently act as a stimulus for further investigation.

Electrolyte abnormalities

Abnormalities in sodium and potassium occur when they are either too low (hyponatraemia – low sodium; hypokalaemia – low potassium) or too high (hypernatraemia – high sodium; hyperkalaemia – high potassium).

Hyponatraemia

Hyponatraemia is defined as a sodium concentration <135 mmol/l. The condition is a source of much confusion among students and doctors alike. The first step in working out why a patient has hyponatraemia is to investigate whether or not the low sodium is a true finding. This can be done by measuring serum osmolality in the laboratory. In some circumstances (eg hyperglycaemia and hyperlipidaemia), a falsely low sodium concentration can be reported. This is known as pseudo-hyponatraemia.

If the osmolality is low (and it will be in the vast majority of cases), it can be assumed that the hyponatraemia is real. The next and most crucial step is to make a detailed assessment of the patient's volume status to decide if they are dehydrated (hypovolaemic), fluid overloaded (hypervolaemic) or normally hydrated (isovolaemic). The likely cause of the hyponatraemia varies depending into which group the patient falls. The diagnosis and potential causes of hyponatraemia are illustrated in the flow diagram in Fig 2.1.

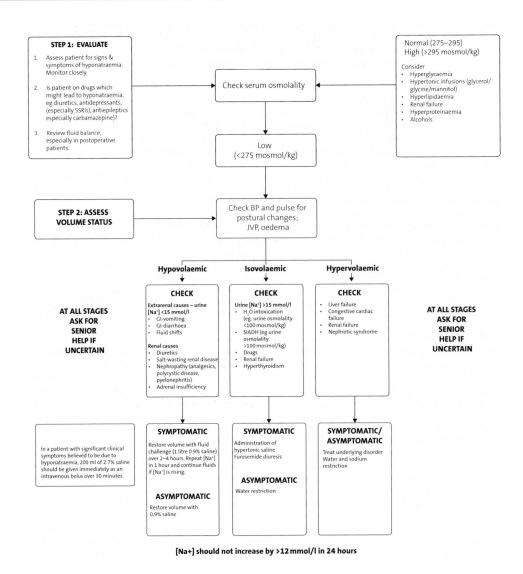

STEP 1: EVALUATE

1. Assess patient for signs & symptoms of hyponatraemia. Monitor closely.

2. Is patient on drugs which might lead to hyponatraemia, eg diuretics, antidepressants, (especially SSRIs), antiepileptics especially carbamazepine)?

3. Review fluid balance, especially in postoperative patients.

Check serum osmolality

Normal (275–295)
High (>295 mosmol/kg)

Consider
- Hyperglycaemia
- Hypertonic infusions (glycerol/glycine/mannitol)
- Hyperlipidaemia
- Renal failure
- Hyperproteinaemia
- Alcohols

Low
(<275 mosmol/kg)

STEP 2: ASSESS VOLUME STATUS

Check BP and pulse for postural changes; JVP, oedema

Hypovolaemic   Isovolaemic   Hypervolaemic

AT ALL STAGES ASK FOR SENIOR HELP IF UNCERTAIN

CHECK

Extrarenal causes – urine [Na⁺] <15 mmol/l
- GI-vomiting
- GI-diarrhoea
- Fluid shifts

Renal causes
- Diuretics
- Salt-wasting renal disease
- Nephropathy (analgesics, polycystic disease, pyelonephritis)
- Adrenal insufficiency

CHECK

Urine [Na⁺] >15 mmol/l
- H₂O intoxication (eg. urine osmolality <100 mosmol/kg)
- SIADH (eg urine osmolality >100 mosmol/kg)
- Drugs
- Renal failure
- Hyperthyroidism

CHECK
- Liver failure
- Congestive cardiac failure
- Renal failure
- Nephrotic syndrome

AT ALL STAGES ASK FOR SENIOR HELP IF UNCERTAIN

In a patient with significant clinical symptoms believed to be due to hyponatraemia, 200 ml of 2.7% saline should be given immediately as an intravenous bolus over 30 minutes.

SYMPTOMATIC

Restore volume with fluid challenge (1 litre 0.9% saline) over 2–4 hours. Repeat [Na⁺] in 1 hour and continue fluids if [Na⁺] is rising.

ASYMPTOMATIC

Restore volume with 0.9% saline

SYMPTOMATIC

Administration of hypertonic saline Furosemide diuresis

ASYMPTOMATIC

Water restriction

SYMPTOMATIC/ ASYMPTOMATIC

Treat underlying disorder Water and sodium restriction

[Na+] should not increase by >12 mmol/l in 24 hours

Fig 2.1: From GAIN. *Hyponatraemia in Adults (on or after 16th birthday)*. GAIN, 2010. Available at: http://www.gain-ni.org/Library/Guidelines/Hyponatraemia_guideline.pdf.

The syndrome of inappropriate antidiuretic hormone secretion (SIADH) is somewhat over-diagnosed as a cause of hyponatraemia. It is in actual fact quite uncommon. SIADH is dealt with separately on page 149.

DON'T FORGET

Hyponatraemia does not mean SIADH!

Hypernatraemia

This is defined as a sodium concentration of more than 145 mmol/l. Hypernatraemia is a very strong stimulus for thirst, so in normal circumstances (healthy patient with access to adequate fluid) it should not develop.

CAUSES OF HYPERNATRAEMIA

Diabetes insipidus
Poor water intake, eg in frail elderly patients who are unable to access water freely, perhaps because they are bed-bound and unable to ask
Administration of excess sodium in intravenous fluids
Administration of drugs containing high concentrations of sodium

For further details on diabetes insipidus, see page 148.

Hypokalaemia

This is defined as a potassium concentration of less than 3.5 mmol/l.

CAUSES OF HYPOKALAEMIA

Drugs:
- diuretic therapy

Intestinal losses:
- excess vomiting (eg pyloric stenosis)
- profuse diarrhoea
- high stoma or fistula output

Renal tubular disease:
- renal tubular acidosis or drug-induced tubular damage

Endocrine causes (eg hyperaldosteronism)

Metabolic alkalosis

Hypokalaemia is associated with characteristic changes on the ECG. This is discussed on page 359.

Hyperkalaemia

This is defined as a potassium concentration of more than 4.5 mmol/l.

CAUSES OF HYPERKALAEMIA

Renal failure

Drugs:
- excess potassium supplementation
- potassium-sparing diuretics
- combination of drugs (eg angiotensin-converting enzyme [ACE] inhibitor and diuretic)

Rhabdomyolysis

Endocrine diseases (eg hypoadrenalism)

Diabetic ketoacidosis

Haemolysis of blood sample in transit (artefactual hyperkalaemia)

Hyperkalaemia is associated with characteristic changes on the ECG. This is discussed on page 359.

DON'T FORGET

Hyperkalaemia is a medical emergency with levels of potassium of more than 6.5 mmol/l requiring immediate attention and lesser levels requiring immediate attention if the ECG is abnormal.

Renal function

The presence of a normal urea and creatinine level is not synonymous with normal renal function. A thin elderly woman may have significant renal impairment despite her creatinine appearing within the 'normal' laboratory range. One must pay attention to the age, sex and muscle bulk of a patient when interpreting the significance of a creatinine level.

For accurate measurement of renal function, estimation of the glomerular filtration rate (GFR) is required. An estimated GFR (eGFR) is now routinely reported by many laboratories to highlight the importance of small increases in creatinine. Rather than reporting precise estimations of GFR for all patients, often laboratories have a cut-off value, so that, if a patient's eGFR falls above the value, the eGFR is simply reported as, for example, >60 ml/min per 1.73 m^2.

DON'T FORGET

A normal GFR is considered to be approximately 100 ml/min per 1.73 m^2.

ESTIMATING KIDNEY FUNCTION

As mentioned above, many laboratories will now report eGFR routinely. If you wish to learn more about the mathematics behind this estimation, the following section explains the formula for calculating eGFR and also creatinine clearance.

ESTIMATED GFR

The eGFR is calculated using the serum creatinine and requires knowledge of the patient's age, sex and race.

eGFR = 186 x $(P_{Cr}/88.4)^{-1.154}$ x $A^{-0.203}$

where P_{Cr} is plasma creatinine concentration (μmol/l) and A is age in years
Correction factors for gender (0.742 female) and for race (1.210 black) are
needed

Computer programs are available for assistance with the mathematics.

EXAMPLE CALCULATION

For a 62-year-old black female patient with a plasma creatinine of 150 μmol/l the
eGFR would be calculated as:

eGFR = 186 x $(150/88.4)^{-1.154}$ x $(62)^{-0.203}$ x 0.742 x 1.210 = 39.3 (in ml/min per
1.73 m^2)

CREATININE CLEARANCE

'Creatinine clearance' provides another useful indication of the GFR and
can be measured in one of two ways.

Method 1
This requires a single blood creatinine value and a 24-h collection of urine.

$$CL_{Cr} = \frac{U_{Cr} \times \dot{U}}{P_{Cr}}$$

where CL_{Cr} is the creatinine clearance (ml/min), U_{Cr} is
the concentration of creatinine in the urine (mmol/l),
$\dot{U}$ is the urine flow rate (ml/min) and P_{Cr} is the
concentration of creatinine in plasma (mmol/l)

Difficulties in this method of calculation arise for two reasons:

1. The plasma creatinine is usually measured in μmol/l, not mmol/l as required by the formula.

2. Urine flow rate is usually measured in litres per 24 h, ie the amount of urine produced in one day (1440 min).

Hence a correction factor of 0.694 is required (1000/1440).

To account for this, use the following modified formula:

$$CL_{Cr} = \frac{U_{cr} \times V \times 0.694}{B_{Cr}}$$

where V = 24-h urine volume (ml)
B_{Cr} = concentration of creatinine in plasma (μmol/l)

EXAMPLE CALCULATION

For a patient with a plasma creatinine of 150 μmol/l, a 24-h urine volume of 2 l and a urinary creatinine concentration of 10 mmol/l, the creatinine clearance would be calculated as:

$$CL_{Cr} = \frac{10 \times 2000 \times 0.694}{150} = 92.5 \text{ (ml/min)}$$

Method 2

This method requires knowledge of the patient's age (A in years), mass (M in kg), sex and serum creatinine concentration (P_{Cr} in mg/dl).

$$CL_{Cr} = \frac{[(140 - A) \times M]}{72 \times P_{Cr}}$$

The formula generates an estimate of creatinine clearance for male patients. For females, the result of this calculation should be multiplied by 0.85.

Difficulties in this method of calculation arise because plasma creatinine is usually measured in μmol/l. To convert from μmol/l to mg/dl, divide by 88.4.

EXAMPLE CALCULATION

For a 66-year-old, 70-kg, female patient with a plasma creatinine of 150 μmol/l, the creatinine clearance would be calculated as:

$$CL_{Cr} = \frac{[(140 - 66) \times 70]}{(72 \times 150 \div 88.4)} = 42.4 \text{ ml/min}$$

Serum urea

The level of urea is reflective of both its production and elimination. Poor dietary intake can lead to a low urea level. Elevations in urea levels occur in renal failure, but are also commonly seen following a gastrointestinal bleed. Blood is effectively an excess protein load which is digested by the bowel.

Plasma osmolarity

Serum osmolarity can be calculated using the results of U&Es with the blood glucose level. Osmolarity is determined by the concentration of osmotically active particles, of which sodium is the most influential. It is calculated as follows.

Plasma osmolarity $= 2 \times (P_{Na} + P_K) + P_{Urea} + P_{Glucose}$
where P_{Na} is plasma sodium, P_K plasma potassium, P_{Urea} plasma urea and $P_{Glucose}$ is plasma glucose, all in mmol/l

Nutritional profile

A nutritional profile comprises measures of magnesium, calcium, phosphate and albumin. In patients with poor nutrition, all these nutrients may be deficient. Commonly deficiencies are seen in patients with poor oral diets (eg alcoholics, hunger strikers), or in patients with malabsorption. Further tests are available to provide blood levels of trace metals such as selenium.

Re-feeding syndrome is the term used to describe the change in blood biochemistry that can occur in patients who begin feeding after a period of starvation. Examples include hunger strikers who start to eat, and patients who have been unable to swallow (eg after a stroke) and begin nasogastric feeding after a period of starvation. Dangerous shifts in many electrolytes (eg phosphate, magnesium and calcium) can occur in such individuals and this can cause problems. Electrolytes should be checked frequently and replaced as necessary.

Urine in acute renal failure

Acute renal failure is a common problem in clinical practice. A common cause of this is renal hypoperfusion. Urine is often analysed for electrolyte content in such patients to enable the differentiation of prerenal uraemia from acute tubular necrosis. Patients with prerenal uraemia would be expected to recover faster than those with acute tubular necrosis when appropriate therapy is initiated.

The key to correct interpretation of urinary electrolytes is understanding that, in prerenal uraemia, normal renal regulatory mechanisms remain intact and attempt to maintain homeostasis. The juxtaglomerular apparatus senses the reduction in renal blood flow and activates the renin–angiotensin–aldosterone system. The end-product, aldosterone, acts to promote sodium reabsorption in the distal convoluted tubule. This results in an increase in the circulating volume. Therefore, in prerenal uraemia, the urinary sodium is low.

In acute tubular necrosis, the normal physiological mechanisms break down. Urinary sodium is therefore high.

It is difficult to interpret urinary sodium levels when a patient is taking a diuretic.

The fractional sodium excretion (FE_{Na}) is sometimes measured in addition. This is simply a measure of the proportion of sodium that is filtered at the glomerulus that ends up in the urine. The FE_{Na} will therefore be low in prerenal uraemia and high in acute tubular necrosis.

The following table summarises the differences.

	PRERENAL URAEMIA	ACUTE TUBULAR NECROSIS
Urinary sodium (mmol/l)	<20	>40
FE_{Na} (%)	<1	>1
Urine concentration	Concentrated	Relatively dilute

Bone profile

In health, bone undergoes a continuous process of remodelling by osteoclasts and osteoblasts. A bone profile is a batch of biochemical blood tests grouped together as they are all relevant to bone disease. It comprises calcium, phosphate and alkaline phosphatase (ALP). Albumin is also included for reasons detailed below. Metabolic bone diseases are associated with characteristic abnormalities on the bone profile. More specialised analyses, eg parathyroid hormone (PTH) or vitamin D levels, can be carried out when clinically relevant.

COMPONENTS OF A BONE PROFILE	
Calcium	Alkaline phosphatase
Phosphate	Albumin

Calcium homeostasis is under hormonal control with PTH being a key regulator. When calcium is low, PTH is released. This acts to raise serum calcium levels by:

- increasing calcium reabsorption from bone
- increasing renal calcium reabsorption
- increasing renal excretion of phosphate
- indirectly increasing absorption of calcium from the gut via effects on vitamin D.

Major metabolic bone diseases

The major bone diseases that a student might be expected to identify from a bone profile are listed in the box below.

MAJOR BONE DISEASES	
Osteoporosis	Bony metastases
Osteomalacia	Hyperparathyroidism
Paget disease of bone	

Typical patterns of results are shown in the following box.

BONE DISEASES	CALCIUM	PHOSPHATE	ALP
Osteoporosis	N	N	N
Osteomalacia	N/↓	↓	↑
Paget disease of bone	N	N	↑
Bony metastases	↑/N	N/↑	↑
Primary hyperparathyroidism	↑	↓	↑
Secondary hyperparathyroidism	N	↑	↑
Tertiary hyperparathyroidism	↑	↓	↑

Corrected calcium

It is important to appreciate that a high proportion of calcium is bound to protein (albumin). However, it is the unbound calcium that is most important physiologically. For this reason when protein (albumin) is low the total calcium level may be misleading and a correction calculation needs to be made. The 'corrected calcium' level refers to the calcium level corrected for the fact that the albumin is abnormal. Corrected calcium can be calculated as follows:

$$P_{Ca}c = P_{Ca} + \frac{(0.1\,(40-Alb))}{4}$$

where $P_{Ca}c$ (in mmol/l) is the corrected calcium level, P_{Ca} (in mmol/l) is the calcium level and Alb is the albumin concentration (g/l).

EXAMPLE CALCULATION

If: Calcium = 1.92 mmol/l
Albumin = 20 g/l

$$P_{Ca}c\ (mmol/l) = 1.92 + \frac{[0.1 \times (40 - 20)]}{4} = 2.42\ mmol/l$$

CAUSES OF HYPERCALCAEMIA

Bone metastases
Multiple myeloma
Hyperparathyroidism
Excessive vitamin D intake

Liver function tests

Liver function tests (LFTs) comprise six measurements: bilirubin, aspartate aminotransferase (AST), alanine aminotransferase (ALT), alkaline phosphatase (ALP), γ-glutamyl transpeptidase (GGT) and albumin. Prothrombin time (PT) which is part of a coagulation screen is an important addition (see page 21).

COMPONENTS OF LIVER FUNCTION TESTS
Bilirubin
Aspartate aminotransferase
Alanine aminotransferase
Alkaline phosphatase
γ-Glutamyl transpeptidase
Albumin

Note that AST and ALP are not tests specific to the liver. AST is also released when muscle (including cardiac muscle) is damaged. ALP is raised in a number of bone diseases, hence its presence in a bone profile.

If these basic LFTs are abnormal, further specific tests may be performed to establish an underlying cause.

TEST	DISEASE	EXPECTED RESULT
Autoantibody screen	Autoimmune hepatitis	Anti-nuclear Anti-smooth muscle Anti-liver/kidney microsomal-I
	Primary biliary cirrhosis	Anti-mitochondrial
	Coeliac disease	Anti-transglutaminase
Iron profile	Haemochromatosis	High iron, ferritin and transferrin saturation Low TIBC
Copper studies	Wilson's disease	Low ceruloplasmin and elevated 24-hour urine copper concentration suggestive
Viral hepatitis 'screen'	Hepatitis	Positive viral tests
α_1-Antitrypsin	α_1-Antitrypsin deficiency	Low level
α-Fetoprotein	Hepatocellular carcinoma	High level
Immunoglobulins	Several liver diseases	Specific pattern of immunoglobulin rise can give a clue to underlying disease but will not be diagnostic

Broadly speaking, disturbances of liver function may be classified into three patterns:

- Hepatitic (parenchymal)
- Cholestatic
- Mixed.

These patterns assist in narrowing the differential diagnosis of altered liver function. An understanding of the different causes allows an appropriate sequence of investigation.

When hepatocellular damage occurs, hepatocytes 'spill out' transaminases (AST and ALT). A rise in these indices alone may be termed a 'transaminitis'.

When there is obstruction to the outflow of bile from the liver, a cholestatic pattern (elevated ALP and GGT) will be seen. The bilirubin level would also be expected to be high.

Bilirubin is conjugated in the liver with the attachment of a glucuronide group. Measured bilirubin may be conjugated (direct bilirubin) or unconjugated (indirect bilirubin). Total bilirubin is the sum of both types.

Confusion sometimes arises in cholestatic liver disease when the AST and ALT are also elevated. This occurs because of back pressure on the liver. In such instances the elevation of ALP and GGT will be out of proportion to that of the transaminases.

In cholestatic jaundice, conjugated bilirubin can be detected in the urine using urinalysis.

CAUSES OF HEPATITIC LFTs

- Viral hepatitis
- Autoimmune hepatitis
- Drugs and toxins
- Alcohol
- Metabolic disorders (eg Wilson's disease)
- Fatty liver
- Malignancy (both primary and metastatic)
- Congestive cardiac failure

CAUSES OF CHOLESTATIC LFTs

Obstruction in the bile duct lumen
- Bile duct gallstone

An abnormal bile duct wall
- Bile duct stricture
- Cholangiocarcinoma

Compression of the bile duct by an extrinsic lesion
- Pancreatic carcinoma
- Nodes at the porta hepatis
- Ampullary carcinoma

One of the functions of the liver is protein synthesis. In a failing liver, synthetic function is often affected. This will manifest as low albumin levels and a raised prothrombin time (since the liver manufactures clotting factors).

C-reactive protein

C-reactive protein (CRP) is a protein produced in the liver. It is an acute phase reactant, being raised in inflammation and infection. It is often thought of in a similar manner to the erythrocyte sedimentation rate (ESR) (see page 17). The CRP and ESR are together termed inflammatory markers. There are a few recognised conditions in which the ESR is raised, but the CRP is normal.

CAUSES OF A RAISED ESR WITH A NORMAL CRP
SLE
Multiple myeloma

The level of the CRP does not necessarily reflect the severity of a disease process.

Urate (uric acid)

Urate is produced during the metabolism of purines, and is excreted by the kidneys. High levels in the blood (hyperuricaemia) can occur through two mechanisms:

- increased purine consumption or uric acid production
- impaired excretion of uric acid.

A modest amount of the body's purines is ingested in food and drink. A patient with a raised urate level may be asymptomatic or may be troubled with gout. It is common practice to measure serum urate levels in any patient with an acute monoarthritis. High levels of urate support a diagnosis of gout. However, urate levels can be normal during an acute attack of gout.

DON'T FORGET
Urate levels may be normal during an acute attack of gout.

Tumour markers

Tumour markers are a selection of blood tests that are commonly elevated in patients with neoplastic disease. Most tumour markers are characteristically associated with a particular type of cancer, as shown in the table.

TUMOUR MARKER	ASSOCIATED TUMOURS
α-Fetoprotein (FP)	Hepatocellular carcinoma; testicular teratoma
Human chorionic gonadotrophin (β-hCG)	Testicular teratoma and seminoma Choriocarcinoma
Prostate-specific antigen (PSA)	Prostate
CA-125	Ovarian
CA-19-9	Pancreatic
Carcinoembryonic antigen (CEA)	Colorectal

However, with the exception of α-FP, β-hCG and PSA, tumour markers are fairly non-specific, and several markers may be elevated with one underlying cancer. Tumour markers should therefore be requested only when the significance of a positive result can be usefully interpreted.

Tumour markers have two chief roles in clinical practice. First, specific markers such as PSA can be used in making a diagnosis. Second, serial measures of tumour markers can be used to monitor disease progress and response to treatment.

DON'T FORGET
Tumour markers are isolated blood tests – interpret them in the context of clinical features and all allied investigations.

Sweat testing

Cystic fibrosis results from a mutation in the gene that encodes the cystic fibrosis transmembrane conductance regulator (CFTR). CFTR is responsible for chloride ion transport across epithelial cells, and abnormalities in its structure result in viscous secretions, particularly in the lung and pancreas.

Abnormal sweat gland function leads to high concentrations of sodium and chloride in the sweat. Indeed, excessively salty tasting sweat was noted to be a clinical feature of cystic fibrosis long before the genetics were fully understood. This feature underlies the diagnostic test for cystic fibrosis – the sweat test.

In this test, sweating is stimulated, and sweat collected for analysis. Sufficient sweat (100 mg) must be collected for the test to be reliable. The test is positive if more than 60 mmol/l chloride is present, and the test should always be repeated before a conclusion is reached. Measurements of sweat sodium concentration are less reliable, but a concentration of greater than 90 mmol/l is in keeping with cystic fibrosis.

There are instances when a false-positive sweat test can occur. The most common of these are listed below.

COMMON CAUSES OF A FALSE-POSITIVE SWEAT TEST
Adrenal insufficiency
Anorexia nervosa
Coeliac disease
Hypothyroidism

Case 2.1

A 49-year-old missionary is brought to your hospital by his wife. He has been vomiting for the past 24 h. He is now very weak. He last ate 2 days previously and has struggled to keep down any liquids since. On examination his mouth is dry, his abdomen is generally uncomfortable and he has reduced skin turgor. After taking his routine blood tests, a 0.9% saline drip is erected before any results are checked. A short time later the following result is available.

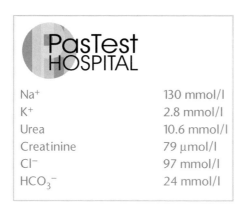

PasTest HOSPITAL	
Na^+	130 mmol/l
K^+	2.8 mmol/l
Urea	10.6 mmol/l
Creatinine	79 µmol/l
Cl^-	97 mmol/l
HCO_3^-	24 mmol/l

1.   Outline the abnormalities on this blood result.

After noting the above results, his intravenous fluid prescription is changed to 1 litre of 0.9% saline containing 40 mmol/l of potassium chloride, to be infused over 6 h.

Two hours later, his U&Es are repeated, and are shown below.

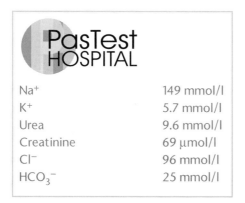

PasTest HOSPITAL	
Na^+	149 mmol/l
K^+	5.7 mmol/l
Urea	9.6 mmol/l
Creatinine	69 µmol/l
Cl^-	96 mmol/l
HCO_3^-	25 mmol/l

The ward doctor is concerned, and a further sample is taken.

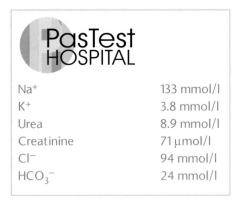

Na^+	133 mmol/l
K^+	3.8 mmol/l
Urea	8.9 mmol/l
Creatinine	71 µmol/l
Cl^-	94 mmol/l
HCO_3^-	24 mmol/l

2. How would you account for the discrepancy between these two blood tests?

Answer 2.1

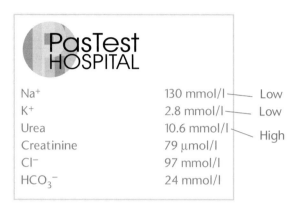

1. Three abnormalities can be seen in the results above:

   - Low sodium (hyponatraemia)
   - Low potassium (hypokalaemia)
   - High urea (uraemia).

The low sodium and low potassium are a consequence of a prolonged period of vomiting combined with very limited oral intake. There has been a substantial loss of electrolytes without any means of replacement until admission to hospital. The patient is clinically dehydrated and the raised urea is a reflection of this.

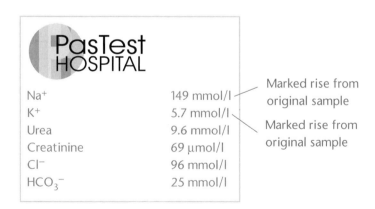

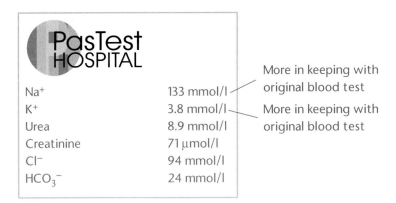

PasTest
HOSPITAL

Na⁺	133 mmol/l	More in keeping with original blood test
K⁺	3.8 mmol/l	More in keeping with original blood test
Urea	8.9 mmol/l	
Creatinine	71 μmol/l	
Cl⁻	94 mmol/l	
HCO₃⁻	24 mmol/l	

2. Looking at the first repeat blood test, the sodium and potassium levels have both risen from the time of admission a few hours previously. There has been a dramatic change in electrolyte levels. The second repeat sample is very different again.

The explanation for these findings is that the first repeat blood sample has been taken from the arm into which fluid is being infused. This is an erroneous sample.

The second repeat sample comes from a 'non-drip' arm, and shows the true state of affairs, ie slowly improving electrolytes from the time of admission.

Case 2.2

A 22-year-old university student is trapped in her house during a fire and when rescued by firefighters has developed substantial burns to the arms and chest. She is admitted to the burns unit. U&Es on her third day are shown.

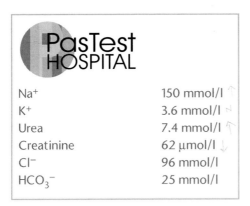

PasTest HOSPITAL	
Na^+	150 mmol/l ↑
K^+	3.6 mmol/l ↗
Urea	7.4 mmol/l ↑
Creatinine	62 μmol/l ↓
Cl^-	96 mmol/l
HCO_3^-	25 mmol/l

What is the main biochemical problem and name some of its causes?

Answer 2.2

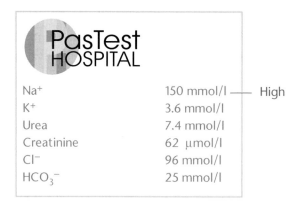

PasTest
HOSPITAL

Na⁺	150 mmol/l	High
K⁺	3.6 mmol/l	
Urea	7.4 mmol/l	
Creatinine	62 µmol/l	
Cl⁻	96 mmol/l	
HCO₃⁻	25 mmol/l	

Hypernatraemia is present. Other components of the U&Es are normal.
A common cause for this observation in hospital medicine is excessive use of
0.9% saline in those patients receiving intravenous fluids. This is one reason
why intravenous fluid prescribing should be considered carefully and regular
U&E samples checked. This is especially important in patients with excessive
fluid losses, such as patients with burns. In this patient, substantial fluid loss
from her burns has led to a water deficit. Consequentially, the sodium
concentration has risen.

Other causes of hypernatraemia are listed on page 59.

Case 2.3

A 76-year-old woman is admitted unwell with vomiting and is found to have a low blood pressure. She had recently been given diclofenac following a complaint of back pain. Her initial blood results included U&Es.

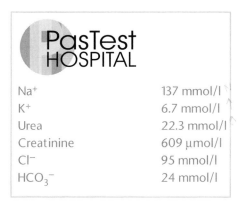

PasTest HOSPITAL	
Na^+	137 mmol/l
K^+	6.7 mmol/l
Urea	22.3 mmol/l
Creatinine	609 µmol/l
Cl^-	95 mmol/l
HCO_3^-	24 mmol/l

1. **What has happened to this patient?**

2. **What immediate treatment is indicated?**

Answer 2.3

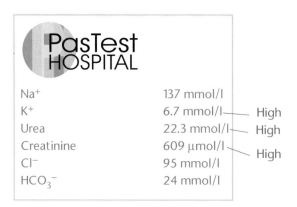

Na⁺	137 mmol/l	
K⁺	6.7 mmol/l	High
Urea	22.3 mmol/l	High
Creatinine	609 μmol/l	High
Cl⁻	95 mmol/l	
HCO₃⁻	24 mmol/l	

1. The urea and creatinine are both grossly elevated indicating that this patient has renal failure. Comparison with previous blood tests would indicate whether this is acute or chronic. As a consequence of the renal failure, serum potassium is dangerously elevated. The rising potassium is a reflection of the failing tubular function of the kidney. In this case it would appear that the use of a non-steroidal anti-inflammatory drug (diclofenac) and vomiting are the causes of an acute deterioration in renal function.

2. Hyperkalaemia can cause fatal dysrhythmias, including cardiac arrest. This requires immediate treatment. Conventional treatment employs insulin and dextrose. Insulin drives potassium into the cells, while glucose prevents hypoglycaemia. Calcium gluconate should be given first to stabilise the myocardium.

    The ultimate treatment is to identify the cause of the renal failure and support the kidneys until function is restored.

Case 2.4

A 46-year-old diplomat is transferred to your care following medical evacuation from Nigeria. In his transfer correspondence it indicates that he has developed renal impairment which as yet has not been investigated in depth.

His U&Es are shown, along with a 24-h urine collection for creatinine clearance.

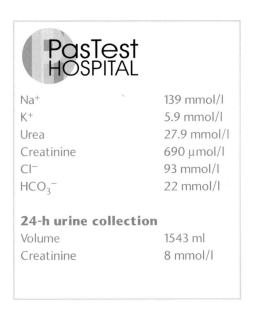

PasTest HOSPITAL

Na^+	139 mmol/l
K^+	5.9 mmol/l
Urea	27.9 mmol/l
Creatinine	690 µmol/l
Cl^-	93 mmol/l
HCO_3^-	22 mmol/l

24-h urine collection

Volume	1543 ml
Creatinine	8 mmol/l

Calculate his creatinine clearance.

Answer 2.4

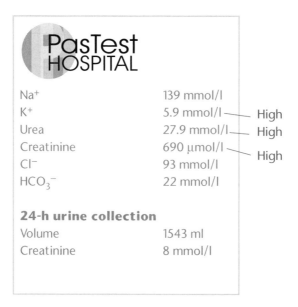

PasTest
HOSPITAL

Na$^+$	139 mmol/l
K$^+$	5.9 mmol/l —— High
Urea	27.9 mmol/l —— High
Creatinine	690 μmol/l —— High
Cl$^-$	93 mmol/l
HCO$_3^-$	22 mmol/l

24-h urine collection

Volume	1543 ml
Creatinine	8 mmol/l

Creatinine clearance can be calculated using the following equation:

$$CL_{Cr} = \frac{U_{Cr} \times V \times 0.694}{B_{Cr}}$$

where V_{Cr} is the concentration of creatinine in urine (in mmol/l), V is the 24-h urine volume (in ml) and B_{Cr} is plasma creatinine in μmol/l

In this case:

$$CL_{Cr} = \frac{8 \times 1543 \times 0.694}{690} = 12.4 \text{ ml/min}$$

The creatinine clearance is 12.4 ml/min. Bearing in mind that the normal creatinine clearance is approximately 100 ml/min, it is clear that this man has significant renal impairment.

Case 2.5

A 34-year-old man is admitted with epigastric discomfort and a single episode of vomiting following a week-long binge of alcohol. His vital signs are within the normal range. Blood tests were taken at the time of admission.

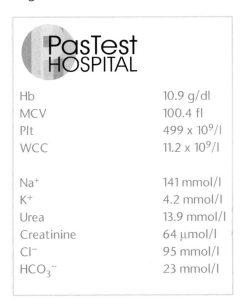

PasTest HOSPITAL	
Hb	10.9 g/dl
MCV	100.4 fl
Plt	499 x 10^9/l
WCC	11.2 x 10^9/l
Na$^+$	141 mmol/l
K$^+$	4.2 mmol/l
Urea	13.9 mmol/l
Creatinine	64 µmol/l
Cl$^-$	95 mmol/l
HCO$_3^-$	23 mmol/l

Explain the elevated urea in the context of the other haematological results.

Answer 2.5

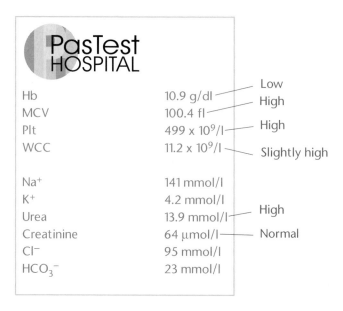

PasTest HOSPITAL		
Hb	10.9 g/dl	Low
MCV	100.4 fl	High
Plt	499 x 10^9/l	High
WCC	11.2 x 10^9/l	Slightly high
Na$^+$	141 mmol/l	
K$^+$	4.2 mmol/l	
Urea	13.9 mmol/l	High
Creatinine	64 μmol/l	Normal
Cl$^-$	95 mmol/l	
HCO$_3$$^-$	23 mmol/l	

This man's U&Es reveal an elevated urea. His creatinine is normal and his clinical history does not suggest dehydration. His full blood count reveals information that helps in interpreting the significance of the elevated urea. His haemoglobin, MCV, white cell count and platelets are all abnormal. The raised MCV most likely represents chronic alcohol use.

During gastrointestinal bleeding, an increase in urea may occur. This is because urea is a breakdown product of digested blood. Similarly during an active bleed, a rise in the white cell count and platelet count may occur.

The combination of the following is suggestive of gastrointestinal bleeding:

- raised urea (with normal creatinine)
- low haemoglobin
- raised white cell count (in the absence of infection)
- raised platelets.

Case 2.6

A 39-year-old man with a history of Crohn's disease and previous extensive small bowel resection is admitted with anorexia and weight loss. His GP is very concerned that he now weighs only 39 kg and has not been able to tolerate much in the way of oral foods for several months. In hospital, attempts were made to start nasogastric feeding, but it could not be tolerated. Total parenteral nutrition (TPN) was therefore commenced. The following table shows his U&Es and nutritional profile over several days following commencement of parenteral feeding.

PasTest HOSPITAL

Date	14/02	15/02	16/02	17/02
Na^+ (mmol/l)	135	135	134	136
K^+ (mmol/l)	3.3	3.4	3.4	3.7
Urea (mmol/l)	2.1	2.2	2.2	2.3
Creatinine (μmol/l)	44	49	47	45
Cl^- (mmol/l)	94	94	93	93
HCO_3^- (mmol/l)	23	22	23	23
Mg^{2+} (mmol/l)	0.39	0.37	0.38	0.51
PO_4^{3-} (mmol/l)	0.70	0.61	0.41	0.40
Total Ca^{2+} (mmol/l)	2.32	2.05	2.12	2.22
Albumin (g/l)	33	32	33	32

Comment on these results.

Answer 2.6

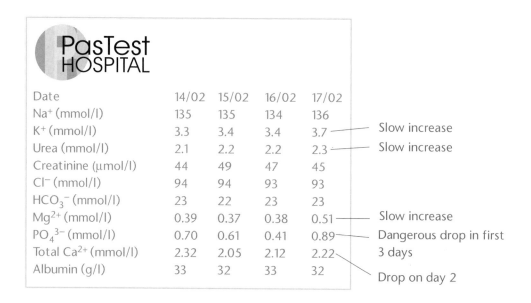

This scenario illustrates the issue of re-feeding in those patients who have been nutritionally depleted for some time. When feeding is commenced, a rapid and precipitous drop often occurs, in particular, in phosphate levels.

Case 2.7

A 72-year-old former engine driver attends his GP complaining of generalised aches and pains. During the consultation you have to speak loudly to be understood. As part of your investigations you request a bone profile. Liver function tests were normal.

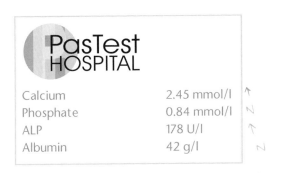

Calcium	2.45 mmol/l	↑
Phosphate	0.84 mmol/l	N
ALP	178 U/l	↑
Albumin	42 g/l	N

On the basis of this test he received a course of treatment for several months. Following treatment his bone profile is repeated and is as follows.

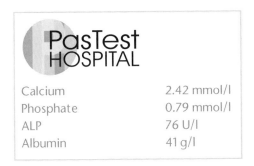

Calcium	2.42 mmol/l
Phosphate	0.79 mmol/l
ALP	76 U/l
Albumin	41 g/l

1. **What bone disease does this patient have?**

2. **What treatment is he likely to have received to explain the change in his bone profile?**

Answer 2.7

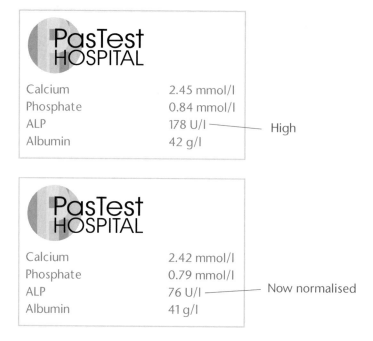

PasTest
HOSPITAL

Calcium	2.45 mmol/l
Phosphate	0.84 mmol/l
ALP	178 U/l — High
Albumin	42 g/l

PasTest
HOSPITAL

Calcium	2.42 mmol/l
Phosphate	0.79 mmol/l
ALP	76 U/l — Now normalised
Albumin	41 g/l

1. This elderly man has Paget's disease of the bone. He has an isolated ALP rise, in the absence of any liver disease. An ALP rise can occur for various reasons, including primary sclerosing cholangitis and bony metastases. However, in the context of this patient's symptoms, with deafness, Paget disease is most likely.

2. The repeat bone profile demonstrates lowering of the ALP after successful treatment. He is likely to have received intravenous bisphosphonate therapy. Note that the majority of patients with Paget's disease are asymptomatic and the disease is often diagnosed incidentally when tests are requested for other reasons.

Case 2.8

A 69-year-old retired nurse complains of generalised aches and pains for the past 5 weeks, sometimes preventing her from sleeping at night. Her past medical history includes hypothyroidism, hypertension and a mastectomy 2 years ago for breast carcinoma. She is a very active member of the Women's Institute and feels less able to complete her daily tasks of late.

Blood tests included a bone profile. Liver function tests were normal.

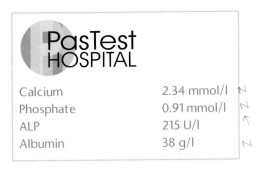

PasTest HOSPITAL		
Calcium	2.34 mmol/l	N
Phosphate	0.91 mmol/l	N
ALP	215 U/l	↑
Albumin	38 g/l	N

Describe the findings on the bone profile and give an explanation.

Answer 2.8

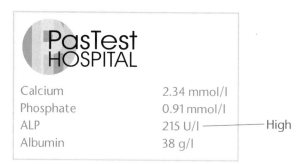

PasTest
HOSPITAL

Calcium	2.34 mmol/l
Phosphate	0.91 mmol/l
ALP	215 U/l ——————High
Albumin	38 g/l

The ALP is significantly raised. The rest of the bone profile is normal. ALP may be high in a number of conditions. It is important to exclude liver disease, but we are told here that the rest of her liver function tests were normal.

Bearing in mind the clinical history, a particular concern in this woman would be bony metastases from breast carcinoma. This can occur a considerable time after treatment of the primary tumour. The calcium may be normal or elevated in the presence of bony metastases.

Case 2.9

A 45-year-old teacher has been complaining of aches and pains for several months. Her colleagues have said that she has not been herself recently, appearing 'under the weather' and sad. She is still menstruating regularly. Among the blood tests requested by her GP was a bone profile.

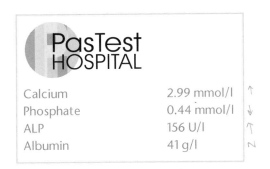

PasTest
HOSPITAL

Calcium	2.99 mmol/l	↑
Phosphate	0.44 mmol/l	↓
ALP	156 U/l	↑
Albumin	41 g/l	N

A further blood test, of great importance in diagnosis, was sent the following day.

1. **What is the additional test likely to be?**

2. **What is the likely diagnosis?**

Answer 2.9

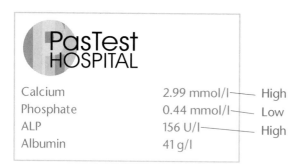

Calcium	2.99 mmol/l	High
Phosphate	0.44 mmol/l	Low
ALP	156 U/l	High
Albumin	41 g/l	

1. The additional test is for parathyroid hormone (PTH).

2. These findings are in keeping with primary hyperparathyroidism.

The excess PTH, most likely from a parathyroid adenoma, is causing excess bone resorption resulting in a high calcium and ALP. Constitutional symptoms include bony aches, low mood and constipation, which can arise due to the hypercalcaemia. Hence the patient with hyperparathyroidism can have problems with 'bones, stones, moans and abdominal groans'.

Note that in primary hyperparathyroidism PTH is generally raised. However, a normal PTH level is also abnormal in a patient with hypercalcaemia and may be indicative of hyperparathyroidism. This is because PTH should normally be suppressed by negative feedback in the setting of hypercalcaemia.

Case 2.10

A 46-year-old office clerk attends a private health clinic complaining of aches in his bones and tenderness over his muscles. This has been troubling him for some time and he is no longer able to walk to work. He has suffered from coeliac disease for many years, but by his own confession finds it hard at times to stick to his gluten-free diet. A 'screen' of tests is taken, some of which are shown below.

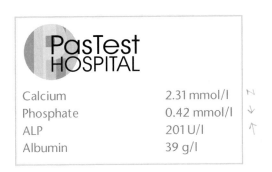

PasTest
HOSPITAL

Calcium	2.31 mmol/l	↗
Phosphate	0.42 mmol/l	↓
ALP	201 U/l	↑
Albumin	39 g/l	

What is the likely diagnosis?

Answer 2.10

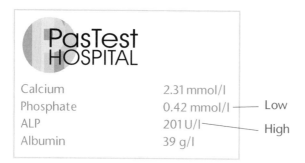

PasTest
HOSPITAL

Calcium	2.31 mmol/l
Phosphate	0.42 mmol/l —— Low
ALP	201 U/l —— High
Albumin	39 g/l

These findings are in keeping with a diagnosis of osteomalacia. Osteomalacia is a metabolic bone disease in which there is a lack of calcium or phosphate (or both) for mineralisation of newly formed osteoid. As a result, bone is 'soft' and unable to withstand the stresses and forces of normal bone. Parathyroid hormone would need to be checked if there was any diagnostic doubt.

It is likely that this patient's coeliac disease is contributing to the development of osteomalacia through malabsorption of calcium.

Case 2.11

A 55-year-old woman is admitted with a fractured neck of femur after a minor trip in the car park of her local supermarket. Looking back through her old records, the admitting doctor notices the following bone profile taken 2 weeks previously.

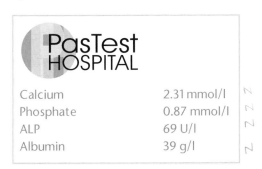

Calcium	2.31 mmol/l	
Phosphate	0.87 mmol/l	
ALP	69 U/l	
Albumin	39 g/l	

What bone disease might you suspect?

Answer 2.11

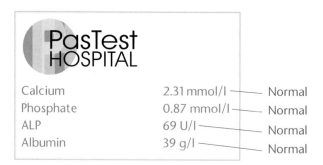

PasTest
HOSPITAL

Calcium	2.31 mmol/l	Normal
Phosphate	0.87 mmol/l	Normal
ALP	69 U/l	Normal
Albumin	39 g/l	Normal

You should suspect osteoporosis given the history of fracture after minimal trauma, and a previously normal bone profile. Osteoporosis is the most common form of metabolic bone disease. It is predominantly found in postmenopausal women and is considered a silent disease. First presentation is often with a low trauma fracture as in this clinical scenario.

Diagnosis of osteoporosis is usually made using dual energy X-ray absorptiometry (DEXA) scan.

Case 2.12

A 47-year-old woman is referred to the regional hepatology outpatient clinic by her GP. She attended her GP on several occasions complaining of tiredness, low mood, altered bowel habit and more recently of itch. On examination a 4-cm smooth hepatomegaly is noted, with xanthelasmata around her eyes.

The referral letter contains the following LFTs:

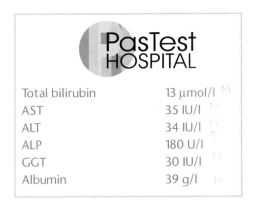

Total bilirubin	13 μmol/l	N
AST	35 IU/l	N
ALT	34 IU/l	N
ALP	180 U/l	↑
GGT	30 IU/l	N
Albumin	39 g/l	N

A blood test taken at the clinic revealed the following:

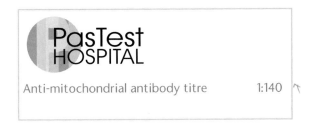

Anti-mitochondrial antibody titre	1:140	↑

1. **Interpret these results.** PBC

2. **Suggest a further investigation.**

Answer 2.12

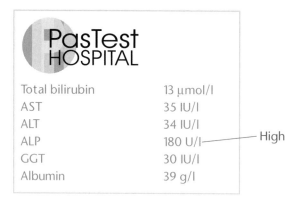

PasTest
HOSPITAL

Total bilirubin	13 µmol/l
AST	35 IU/l
ALT	34 IU/l
ALP	180 U/l —— High
GGT	30 IU/l
Albumin	39 g/l

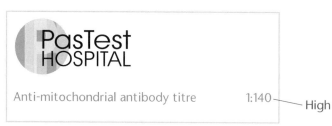

PasTest
HOSPITAL

Anti-mitochondrial antibody titre	1:140 —— High

1. The only abnormality on the liver biochemistry is a raised ALP. ALP may be raised in bone as well as liver disease (see page 70). An isolated ALP rise may be seen in both primary sclerosing cholangitis (PSC) and early primary biliary cirrhosis (PBC). The normal albumin suggests that the synthetic function of the liver remains intact. The immunological tests are the diagnostic key in this case. A substantially raised anti-mitochondrial antibody (AMA) is observed. Ninety-five per cent of patients with PBC will have a positive antibody for AMA-M2. In PSC the presence of autoantibodies is uncommon.

2. The most useful investigation to confirm and assess the extent of disease would be a liver biopsy.

Case 2.13

A 68-year-old woman was admitted with itch, lethargy and discoloration of the skin over the past month. On examination she is icteric and cachexic. There are no stigmata of chronic liver disease. Nursing staff indicate that there is discoloration of her urine.

Her admission bloods include LFTs.

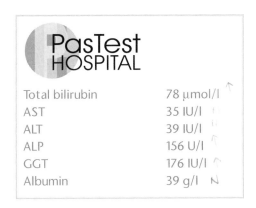

PasTest HOSPITAL

Total bilirubin	78 μmol/l ↑
AST	35 IU/l
ALT	39 IU/l
ALP	156 U/l ↑
GGT	176 IU/l ↑
Albumin	39 g/l N

1. **Outline the abnormalities seen on the liver function tests.** ↑ AU bili

2. **What would be your next choice of investigation?** USS

3. **What are the potential causes of these results?** CA pancreas other causes biliary obs

Answer 2.13

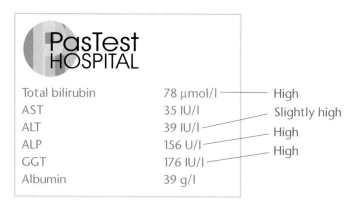

Total bilirubin	78 µmol/l	High
AST	35 IU/l	Slightly high
ALT	39 IU/l	High
ALP	156 U/l	High
GGT	176 IU/l	
Albumin	39 g/l	

1. The LFTs show an elevated bilirubin with cholestatic LFTs.

2. An ultrasound scan of the abdomen is the next most important investigation. This will confirm the presence of obstruction and may identify the underlying cause. This can then act as a guide for further investigations.

3. The causes of cholestatic jaundice are listed on page 73.

Case 2.14

A 34-year-old labourer is admitted with right upper quadrant discomfort, fever and sweats. He returned from a project overseas 3 weeks earlier. On examination he is tender to palpitation over the right hypochondrium making complete examination difficult. A spiking fever pattern is seen on his observation chart. His LFTs are as follows.

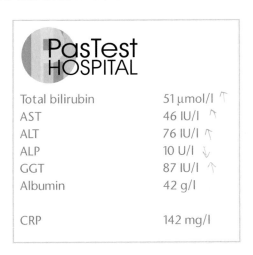

PasTest HOSPITAL	
Total bilirubin	51 μmol/l ↑
AST	46 IU/l ↑
ALT	76 IU/l ↑
ALP	10 U/l ↓
GGT	87 IU/l ↑
Albumin	42 g/l
CRP	142 mg/l

1. **What investigation does this patient need as soon as possible based on his clinical history and blood tests?** *hepatitic picture hepatitis screen ? viral hepatitis*

2. **What is the likely diagnosis?**

Answer 2.14

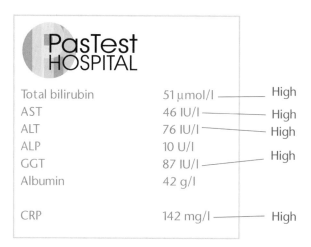

PasTest
HOSPITAL

Total bilirubin	51 µmol/l	High
AST	46 IU/l	High
ALT	76 IU/l	High
ALP	10 U/l	
GGT	87 IU/l	High
Albumin	42 g/l	
CRP	142 mg/l	High

1. The bilirubin and transaminases are raised. The CRP is highly elevated. He requires an ultrasound scan of the abdomen to investigate an infective cause for his symptoms.

2. Viral hepatitis, a liver abscess or cholangitis are all potential causes.

Case 2.15

A 32-year-old man is recalled by his occupational health department following a recent 'medical' before transfer to an overseas operation within the company. He is teetotal. He cannot understand what all the fuss is about as he feels fine.

The blood results of concern are shown.

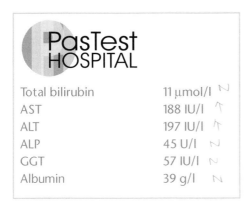

PasTest HOSPITAL		
Total bilirubin	11 µmol/l	N
AST	188 IU/l	↑
ALT	197 IU/l	↑
ALP	45 U/l	N
GGT	57 IU/l	N
Albumin	39 g/l	N

1. **What pattern of LFTs is demonstrated?** *hepatic picture*
2. **What further blood tests may help in coming to a diagnosis?**

Answer 2.15

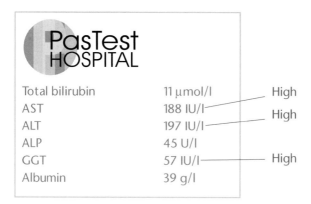

PasTest
HOSPITAL

Total bilirubin	11 μmol/l	High
AST	188 IU/l	High
ALT	197 IU/l	
ALP	45 U/l	
GGT	57 IU/l	High
Albumin	39 g/l	

1. This patient has a parenchymal LFT derangement. Both the ALT and AST are markedly elevated.

2. A set of 'screening' investigations should be performed next to further investigate the situation. See Page 71 for details.

This patient had hepatitis C. Not infrequently hepatitis C is diagnosed incidentally when LFTs are checked for some other reason.

Case 2.16

A 37-year-old manual worker is admitted with generalised abdominal discomfort, vomiting and shakiness. On examination there is a 4-cm mildly tender hepatomegaly. He is sweaty to the touch. Some blood tests are requested.

PasTest HOSPITAL

Hb	13.4 g/dl
MCV	105.6 fl
Plt	124 x 10^9/l
WCC	5.6 x 10^9/l
Na$^+$	142 mmol/l
K$^+$	3.4 mmol/l
Urea	2.1 mmol/l
Creatinine	58 µmol/l
Cl$^-$	105 mmol/l
HCO$_3^-$	26.7 mmol/l
Mg^{2+}	0.42 mmol/l
PO$_4^{3-}$	0.32 mmol/l
Total Ca^{2+}	2.36 mmol/l
Total bilirubin	14 µmol/l
AST	32 IU/l
ALT	33 IU/l
ALP	67 U/l
GGT	145 IU/l
Albumin	30 g/l

1. **Outline the abnormalities on this set of blood results.**

2. **Explain the likely cause of the LFT abnormalities given the abnormalities in the other results.**

Answer 2.16

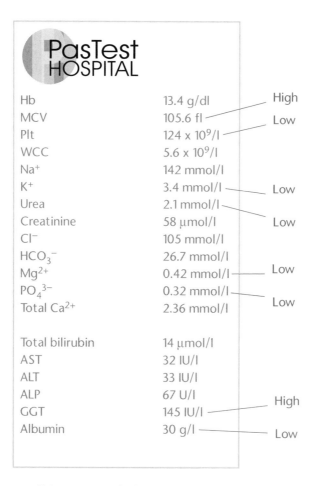

PasTest
HOSPITAL

Hb	13.4 g/dl	High
MCV	105.6 fl	Low
Plt	124 x 10^9/l	
WCC	5.6 x 10^9/l	
Na$^+$	142 mmol/l	
K$^+$	3.4 mmol/l	Low
Urea	2.1 mmol/l	
Creatinine	58 µmol/l	Low
Cl$^-$	105 mmol/l	
HCO$_3$$^-$	26.7 mmol/l	
Mg^{2+}	0.42 mmol/l	Low
PO$_4$$^{3-}$	0.32 mmol/l	
Total Ca^{2+}	2.36 mmol/l	Low
Total bilirubin	14 µmol/l	
AST	32 IU/l	
ALT	33 IU/l	
ALP	67 U/l	
GGT	145 IU/l	High
Albumin	30 g/l	Low

1. The abnormalities seen include:

   - a raised MCV, with a slightly low platelet count
   - low values for urea, potassium, magnesium and, in particular, phosphate
   - a raised GGT
   - a low albumin.

2. The findings on these simple blood tests are classic for an individual who has consumed large quantities of alcohol for a significant time period.

Case 2.17

A 44-year-old woman with primary biliary cirrhosis has been attending hepatology outpatients for many years. Over the past 18 months she has been feeling less well in herself and her frequency of attendance for review has increased at the insistence of her physician. On examination she is jaundiced and her abdomen is mildly distended with a 3-cm hepatomegaly.

Her recent blood results are shown.

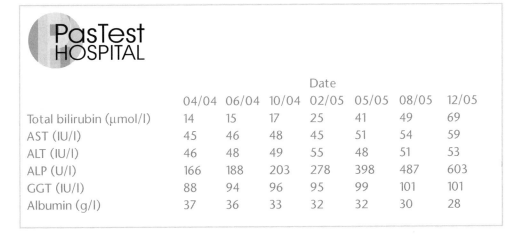

				Date			
	04/04	06/04	10/04	02/05	05/05	08/05	12/05
Total bilirubin (µmol/l)	14	15	17	25	41	49	69
AST (IU/l)	45	46	48	45	51	54	59
ALT (IU/l)	46	48	49	55	48	51	53
ALP (U/l)	166	188	203	278	398	487	603
GGT (IU/l)	88	94	96	95	99	101	101
Albumin (g/l)	37	36	33	32	32	30	28

Give a summary of the findings.

Answer 2.17

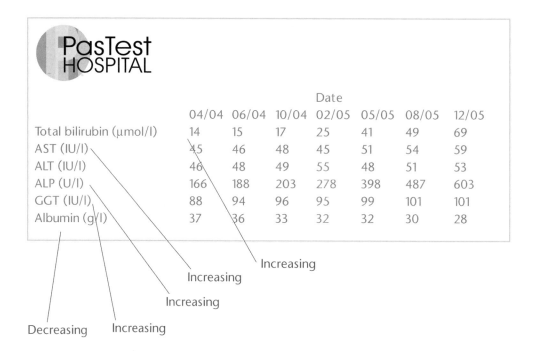

PasTest
HOSPITAL

	Date						
	04/04	06/04	10/04	02/05	05/05	08/05	12/05
Total bilirubin (µmol/l)	14	15	17	25	41	49	69
AST (IU/I)	45	46	48	45	51	54	59
ALT (IU/I)	46	48	49	55	48	51	53
ALP (U/I)	166	188	203	278	398	487	603
GGT (IU/I)	88	94	96	95	99	101	101
Albumin (g/l)	37	36	33	32	32	30	28

Increasing

Increasing

Increasing

Decreasing   Increasing

The course of primary biliary cirrhosis is variable. Patients may live with stable LFTs for a number of years. Decompensation may occur at any time with deterioration in the liver's synthetic function.

The chart shows LFTs over a period of 20 months. Initially only a moderately elevated ALP is seen in April 2004. Over the ensuing months the ALP continues to rise, and with this the albumin falls reaching a low of 28 g/l in December 2005.

The prothrombin time should also be checked. One would expect it to be raised indicating impaired production of clotting factors by the failing liver.

Case 2.18

A patient is referred to a psychiatrist for investigation of bizarre thoughts. She has occasional involuntary movements. The psychiatrist requests a series of blood tests as part of her initial screening tests, and the following results are obtained.

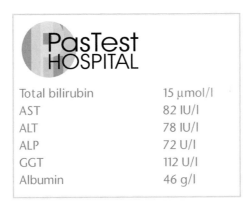

PasTest HOSPITAL	
Total bilirubin	15 µmol/l
AST	82 IU/l
ALT	78 IU/l
ALP	72 U/l
GGT	112 U/l
Albumin	46 g/l

What disease could account for the presentation and the blood test abnormalities? How would you investigate it further?

Answer 2.18

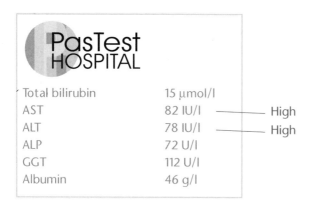

PasTest HOSPITAL		
Total bilirubin	15 μmol/l	
AST	82 IU/l	High
ALT	78 IU/l	High
ALP	72 U/l	
GGT	112 U/l	
Albumin	46 g/l	

The blood tests show very mild elevations in AST and ALT. These are very minor and non-specific findings and could be caused by a variety of conditions, including viral hepatitis and drug-induced hepatitis. The only condition that meaningfully links a psychiatric disorder with these abnormal liver function tests is, however, Wilson's disease – a condition associated with copper overload. Tests that could be performed to investigate further include: serum copper level, serum ceruloplasmin level, slit-lamp examination of the eyes to look for copper deposition, 24-hour urinary collection for copper measurement and liver biopsy.

Case 2.19

A 38-year-old woman complains of a rash over her face and nose for several weeks and a recent problem with pain and swelling in the joints of her hands. She is married but without children. A number of blood tests were sent – some of which are shown below.

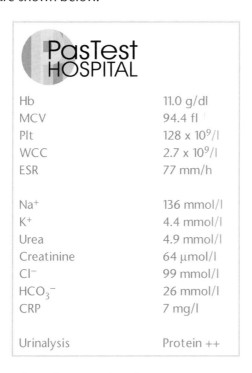

PasTest
HOSPITAL

Hb	11.0 g/dl
MCV	94.4 fl
Plt	128 x 10^9/l
WCC	2.7 x 10^9/l
ESR	77 mm/h
Na$^+$	136 mmol/l
K$^+$	4.4 mmol/l
Urea	4.9 mmol/l
Creatinine	64 µmol/l
Cl$^-$	99 mmol/l
HCO$_3^-$	26 mmol/l
CRP	7 mg/l
Urinalysis	Protein ++

1. **Summarise the results shown.**

2. **Using the clinical information what is the most likely diagnosis?**

Answer 2.19

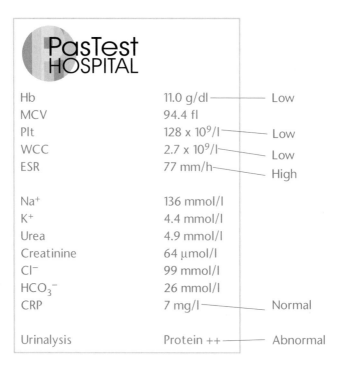

PasTest
HOSPITAL

Hb	11.0 g/dl	Low
MCV	94.4 fl	
Plt	128 x 10^9/l	Low
WCC	2.7 x 10^9/l	Low
ESR	77 mm/h	High
Na$^+$	136 mmol/l	
K$^+$	4.4 mmol/l	
Urea	4.9 mmol/l	
Creatinine	64 μmol/l	
Cl$^-$	99 mmol/l	
HCO$_3$$^-$	26 mmol/l	
CRP	7 mg/l	Normal
Urinalysis	Protein ++	Abnormal

1. There are a number of abnormalities on this set of results:

   - the haemoglobin is slightly low

   - the platelet count is slightly below normal

   - the WCC is low

   - the ESR is raised, with a normal CRP

   - protein is noted in the urine.

2. The CRP is normal. This would go against an infectious cause for a raised ESR and be more suggestive of inflammation of some description. There are only a few conditions in which the ESR is elevated but the CRP remains normal. One such condition is systemic lupus erythematosus (SLE) which this patient's clinical features and blood test abnormalities are in keeping with.

Case 2.20

A 77-year-old patient with dementia was admitted generally unwell. No history was obtained. He was pyrexic and appeared a little short of breath. Examination was difficult, although there was the impression of reduced breath sounds at the right lung base. Urinalysis was normal. Blood tests were taken.

PasTest
HOSPITAL

Hb	13.9 g/dl
MCV	95.5 fl
Plt	188 x 10^9/l
WCC	9.7 x 10^9/l
Na$^+$	142 mmol/l
K$^+$	4.4 mmol/l
Urea	4.6 mmol/l
Creatinine	75 µmol/l
Cl$^-$	100 mmol/l
HCO$_3^-$	24 mmol/l
CRP	156 mg/l

How do these tests help in the management of this patient?

Answer 2.20

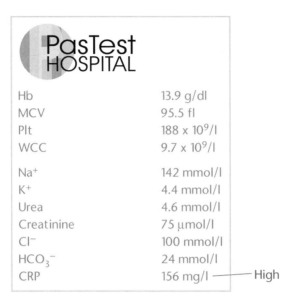

PasTest
HOSPITAL

Hb	13.9 g/dl
MCV	95.5 fl
Plt	188 x 10⁹/l
WCC	9.7 x 10⁹/l
Na⁺	142 mmol/l
K⁺	4.4 mmol/l
Urea	4.6 mmol/l
Creatinine	75 μmol/l
Cl⁻	100 mmol/l
HCO_3^-	24 mmol/l
CRP	156 mg/l ——— High

Establishing a diagnosis in elderly people can be difficult by clinical assessment
alone, especially when no history is available. It is often necessary to place
greater emphasis on investigations. Although, in this case, the FBP and U&Es are
normal, the CRP is significantly raised. In the presence of infection one might
expect the WCC to be raised too, but this is not always the case. An infection is
likely to be the cause of the patient's illness. A urinary tract infection and
pneumonia are the most common causes of these findings in clinical practice.
Given the normal urinalysis and abnormal examination findings in the chest,
pneumonia is the most likely diagnosis.

Case 2.21

A 34-year-old woman with acute lymphoblastic leukaemia (ALL) is receiving chemotherapy within the haematology suite of the hospital. Several days into treatment she complains of an intensely sore right knee. On examination there is an effusion and she is unable to extend the knee fully due to pain. She has no pre-existing joint disease. Fluid was aspirated from the knee and sent for analysis along with blood samples.

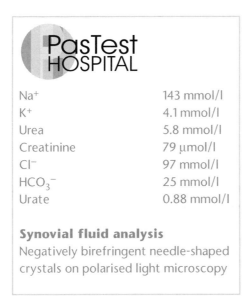

PasTest
HOSPITAL

Na$^+$	143 mmol/l
K$^+$	4.1 mmol/l
Urea	5.8 mmol/l
Creatinine	79 μmol/l
Cl$^-$	97 mmol/l
HCO$_3$$^-$	25 mmol/l
Urate	0.88 mmol/l

Synovial fluid analysis
Negatively birefringent needle-shaped crystals on polarised light microscopy

Interpret these results (see page 496 for details of synovial fluid analysis).

Answer 2.21

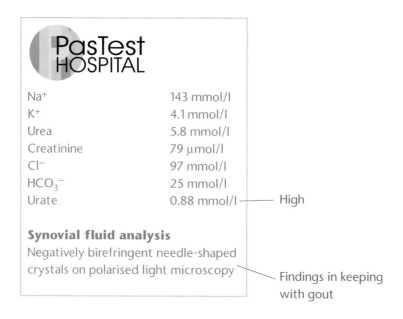

PasTest
HOSPITAL

Na$^+$	143 mmol/l
K$^+$	4.1 mmol/l
Urea	5.8 mmol/l
Creatinine	79 μmol/l
Cl$^-$	97 mmol/l
HCO$_3^-$	25 mmol/l
Urate	0.88 mmol/l ——— High

Synovial fluid analysis
Negatively birefringent needle-shaped
crystals on polarised light microscopy ——— Findings in keeping
with gout

Hyperuricaemia may occur due to excess purine metabolism. This includes those suffering from haematological malignancies in which there is increased cell turnover, especially following cell lysis from chemotherapy.

The presence of negatively birefringent crystals from the joint aspiration confirms gout.

Case 2.22

A 32-year-old woman with diabetes is admitted for treatment of a large abscess. The patient is reluctant to undergo surgical intervention and medical treatment is pursued initially. Four days into her care she becomes more unwell and her treatment is changed. A further 3 days on, when her condition remains poor, she agrees to surgical intervention. Below is a chart of her CRP throughout this period.

PasTest
HOSPITAL

DAY	CRP (mg/l)
1	356
2	345
3	387
4	444
5	467
6	499
7	550
8	422
9	302
10	143
11	121

Try to explain the trend in the results.

Answer 2.22

PasTest HOSPITAL

DAY	CRP (mg/l)	
1	356	
2	345	
3	387	
4	444	
5	467	
6	499	
7	550	CRP rising until this day; thereafter falling
8	422	
9	302	
10	143	
11	121	

Some of the most rewarding data to interpret are those collated over a period of time when trends can be observed. This scenario illustrates the value of CRP in both supporting a clinical diagnosis and monitoring its response to treatment. On admission this patient's CRP is significantly raised, as one may expect in the presence of an abscess. With the commencement of antibiotics, one might hope for the CRP to improve as the abscess is treated. The worsening of her clinical state and the rising CRP suggest that either the antibiotics are ineffective against the causative organism or they are unable to penetrate the abscess. Day 4 sees a change in treatment, no doubt to an alternative antimicrobial. However, the CRP remains stubbornly high. It is only in the days following surgical intervention that the CRP begins to decrease, reflecting the successful treatment of the abscess.

Case 2.23

A 58-year-old man complains of an exquisitely tender great toe. It is red, swollen and impossible to examine fully because of pain. No other joints are affected. He has a history of hypertension and a previous myocardial infarction at 49 years of age. He drinks 14 units of alcohol a week. To his knowledge he does not have any kidney problems. Blood tests are shown.

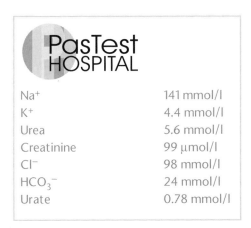

PasTest
HOSPITAL

Na^+	141 mmol/l
K^+	4.4 mmol/l
Urea	5.6 mmol/l
Creatinine	99 µmol/l
Cl^-	98 mmol/l
HCO_3^-	24 mmol/l
Urate	0.78 mmol/l

Does this man have gout? Justify your answer.

Answer 2.23

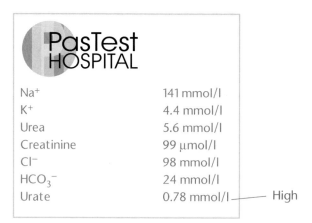

PasTest
HOSPITAL

Na$^+$	141 mmol/l
K$^+$	4.4 mmol/l
Urea	5.6 mmol/l
Creatinine	99 μmol/l
Cl$^-$	98 mmol/l
HCO$_3$$^-$	24 mmol/l
Urate	0.78 mmol/l ——— High

The clinical history is one of podagra (gout of the great toe). The elevated urate in the blood supports this diagnosis. Definitive diagnosis of gout depends on the detection of crystals of sodium urate in synovial fluid (see page 496). However, not all joints with acute gout are amenable to aspiration and one must rely on a clinical impression and supportive blood tests. Remember that the serum urate level can be normal in acute gout.

This patient may well be taking a thiazide diuretic for hypertension. This would place him at higher risk for gout.

Case 2.24

A 67-year-old man attends outpatients with a complaint of constipation and vague abdominal discomfort. Abdominal examination and proctoscopy were normal. Imaging investigations and endoscopy have been arranged. CEA levels were also requested, along with routine blood tests.

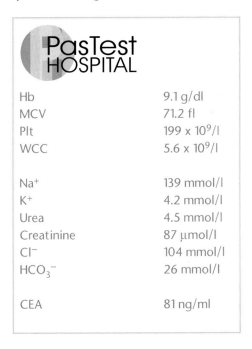

PasTest
HOSPITAL

Hb	9.1 g/dl
MCV	71.2 fl
Plt	199 x 10^9/l
WCC	5.6 x 10^9/l
Na$^+$	139 mmol/l
K$^+$	4.2 mmol/l
Urea	4.5 mmol/l
Creatinine	87 μmol/l
Cl$^-$	104 mmol/l
HCO$_3$$^-$	26 mmol/l
CEA	81 ng/ml

What underlying diagnosis unites all the abnormalities observed?

Answer 2.24

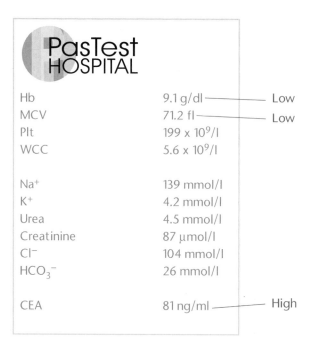

PasTest
HOSPITAL

Hb	9.1 g/dl	Low
MCV	71.2 fl	Low
Plt	199 x 10⁹/l	
WCC	5.6 x 10⁹/l	
Na⁺	139 mmol/l	
K⁺	4.2 mmol/l	
Urea	4.5 mmol/l	
Creatinine	87 µmol/l	
Cl⁻	104 mmol/l	
HCO₃⁻	26 mmol/l	
CEA	81 ng/ml	High

The key findings on this patient's blood tests are a microcytic anaemia (see page 4) and a raised CEA. Given his symptoms, these results should arouse a great deal of suspicion of colorectal carcinoma. Although proctoscopy was normal this visualises only a very small percentage of the large bowel and further imaging is required. In this case the tumour marker merely adds weight to a clinical suspicion.

Case 2.25

A 55 year old with haemophilia attends her routine 6-monthly review at hepatology outpatients. She has been attending for several years after contracting hepatitis C from a blood transfusion. The doctor notes that she has not attended for 8 months, and requests a number of blood tests.

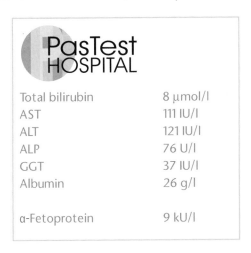

PasTest HOSPITAL

Total bilirubin	8 µmol/l
AST	111 IU/l
ALT	121 IU/l
ALP	76 U/l
GGT	37 IU/l
Albumin	26 g/l
α-Fetoprotein	9 kU/l

What would you infer from these results?

Answer 2.25

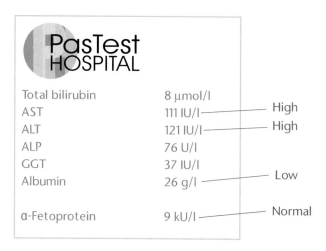

PasTest
HOSPITAL

Total bilirubin	8 μmol/l	
AST	111 IU/l	High
ALT	121 IU/l	High
ALP	76 U/l	
GGT	37 IU/l	
Albumin	26 g/l	Low
α-Fetoprotein	9 kU/l	Normal

This patient most likely has liver cirrhosis secondary to hepatitis C. Her regular attendance at an outpatient clinic is at least in part for surveillance for hepatocellular carcinoma. Her α-FP level is within normal limits, indicating a low likelihood of this tumour being present. An annual surveillance ultrasound of the liver will be used in conjunction with α-FP measurements to seek out a hepatocellular carcinoma. A significant percentage of tumour markers are performed for monitoring so you should expect to interpret some normal results.

Case 2.26

A 44-year-old reformed intravenous drug user with known hepatitis C is well known to the local hepatologists. He has been attending on a regular basis and is enrolled in the hepatocellular carcinoma surveillance programme. Below are an overview of his blood tests.

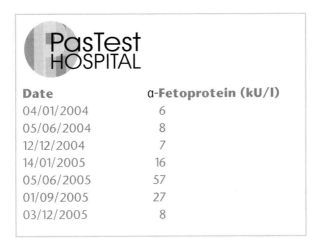

Date	α-Fetoprotein (kU/l)
04/01/2004	6
05/06/2004	8
12/12/2004	7
14/01/2005	16
05/06/2005	57
01/09/2005	27
03/12/2005	8

What may explain the pattern in these results?

Answer 2.26

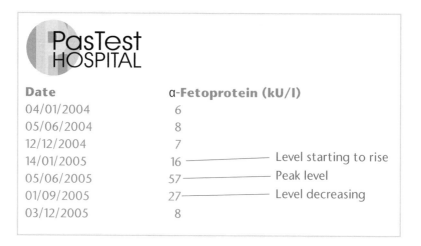

One important role of α-AFP measurement is demonstrated well in this patient with hepatitis C. It is one of the more specific tumour markers and can be used with some degree of confidence to monitor patients with liver cirrhosis who have a substantially increased risk of developing hepatocellular carcinoma (HCC). Identifying a patient who has developed HCC early may allow successful treatment to be instigated. The level in January 2005 is higher than 6 months previously but is not dramatically elevated. However, 6 months later it has increased substantially. This suggests the development of HCC, and ultrasound and/or other cross-sectional imaging would be merited. The encouraging downward trend in the following 6 months would indicate that the tumour has been successfully treated.

Case 2.27

A 55-year-old senior civil servant plucks up the courage to attend his GP after complaints of a poor urinary stream, frequency and nocturia. He is concerned as his father had 'prostate problems', On rectal examination an enlarged prostate was felt. Later that week his renal function and prostate-specific antigen tests come back.

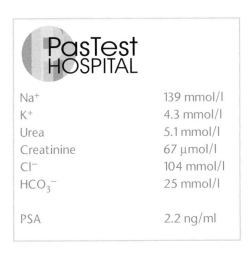

PasTest
HOSPITAL

Na$^+$	139 mmol/l
K$^+$	4.3 mmol/l
Urea	5.1 mmol/l
Creatinine	67 µmol/l
Cl$^-$	104 mmol/l
HCO$_3^-$	25 mmol/l
PSA	2.2 ng/ml

Does this patient have anything to worry about?

Answer 2.27

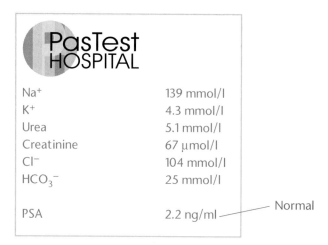

PasTest
HOSPITAL

Na$^+$	139 mmol/l
K$^+$	4.3 mmol/l
Urea	5.1 mmol/l
Creatinine	67 µmol/l
Cl$^-$	104 mmol/l
HCO$_3^-$	25 mmol/l
PSA	2.2 ng/ml —— Normal

Of all the tumour markers available, probably the most commonly requested is the PSA. It is sometimes used in an attempt to identify the presence of prostatic carcinoma, but more usefully in monitoring the disease and treatment response. This patient has obstructive urinary symptoms and an enlarged prostate, but this does not mean that he has prostate carcinoma. Likewise a normal PSA does not exclude the presence of this tumour. However, this man most likely has benign prostatic hypertrophy. There are a number of causes of a raised PSA, as shown below.

CAUSES OF RAISED PSA

Prostate carcinoma
Instrumentation of prostate (including urinary catheterisation)
Urinary tract infection
Recent ejaculation

Case 2.28

A 28-year-old media studies student attends A&E with a swollen left testicle. He is sexually active, with multiple sexual partners in the last 6 months. The A&E officer is concerned, and arranges admission. Ultrasound of the scrotum and blood tests were requested.

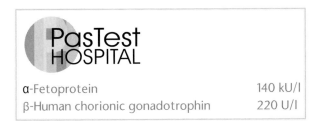

α-Fetoprotein	140 kU/l
β-Human chorionic gonadotrophin	220 U/l

Can these results be explained by a diagnosis of epididymo-orchitis?

Answer 2.28

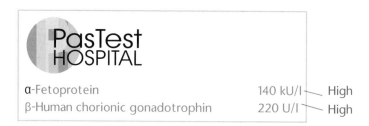

PasTest
HOSPITAL

α-Fetoprotein	140 kU/l	High
β-Human chorionic gonadotrophin	220 U/l	High

α-Fetoprotein is one of the few tumour markers with a good specificity for two different tumours – hepatocellular carcinoma and testicular teratoma. Similarly testicular teratoma is unique in characteristically causing high levels of two tumour markers – α-FP and β-hCG. Both tumour markers are significantly elevated here indicating a high probability of testicular malignancy. Following treatment, these markers should be checked again and should have decreased.

Case 2.29

A 55-year-old woman is admitted under the care of the surgical team with a distended abdomen. She admits that it has become increasingly large over the past few weeks, but was scared to come to hospital. She has no complaints of abdominal pain and her bowel habit is normal. The enthusiastic junior doctor who admitted the patient included in the notes that she has sent blood for CEA, CA-125 and CA-19-9.

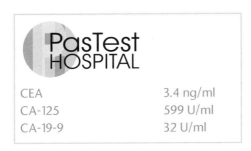

PasTest
HOSPITAL

CEA	3.4 ng/ml
CA-125	599 U/ml
CA-19-9	32 U/ml

What do these blood results tell you?

Answer 2.29

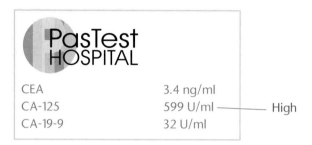

PasTest
HOSPITAL

CEA	3.4 ng/ml
CA-125	599 U/ml ——— High
CA-19-9	32 U/ml

It is not uncommon (though not particularly good practice), especially in puzzling clinical cases, to request a host of blood tests. Tumour markers for intra-abdominal pathology are sometimes used in this manner. However, due to the non-specific nature of these results, abnormal results can sometimes add to the diagnostic conundrum. The abnormal marker in this case is CA-125. This is most closely associated with ovarian malignancy. The clinical history is certainly in keeping with this, as the distended abdomen may reflect both tumour bulk and/or the presence of malignant ascites.

ENDOCRINOLOGY

ENDOCRINOLOGY

Endocrine disorders can be divided into primary and secondary disorders. In a primary endocrine gland disorder, the problem lies within the endocrine gland itself. Thus, in primary hyperthyroidism, the principal problem is an overactive thyroid gland. Secondary endocrine diseases arise when there is a problem with the hormones controlling the activity of the target gland, such as the overproduction of a hormone by the pituitary gland.

Thyroid hormones

Normally, thyrotrophin-releasing hormone (TRH) is released from the hypothalamus and stimulates the pituitary gland to release thyroid-stimulating hormone (TSH). This hormone then acts on the thyroid gland and results in the liberation of thyroxine (T_4) and triiodothyronine (T_3) into the circulation. These hormones exert negative feedback on both the hypothalamus and pituitary, and result in a reduction in the production of TRH and TSH. Most of the T_3 and T_4 in the body is carried by carrier proteins (principally thyroxine-binding globulin, TBG). A small percentage is present in unbound form, and it is this that is physiologically active. In clinical practice, the commonly measured hormones are TSH, free T_4 and T_3. Total T_4 (ie bound and unbound forms) is sometimes given.

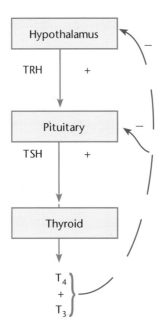

Fig 3.1

Hyperthyroidism

In primary hyperthyroidism (eg with Graves' disease), the thyroid gland autonomously produces thyroid hormones. The levels of T_3 and T_4 therefore rise. Normal negative feedback continues, and the level of TSH will be low. In T_3 thyrotoxicosis, the T_3 level may be elevated in isolation.

In secondary hyperthyroidism (eg due to a pituitary tumour secreting TSH), the levels of T_3 and T_4 will again be high, but this time the TSH level will be inappropriately normal or high.

DON'T FORGET

The finding of a normal TSH level in the setting of raised T_3 and T_4 should raise suspicions of a pituitary lesion, since in normal circumstances the TSH level will be suppressed.

Hypothyroidism

In primary hypothyroidism (eg with Hashimoto's thyroiditis), the thyroid gland is defective. The levels of T_3 and T_4 are low. As a result of reduced negative feedback, the TSH level will be high.

In secondary hypothyroidism (eg destructive pituitary tumour), the levels of T_3 and T_4 will again be low, but this is because of low TSH levels.

Sick euthyroid syndrome

Caution should be taken when interpreting thyroid function tests in a patient with an acute illness. This is because thyroid function tests are often abnormal during the acute phase of an illness, but normalise on its resolution. This phenomenon is known as the sick euthyroid syndrome, indicating that the patient is euthyroid (ie normal thyroid function), but that he or she has an intercurrent illness. The common picture in sick euthyroid syndrome is one of low T_3 and T_4 with low or normal TSH.

DON'T FORGET

Be cautious when interpreting thyroid function tests in an acutely unwell patient.

SUMMARY OF HORMONE CHANGES IN VARIOUS THYROID DISEASE STATES		
	T_3/T_4	TSH
Primary hyperthyroidism	↑	↓
T_3 thyrotoxicosis	Only T_3 ↑	↓
Secondary hyperthyroidism	↑	↑
Primary hypothyroidism	↓	↑
Secondary hypothyroidism	↓	↓
Sick euthyroid syndrome	↓	↓

Variations in thyroxine-binding globulin levels

Care must be taken when interpreting free and total T_4 levels. This is because the level of TBG can vary in various states. Always remember that it is the level of free hormone that is important physiologically. Factors influencing the level of TBG are listed below.

INCREASE TBG	DECREASE TBG
High oestrogen states, eg pregnancy, oral contraceptive pill use	High corticosteroid levels
Hypothyroidism	Protein deficiency states: low intake (malnutrition); low synthesis (chronic liver disease); increased losses (nephrotic syndrome)
	Thyrotoxicosis

Adrenal hormones

Normally, corticotrophin-releasing hormone (CRH) is released from the hypothalamus and stimulates the pituitary gland to release adrenocorticotrophic hormone (ACTH). This hormone then acts on the adrenal cortex and results in the release of glucocorticoids. Glucocorticoids exert negative feedback on both the hypothalamus and pituitary, and result in a reduction in the production of CRH and ACTH.

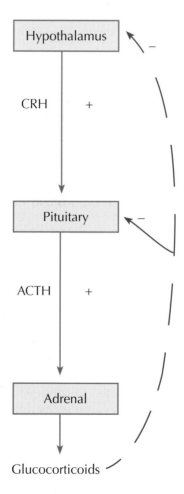

Fig 3.2

Cushing syndrome

Cushing syndrome results from glucocorticoid excess. It is seen most commonly in patients receiving glucocorticoid treatment, eg for chronic severe asthma. Endogenous forms of Cushing syndrome have several causes which are listed below.

ENDOGENOUS CAUSES OF CUSHING SYNDROME

Primary adrenal disease
- Adrenal tumour (adenoma or carcinoma)

ACTH excess
- From the pituitary gland (Cushing disease)
- From an ACTH-producing tumour

In primary adrenal disease causing Cushing syndrome, the adrenal gland autonomously produces adrenal hormones. Normal negative feedback continues, and the level of ACTH will be low.

In instances of secondary hyperadrenalism (eg due to a pituitary tumour), the ACTH level will be normal or high.

There are several methods for diagnosing Cushing syndrome:

1. **Measure free cortisol in a 24-hour urine collection**

   An elevated level of free cortisol in the urine is in keeping with Cushing syndrome. An abnormal test should be followed up by a repeat test in the first instance.

2. **Measure cortisol in a late-night salivary sample**

   In people with a normal sleep pattern (sleeping through the night), the cortisol level should reach a nadir at night. In patients with Cushing syndrome, cortisol levels may be elevated even at this time, and elevated levels of cortisol can be measured in saliva. As with urinary free cortisol, an abnormal test should be followed up by a repeat test in the first instance.

3. **Perform a 1 mg overnight dexamethasone suppression test**

   In healthy individuals, taking 1 mg dexamethasone will have a negative feedback effect on the pituitary gland, thereby decreasing ACTH and hence cortisol production. In patients with Cushing syndrome, cortisol production will not be affected, and hence a cortisol test the morning after dosing will reveal abnormally elevated cortisol levels.

4. Perform a 2 mg 48-hour dexamethasone suppression test (low-dose dexamethasone suppression test)

The rationale for this test is similar to that for the overnight suppression test. For this test, however, 0.5 mg dexamethasone is given 6-hourly for 48 hours. A cortisol level taken 6 hours after the last dose will reveal an abnormally elevated level in patients with Cushing syndrome.

Other more specialised tests can also be used to confirm the diagnosis and to help differentiate between the causes of Cushing syndrome.

Nieman LK, Biller BM, Findling JW, et al. The diagnosis of Cushing's syndrome. *J Clin Endocrinol Metab* 2008;**93**:1526–40.

Primary hyperaldosteronism

The measurement of aldosterone and renin levels is important in patients suspected of having primary hyperaldosteronism. In this condition, aldosterone levels are elevated and renin levels are suppressed (due to negative feedback mechanisms). Measuring these hormones is fraught with difficulty because the levels vary depending on posture (lying or standing, for example), and can be affected by a variety of drugs. The particular way in which the hormones are measured and the units of measurement vary between laboratories, so take care when interpreting results that you understand what is being reported.

In order to screen carefully selected patients for the presence of primary hyperaldosteronism, increasing emphasis is being placed on the ratio between aldosterone and renin levels (the aldosterone:renin ratio or ARR). If plasma aldosterone concentration is given in nanograms/decilitre and plasma renin activity in nanograms/millilitre per hour, then an accepted cut-off for an abnormal ARR is 30. If the ARR is above this level, the patient may well have the condition and further investigations would be warranted.

There are several tests available to confirm or refute the diagnosis in patients with an abnormal ARR. One test that is commonly used is the 'saline suppression test'. The specifics of this test are beyond the scope of this book, but, in principle, an infusion of saline should reduce blood aldosterone levels. Failure of aldosterone levels to suppress after administration of saline makes the diagnosis of primary hyperaldosteronism more likely.

If the diagnosis seems likely, imaging should be performed to visualise the adrenal glands. If unilateral adrenal gland disease appears likely, blood can be sampled from the adrenal veins in an attempt to prove that aldosterone is being produced in excess from an adrenal gland.

Funder JW, Carey RM, Fardella C, et al. Case detection, diagnosis, and treatment of patients with primary aldosteronism: An Endocrine Society Clinical Practice Guideline. *J Clin Endocrinol Metab* 2010;**93**:3266–81.

Hypoadrenalism

In primary hypoadrenalism (eg Addison's disease), the adrenal gland itself is defective. As a result of reduced negative feedback, the ACTH level will be high.

In secondary hypoadrenalism, ACTH levels will be low.

Short Synacthen® test

Synacthen®, or SYNthetic ACTH, is used to stimulate the adrenal gland. Normally, an injection of Synacthen® will result in an increase in circulating cortisol levels. If the patient has a primary adrenal disease, the Synacthen® will not have its normal effect, and the rise in cortisol levels will be poor. A cortisol level of less than 600 nmol/l 30 min after Synacthen® has been administered is in keeping with failure of the adrenal gland. The Synacthen® test will be normal in cases of secondary hypoadrenalism.

Insulin tolerance test

This test is used in specialist centres to assess adrenal function as well as to assess for growth hormone deficiency.

Several criteria must be met before this test can be attempted.

CRITERIA TO BE MET BEFORE PERFORMING AN INSULIN TOLERANCE TEST
Cortisol level >100 nmol/l
Normal thyroid function
No cardiovascular disease
No epilepsy or other seizure activity or blackouts

The essence of the test is to induce hypoglycaemia (blood glucose must fall to less than 2.2 mmol/l) in a carefully controlled environment. In a normal patient, a stress response will occur with a rise in cortisol and growth hormone levels. Normally, the cortisol level should rise to more than 550 nmol/l, and the growth hormone level to more than 20 mU/l.

Phaeochromocytomas

These tumours are associated with excess circulating catecholamines. Diagnosis relies on the demonstration of excessive amounts of catecholamine breakdown products in the plasma (free metanephrines) or urine (fractional metanephrines).

If levels are extremely high, phaeochromocytoma is likely. If levels are only slightly high, a 'clonidine suppression test' can be performed. Plasma free metanephrines are measured after dosing with clonidine, and would be expected to be suppressed in people without a phaeochromocytoma.

If the diagnosis seems likely, an attempt should be made to visualise the tumour. This can be done using MRI or CT. Alternatively, radionuclide scanning or positron emission tomography (PET) may be necessary.

Lenders JW, Eisenhofer G, Mannelli M, Pacak K. Phaeochromocytoma. *Lancet* 2005;**366**:665–75.

The thirst axis

Psychogenic polydipsia and diabetes insipidus

The combination of passing excessive volumes of urine (polyuria) with excessive thirst (polydipsia) is common. The water deprivation test is used to differentiate between two major causes – psychogenic polydipsia and diabetes insipidus (DI).

Patients with psychogenic polydipsia simply drink fluid in excess for psychological or psychiatric reasons.

In DI, there is a problem with antidiuretic hormone (ADH). ADH normally acts on the collecting ducts in the kidney to stimulate water reabsorption. If ADH does not function properly, too much urine is passed. In turn the patient becomes relatively dehydrated and drinks to compensate for this.

MEMORY AID

Diuretic medications increase urine volume.
Therefore, antidiuretic hormone (ADH) does the opposite, and acts to conserve water.

There are two forms of DI – cranial and nephrogenic. In cranial DI, there is a problem with the release of ADH from the hypothalamus. Blood levels of ADH are low. In nephrogenic DI, there is sufficient ADH in the system, but it fails to exert its effects on the kidney.

The water deprivation test restricts patients' intake of water. If they have psychogenic polydipsia, reducing water intake will solve their problem and they will gradually return to normal. However, with DI, water restriction will result in a worsening state of dehydration.

The test involves forbidding the patient to drink after waking. Blood and urine osmolalities are tested each hour for a period of 8 h. In health (or psychogenic polydipsia), one would expect the patient to retain water and to pass concentrated urine (with a high urine osmolality). In DI, the urine osmolality does not rise, and the patient becomes dehydrated with a rise in serum osmolality.

To differentiate between the two forms of DI, patients are then given a dose of a synthetic ADH compound called desmopressin. This will correct the problem in cranial DI, but will have no effect in nephrogenic DI.

Syndrome of inappropriate ADH secretion (SIADH)

In this condition, there is a state of excessive ADH production. SIADH has many causes, the most common of which are listed in the table.

COMMON CAUSES OF SIADH	

Intrathoracic causes:
  • Infection
  • Tumour
Intracranial causes:
  • Infection
  • Tumour
  • Head injury
	Medications:
	  • Carbamazepine
	  • Antipsychotics

SIADH is, in essence, the opposite of DI. Excessive ADH action results in retention of water, with the subsequent development of dilute serum and concentrated urine.

For a person to be labelled with the diagnosis of SIADH the following criteria should be met:

1. Clinically isovolaemic

2. Normal renal function

3. Normal adrenal function

4. Normal thyroid function

5. Normal pituitary function

6. Absence of diuretic therapy

7. Low serum osmolality (<275 mosmol/kg)

8. Inappropriately concentrated urine (>100 mosmol/kg)

For a reference see the GAIN hyponatraemia document in Chapter 2, page 58.

Hyperprolactinaemia

There are many causes of a raised serum prolactin level (see box below). Very high levels (>5000 mU/l) strongly suggest a prolactin-secreting pituitary tumour.

COMMON CAUSES OF HYPERPROLACTINAEMIA

Physiological:
- Pregnancy
- Lactation

Prolactin-secreting pituitary tumour

Medications:
- Phenothiazine antipsychotics
- Most antiemetics

Polycystic ovarian syndrome

Following a seizure

Primary hypothyroidism

Hyperglycaemia

The diagnosis of diabetes mellitus and related hyperglycaemic states relies on accurate interpretation of blood glucose readings. A patient's glycaemic status can be classed as one of the following:

- Normal
- Impaired fasting glucose
- Impaired glucose tolerance
- Diabetes mellitus
- Gestational diabetes mellitus.

In some circumstances, diabetes will be suspected clinically, particularly if the patient is symptomatic from hyperglycaemia. In other instances, hyperglycaemia will be detected incidentally when a blood glucose level is checked. Typical symptoms are shown in the box below.

SYMPTOMS OF DIABETES MELLITUS
Polyuria
Polydipsia
Weight loss
Fatigue
Blurring of vision
Symptoms related to a complication of diabetes such as a cutaneous abscess

An oral glucose tolerance test (OGTT) is often used in differentiating between these various states. This test involves giving the patient a 75 g glucose load by mouth, after they have been fasting. The plasma glucose level is measured at baseline and after 2 h.

Diabetes mellitus may be diagnosed in a variety of ways. Any one of the following is sufficient:

1. A single random plasma glucose of more than 11.1 mmol/l in a patient with symptoms

2. Two separate random plasma glucose samples of more than 11.1 mmol/l in a patient without symptoms

3. A single fasting plasma glucose of more than 7.0 mmol/l in a patient with symptoms

4. Two separate fasting plasma glucose samples of more than 7.0 mmol/l in a patient without symptoms

5. A plasma glucose level of 11.1 mmol/l or more 2 h after a glucose load in an OGTT. An OGTT is generally performed only if borderline results are obtained on random or fasting samples.

DON'T FORGET

If a patient is asymptomatic, two blood tests are required before diabetes mellitus can be diagnosed.

Patients with **normoglycaemia** (ie definitely not diabetic) have a fasting plasma glucose of less than 6.1 mmol/l. Two hours following a glucose load in an OGTT, the plasma glucose will be less than 7.8 mmol/l.

'Impaired fasting glucose' and **'impaired glucose tolerance'** are terms used to describe states of glycaemic control that lie somewhere between normal and frank diabetes mellitus. The terms are not mutually exclusive. It is therefore possible for a patient to have both impaired fasting glucose and impaired glucose tolerance. Alternatively, they may have one or other of the terms attached to them in isolation. The significance of labelling a patient with one of these terms lies with the fact that such patients have an increased risk of developing diabetes mellitus in the future. The diagnostic criteria are shown in the table below.

	NORMAL	IMPAIRED FASTING	IMPAIRED GLUCOSE TOLERANCE	DIABETES MELLITUS
Fasting plasma glucose (mmol/l)	<6.1	6.1–6.9	Not necessary for diagnosis	≥7.0
Plasma glucose 2 hours after glucose load in OGTT (mmol/l)	<7.8	Not necessary for diagnosis	7.8–11.0	≥11.1

Gestational diabetes mellitus describes diabetes that is of new onset in pregnancy, or that is first noted during pregnancy. The principles of diagnosis are identical to those above. The term may be used if a woman fits the criteria for impaired glucose tolerance or diabetes mellitus while pregnant. All such women should have an OGTT at least 6 weeks after delivery, and be re-classified as necessary. The significance of gestational diabetes mellitus again relates to the fact that such patients have a reasonable chance of having a 'large-for-dates' foetus, and that they have a chance of developing diabetes mellitus in later life.

Glycated haemoglobin

Random blood glucose measurements are useful for monitoring variations on a day-to-day basis, however, the inevitable variation makes interpretation of long-term trends difficult. For this reason measurement of glycated haemoglobin (HbA1 or HbA1c) is often used.

Glycated haemoglobin is the product of the reaction between glucose and haemoglobin A (the main type of haemoglobin in most adults). The higher the average blood glucose level, the higher the glycated haemoglobin level will be. As red blood cells have an average life-span of around 60 days, glycated haemoglobin estimation provides information on the glycaemic control over this time period.

The Diabetes Control and Complications Trial (DCCT) provided evidence that well-controlled diabetes was associated with fewer microvascular complications (*N Engl J Med* 1993; **329**: 977–86). For most patients, a target HbA1c of between 6.5 and 7.5% will be adequate. A slightly less ambitious target of between 7 and 8% may prove adequate for some patients, and reduce the risk of hypoglycaemic attacks when compared with a more intensive treatment regimen.

Glycated haemoglobin is reliable only when normal haemoglobin is present in red blood cells that have normal life-spans. If a haemoglobin disorder is present, or in patients who have red cells with shortened life-spans (eg haemolytic anaemia), measurement of fructosamine levels may be used instead to measure glycaemic control. Fructosamine is a glycated plasma protein, and provides information on glucose levels over the previous 1–3 weeks.

Hypoglycaemia

Hypoglycaemia describes a plasma glucose that is lower than normal (less than 3.5 mmol/l). The most common cause is an imbalance between intake and insulin requirements in a patient with type 1 diabetes mellitus (eg the patient who takes normal insulin without eating lunch). Other causes of hypoglycaemia are listed in the box on page 154.

CAUSES OF HYPOGLYCAEMIA

Imbalance between insulin and calorie intake in type 1 diabetes
Excess exogenous insulin administration
As a side effect of anti-hyperglycaemic medication
Insulinoma
Liver failure
Alcohol ingestion

A fairly common clinical scenario is the patient who presents with hypoglycaemia of unknown cause. Endogenous insulin (ie insulin derived from an insulinoma) can be differentiated easily from exogenous insulin (ie a patient with Munchausen syndrome who administers insulin to themselves in an attempt to seek medical attention) with a little knowledge of insulin physiology.

Normal physiological insulin is manufactured in the body from proinsulin which in turn is derived from pre-proinsulin. Each protein precursor is cleaved to yield its product. This cleavage process generates a 'waste' chain of amino acids called C-peptide.

If hypoglycaemia is due to excess endogenous insulin from an insulinoma, one would expect high insulin and C-peptide levels in a patient who is hypoglycaemic.

Exogenous insulin does not contain C-peptide. Therefore, a hypoglycaemic patient with raised levels of insulin in the blood but normal/low levels of C-peptide is likely to have been given insulin.

Acromegaly

Acromegaly is associated with an elevated level of growth hormone (GH), usually due to a pituitary tumour. Measuring the level is not a reliable method of making this diagnosis. Insulin-like growth factor I (IGF-I) levels can be used as a marker of average GH levels and, if raised, is suggestive of acromegaly. The definitive test for the diagnosis is a glucose tolerance test, exactly like that used in the investigation of hyperglycaemia. The test is performed in the same manner, but GH levels are measured. Failure of the GH level to fall below 1mU/l is in keeping with a diagnosis of acromegaly.

DON'T FORGET

Acromegaly is diagnosed if the GH level is >1 mU/l during a glucose tolerance test.

Case 3.1

A 21-year-old woman is referred to the medical clinic because of abnormal thyroid function results noted by her GP. There is no personal or family history of thyroid disease, and she is on no medication, but the GP requested the test because the patient had been feeling generally unwell recently. Clinical examination is unremarkable. The thyroid function tests are repeated and the following results are obtained.

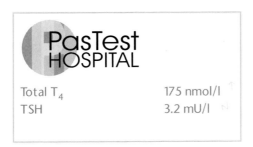

PasTest
HOSPITAL

Total T$_4$	175 nmol/l
TSH	3.2 mU/l

1. **How would you interpret these tests?**

2. **What two tests should be ordered?**

Answer 3.1

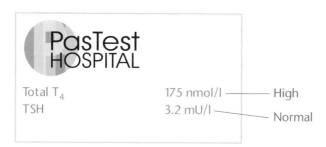

PasTest
HOSPITAL

Total T$_4$	175 nmol/l	High
TSH	3.2 mU/l	Normal

1. Care should be taken when interpreting these results. Note that the TOTAL T$_4$ level is given, not the FREE T$_4$ level. It is the free level that is important physiologically. It is impossible to make any further comments on these tests other than to say that the total T$_4$ level is raised, and the TSH is normal.

2. First, the free T$_4$ level should be measured. In this case it was normal (result not shown), indicating normal thyroid function. The patient therefore has an elevated total T$_4$ level with a normal free T$_4$ level. The reason for this is increased levels of TBG. The most likely reason for this is a high oestrogen state (eg pregnancy or use of the oral contraceptive pill). Since the question states that the patient is not on any medication, the most likely diagnosis here is pregnancy. The second test that should be performed is therefore a pregnancy test.

Case 3.2

A 64-year-old woman is admitted with palpitations. She feels that these have been intermittent over the last month. Examination reveals an anxious woman with an irregularly irregular pulse at 120 beats/min. ECG confirms the suspicions of atrial fibrillation. As part of her initial investigations, the following blood test is returned.

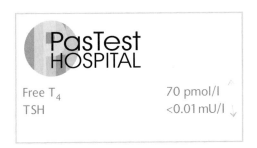

PasTest
HOSPITAL

Free T$_4$	70 pmol/l
TSH	<0.01 mU/l

What is the underlying cause of the atrial fibrillation?

Answer 3.2

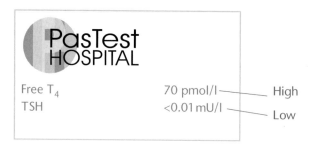

PasTest
HOSPITAL

Free T$_4$	70 pmol/l	High
TSH	<0.01 mU/l	Low

This woman has primary hyperthyroidism. Her overactive thyroid gland is producing thyroid hormones in excess. Normal negative feedback mechanisms still function, however, so the TSH level is suppressed.

It is not uncommon for atrial fibrillation to be the only evidence of hyperthyroidism, so always remember to check thyroid function in such patients.

Case 3.3

A patient is reviewed at the chest clinic. He was treated over 1 year ago for pulmonary tuberculosis. He now complains of lethargy. Clinical examination reveals no chest abnormalities, but he is found to have significant postural hypotension. A urea and electrolyte (U&E) blood test is sent and, on the basis of the results, the following test is arranged.

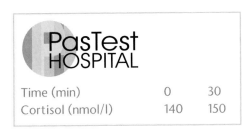

PasTest HOSPITAL		
Time (min)	0	30
Cortisol (nmol/l)	140	150

1. **What is the test, and what does it demonstrate in this case?**

2. **What were the likely abnormalities on the U&Es that raised suspicions of this disorder?**

3. **What is the likely underlying disease?**

Answer 3.3

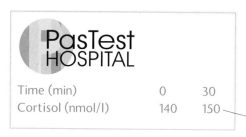

Time (min)	0	30
Cortisol (nmol/l)	140	150

Poor rise in cortisol post-injection with Synacthen

1. This is a short Synacthen® test. The cortisol level fails to rise to more than 600 nmol/l 30 min after injection with Synacthen®. This indicates primary hypoadrenalism (ie a problem with the adrenal gland itself).

2. A low sodium and raised potassium level are commonly found. The glucose level would also be expected to be low.

3. The underlying disease is primary hypoadrenalism, probably due to autoimmune adrenalitis or tuberculosis affecting the adrenal gland.

Case 3.4

A patient is referred to the endocrine clinic complaining of excess thirst and of passing excessive amounts of urine. A random blood glucose level is 4.2 mmol/l. He is admitted to hospital and a water deprivation test is arranged. The results are shown.

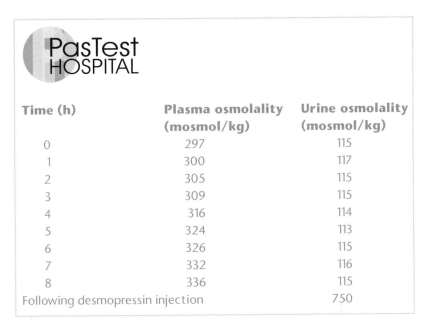

PasTest
HOSPITAL

Time (h)	Plasma osmolality (mosmol/kg)	Urine osmolality (mosmol/kg)
0	297	115
1	300	117
2	305	115
3	309	115
4	316	114
5	324	113
6	326	115
7	332	116
8	336	115
Following desmopressin injection		750

1. **What is your interpretation of the blood glucose level?**
2. **What is the diagnosis?**

Answer 3.4

**PasTest
HOSPITAL**

Time (h)		Plasma osmolality (mosmol/kg)		Urine osmolality (mosmol/kg)
0		297		115
1		300		117
2		305		115
3	Increasing plasma	309		115
4	osmolality with	316		114
5	time	324	No change in	113
6		326	urine osmolality	115
7		332	with time	116
8		336		115
Following desmopressin injection				750

Increase in urine osmolality following
desmopressin injection

1. The random blood glucose level is normal. The patient therefore does not have diabetes mellitus. It is important to exclude this diagnosis, since it can also present with polydipsia and polyuria.

2. The diagnosis is cranial diabetes insipidus. The patient has a problem producing ADH. When deprived of water, he is unable to concentrate the urine. The plasma rapidly becomes more concentrated. Following an injection of synthetic ADH (desmopressin), the urine osmolality increases. This shows that the kidney is still sensitive to the effects of ADH, and excludes nephrogenic diabetes insipidus as the diagnosis.

Case 3.5

A 57-year-old man is referred to the hypertension clinic. Two tests are performed in order to screen for an endocrine cause of hypertension.

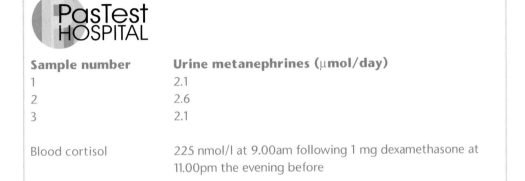

	PasTest HOSPITAL
Sample number	**Urine metanephrines (μmol/day)**
1	2.1
2	2.6
3	2.1
Blood cortisol	225 nmol/l at 9.00am following 1 mg dexamethasone at 11.00pm the evening before

How would you interpret these results?

Answer 3.5

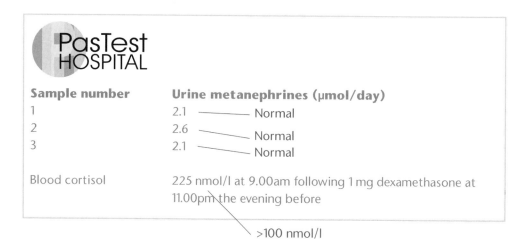

PasTest HOSPITAL

Sample number	Urine metanephrines (µmol/day)
1	2.1 ——————— Normal
2	2.6 ——————— Normal
3	2.1 ——————— Normal

Blood cortisol 225 nmol/l at 9.00am following 1 mg dexamethasone at 11.00pm the evening before

>100 nmol/l

Three separate 24-h urine collections for urinary metanephrines have been taken. The metanephrine levels are normal in each. This excludes phaeochromocytoma as a cause of the hypertension with some certainty.

The second test shows the results of an overnight dexamethasone suppression test. The morning cortisol level is greater than 100 nmol/l, suggesting a diagnosis of Cushing syndrome.

Case 3.6

A patient is referred to the endocrine clinic after having been assessed in the eye A&E. The registrar arranges for a glucose tolerance test to be carried out.

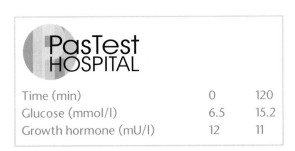

PasTest HOSPITAL			
Time (min)		0	120
Glucose (mmol/l)		6.5	15.2
Growth hormone (mU/l)		12	11

1. **What two diagnoses can be made on the basis of this test?**
2. **Why do you think the patient was seen in the eye A&E?**

Answer 3.6

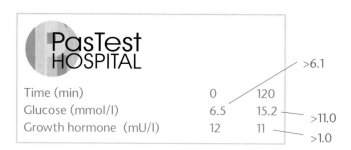

1. The two diagnoses that can be made from this one test are: diabetes mellitus and acromegaly.

   The glucose level before the start of the test is elevated in keeping with the label of impaired fasting glucose. However, the abnormally high glucose level 2 h after the glucose load confirms the diagnosis of diabetes mellitus.

   The growth hormone level is greater than 2.0 µg/l at all stages of the test, allowing the diagnosis of acromegaly to be made.

2. The most common cause of acromegaly is a pituitary tumour. This commonly extends in an upward direction and can compress the optic chiasma, causing a bitemporal hemianopia. Loss of temporal visual fields is the probable reason for presentation at the eye A&E.

TOXICOLOGY

4

TOXICOLOGY

Poisoning is one of the most common causes of admission to hospital. It is most often deliberate, but can also be accidental, sometimes due to the accumulation of prescribed medications.

The management of a poisoned patient largely involves supportive care, allowing the body to excrete or metabolise a drug naturally. In certain circumstances, antidotes may be necessary along with the use of other methods designed to clear the drug more quickly from the body.

It is important that you are able to assimilate data of a variety of types when treating a poisoned patient.

Paracetamol

Paracetamol (called acetaminophen in the USA) is one of the most common drugs taken in overdose. This reflects its ready availability and ubiquitous use. When taken in overdose, paracetamol depletes antioxidant stores in hepatocytes and can result in liver damage. If a patient takes a significant quantity of paracetamol and is delayed in their presentation to hospital, the following abnormalities may be apparent:

1. Elevated liver enzymes, particularly aspartate aminotransferase (AST) and alanine aminotransferase (ALT). Bilirubin levels will also rise. These changes occur because of liver cell damage. Further details on liver tests can be found on page 70.

2. Elevated prothrombin time (PT) (and international normalised ratio [INR], because this is calculated from the PT). This occurs because of impaired liver synthesis of clotting factors. Further details on PT and INR can be found on page 21.

3. Impaired kidney function (elevated urea and creatinine). This can arise secondary to liver impairment (hepatorenal syndrome) or sometimes as a direct effect of paracetamol metabolites on the kidney.

4. Metabolic acidosis mainly due to liver failure. This will be a high anion gap metabolic acidosis. For further details, refer to page 428.

Administration of an antidote, *N*-acetylcysteine, can help patients after a significant paracetamol overdose. This agent replenishes liver antioxidant stores.

On most occasions in clinical practice, patients present to hospital within a few hours of taking an overdose. Although N-acetylcysteine is a fairly safe and effective drug, anaphylaxis has been reported after its administration. It is therefore routine practice to weigh up whether or not a patient requires antidote administration. This is done by measuring blood paracetamol levels and using the nomogram in Fig 4.1 (which can be found in the *British National Formulary*).

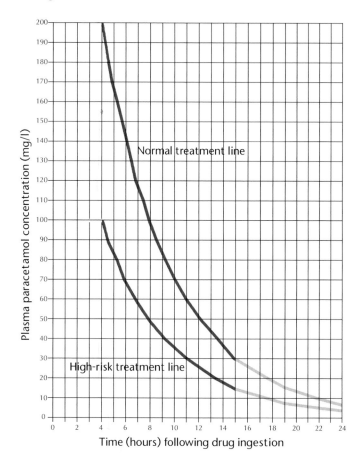

Fig 4.1

Timing of the overdose is critical because blood levels are interpretable only if the time of drug ingestion is known. You will note that the lines on the nomogram start at 4 hours – blood levels taken within 4 hours of ingestion are meaningless because absorption will be incomplete, and levels could rise if blood is re-sampled later. Once timing has been established and the post-4-hour blood levels measured, plot the patient's data on the nomogram. Decide on whether the 'normal' or 'high-risk' treatment line should be used (see below). If the patient's level lies above the relevant line at the time point chosen, then they are deemed to be at significant risk of liver injury, and the antidote should be administered. If their level is below the treatment line, the risk of liver damage is small and treatment is not generally required.

As mentioned, knowledge of the time of ingestion is critical. It is, however, acknowledged that it is often extremely difficult to be certain about this, because patients who have taken an overdose are often intoxicated, drowsy or generally uncooperative. One should collect information from every available source, and generally speaking one should have a low threshold for treatment if details are sketchy. Another point of note is that the nomogram curves flatten considerably towards the right side of the chart. The differences in blood levels between whom to treat and whom not to treat if presentation is delayed are very small, and generally treatment should be instigated in all cases of delayed presentation. Patients who have taken a potentially lethal quantity of paracetamol (>12 g in most circumstances) but who present earlier than 4 hours should generally receive treatment, which can be stopped if their post-4-hour drug level suggests that treatment is not required. In addition, patients who have taken a staggered overdose should generally be treated regardless of the blood level.

DON'T FORGET

Always check plasma paracetamol levels at least 4 h after ingestion.

In routine circumstances, the 'normal' treatment line should be used. Some patients are deemed 'high risk' for liver damage, and for them the 'high-risk treatment line' should be used (see box for details). Such patients are presumed to have lower than normal antioxidant stores.

PATIENTS AT HIGH RISK IN PARACETAMOL OVERDOSE

On hepatic enzyme-inducing drugs
(eg phenytoin, rifampicin, carbamazepine)
Alcoholics
Malnutrition (including anorexia nervosa)
Patients with AIDS

MEMORY AID

Always assess paracetamol overdose patients for high-risk status.

Salicylate

Salicylates (such as aspirin) are found in a wide variety of preparations commonly available in households and are therefore taken reasonably commonly in overdose. Two main types of data can be useful in salicylate poisoning:

1. **Salicylate levels**: the higher the level, the greater the likelihood of symptoms and organ damage, and the more likely it will be that specific treatments will be required to increase clearance of salicylate from the body. The absorption of salicylates can be slow. It is therefore good practice to repeat blood levels at intervals until they start to fall.

2. **Abnormalities of acid–base balance**: see Chapter 13 for detailed information about the interpretation of acid–base abnormalities. Significant salicylate overdose produces a characteristic pattern of acid–base disturbance. The respiratory centre in the brain is stimulated, causing patients to hyperventilate and 'blow off' carbon dioxide. The levels of the acidic gas carbon dioxide therefore fall, resulting in a respiratory alkalosis. At the same time, however, a metabolic acidosis develops due to the production of a variety of acids. Levels of the alkaline substance bicarbonate fall, and the pH becomes acidic. The overall effect on a particular patient is hard to predict. Either alkalosis or acidosis can predominate, or alternatively the pH can remain neutral due to opposing respiratory and metabolic effects.

Opiates

Significant opiate poisoning will have a variety of effects on the patient. From a data interpretation perspective, however, the one piece of data that can provide a clue to the fact that opiates have been taken is the respiratory rate. Opiates suppress respiratory drive, so, if a patient has taken a cocktail of unknown drugs and the respiratory rate is slow, it would be reasonable to assume that they have taken an opiate and to administer the antidote (naloxone).

Tricyclic antidepressants

Tricyclic antidepressants (TCAs) such as amitriptyline are extremely dangerous when taken in overdose. The two major clinical complications that can arise are:

1. Cardiac toxicity – this can cause hypotension, arrhythmias and cardiac arrest

2. Seizures.

It would seem logical that one should measure blood levels of these drugs to predict which patients are likely to develop problems. This is, however, not part of routine management, and the following two tests are much more useful:

1. An electrocardiograph (ECG). Please see Chapter 10 for more information on ECG interpretation. There are two major signs on the ECG that indicate that a significant TCA overdose has been taken:

    (a) QRS broadening: the normal QRS width is <120 ms (three small squares on ECG paper). In the setting of TCA overdose, any QRS widening over 100 ms is significant. The broader the QRS complex, the higher the risk of cardiac arrhythmia and seizure.

    (b) Abnormally tall T wave in lead aVR, as shown in Fig 4.2.

2. Arterial blood gas analysis: see Chapter 13 for detailed information about the interpretation of acid–base abnormalities. A metabolic acidosis can occur in significant TCA overdose and should be treated with sodium bicarbonate. A respiratory acidosis may also occur.

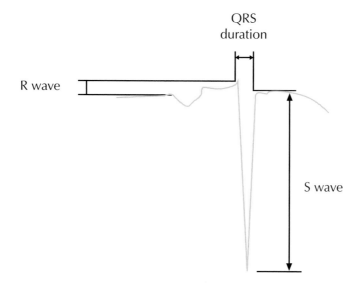

Normal aVR

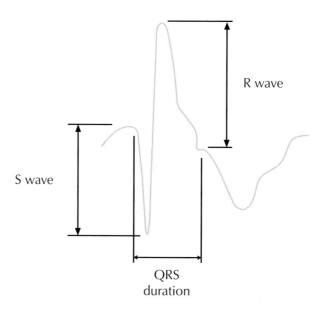

Abnormal aVR

Fig 4.2

Drugs with a low therapeutic ratio

The therapeutic ratio is the ratio between the dose of a drug needed to cause a toxic effect and the dose required to produce the intended effect. Drugs with a low therapeutic ratio thus have a small difference between helpful blood levels for treatment and toxic levels. The plasma levels of such medications can be easily measured by a hospital laboratory. For details of antibiotic drug level interpretation, please refer to page 219. For other drugs, an estimation of the steady-state drug level is most helpful, so blood is generally sampled at a fixed time point following drug ingestion.

EXAMPLES OF DRUGS WITH NARROW THERAPEUTIC RATIOS

Digoxin
Theophylline
Lithium
Phenytoin
Antibiotics, eg gentamicin, vancomycin, tobramycin

From a data interpretation perspective, digoxin deserves special mention because of its effects on the ECG. Ingestion of digoxin can cause down-sloping ST segment depression as shown in Fig 4.3 (see Chapter 10 for further details on ECG interpretation). In addition, digoxin toxicity can cause virtually any type of cardiac arrhythmia.

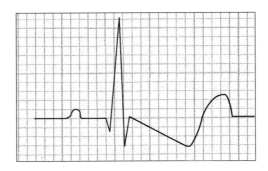

Fig 4.3

Urine testing for drug metabolites

A number of drugs can be detected in urine. A urine drug screen is often requested when a patient presents with unusual symptoms and there is a suspicion of potential drug use.

TYPICAL COMPONENTS OF URINE 'DRUGS' SCREEN

Amphetamines, barbiturates, benzodiazepines, methadone, cannabinoids, cocaine metabolites, LSD and opiates

Case 4.1

A 72-year-old woman is admitted complaining of poor appetite, nausea and vomiting. She also complains of intermittent palpitations and visual disturbance. She had a stomach upset one week previously and had been off her food and consumed little fluid. Her medical history includes hypertension, atrial fibrillation and vertigo. She is unable to recall her medications. An ECG was reported as having ST-segment abnormalities, but the house officer did not feel that this was significant.

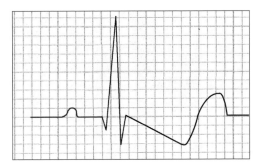

PasTest
HOSPITAL

Hb	12.5 g/dl
MCV	95.7 fl
Plt	293 $\times 10^9$/l
WCC	6.7 $\times 10^9$/l
Na$^+$	139 mmol/l
K$^+$	3.1 mmol/l
Urea	15.6 mmol/l
Creatinine	298 μmol/l
Cl$^-$	104 mmol/l
HCO$_3^-$	27 mmol/l
Digoxin level	2.9 nmol/l

Explain the full significance of these results.

Answer 4.1

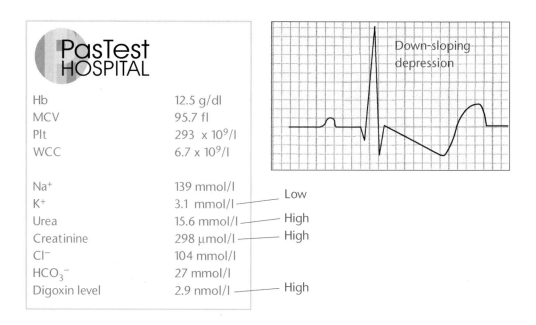

PasTest
HOSPITAL

Hb	12.5 g/dl
MCV	95.7 fl
Plt	293 x 10⁹/l
WCC	6.7 x 10⁹/l

Na⁺	139 mmol/l	
K⁺	3.1 mmol/l	Low
Urea	15.6 mmol/l	High
Creatinine	298 μmol/l	High
Cl⁻	104 mmol/l	
HCO₃⁻	27 mmol/l	
Digoxin level	2.9 nmol/l	High

Down-sloping depression

This patient has been prescribed digoxin for atrial fibrillation, and has digoxin toxicity. Digoxin is a drug with a narrow therapeutic ratio and a normal therapeutic range of 0.8–2.0 nmol/l. A level as high as 2.9 nmol/l is enough for the symptoms described in this elderly patient. Digoxin levels can accumulate rapidly in patients with renal impairment. It is likely that this woman has become dehydrated following a bout of gastroenteritis. Renal impairment has caused the rise in plasma digoxin resulting in toxicity. Hypokalaemia is also present. This can exacerbate the symptoms of digoxin toxicity.

This iatrogenic problem is simply treated. Fluid resuscitation with the replacement of potassium intravenously and the exclusion of digoxin is appropriate in this case. The ECG shows down-sloping ST-segment depression ('reverse tick') often seen in patients on digoxin, and would have been a clue here that the patient was taking this drug.

Case 4.2

A 20-year-old law student attends A&E feeling unwell after a car journey back to Belfast from Dublin, having been to visit his girlfriend over the weekend. He has a headache and informs you that he had great difficulty concentrating on the final part of his trip. He does admit to having a 'big weekend' while in Dublin. On examination his pulse is bounding in character.

His various investigations are shown. The arterial blood gas was sampled with the patient breathing room air.

PasTest
HOSPITAL

Na$^+$	140 mmol/l
K$^+$	4.2 mmol/l
Urea	4.8 mmol/l
Creatinine	76 µmol/l
Cl$^-$	105 mmol/l
HCO$_3$$^-$	23 mmol/l
pH	7.41
PaO$_2$	13.8 kPa
PaCO$_2$	4.3 kPa
HCO$_3$$^-$	24.3 mmol/l
Carboxyhaemoglobin	17%
Alcohol	nil
Urine – trace of cannabinoids	

Describe the abnormalities seen and explain the cause of this man's symptoms.

Answer 4.2

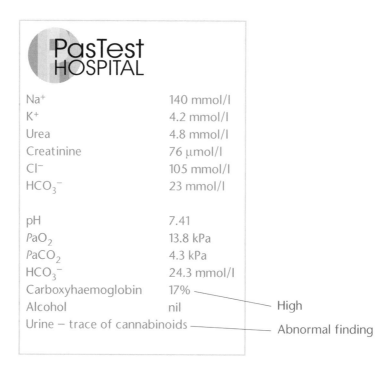

PasTest
HOSPITAL

Na+	140 mmol/l
K+	4.2 mmol/l
Urea	4.8 mmol/l
Creatinine	76 μmol/l
Cl−	105 mmol/l
HCO₃−	23 mmol/l
pH	7.41
PaO_2	13.8 kPa
$PaCO_2$	4.3 kPa
HCO₃−	24.3 mmol/l
Carboxyhaemoglobin	17% ——— High
Alcohol	nil
Urine − trace of cannabinoids ——— Abnormal finding	

On first inspection, one might suspect that illicit drug use could provide the explanation for this patient's symptoms. However, another diagnosis may be more likely − carbon monoxide poisoning. This student developed symptoms following a car journey of several hours. Typically, students, elderly people and socially deprived people are most susceptible to exposure to carbon monoxide from poorly maintained fires and motor cars. Carbon monoxide poisoning can be diagnosed by measuring carboxyhaemoglobin in an arterial blood gas sample. This patient's carboxyhaemoglobin is elevated, in keeping with the clinical suspicion. It is entirely appropriate that a urine drug screen has been performed, although the patient should be informed if this is being sent. A trace of cannabinoids suggests recent use of cannabis. This is, however, unlikely to be the explanation for this recent onset of symptoms.

Case 4.3

A 25-year-old shop assistant is brought to hospital by her colleague at 16:30 hours after she admitted to taking an overdose of paracetamol. She regrets the incident and is able to tell you clearly that she has taken one packet of 16 tablets during her lunch break between 12:00 and 12:30 hours. She feels fine and wishes to go home. No other medications or alcohol was taken. She has no health problems and is on no prescribed medications except the oral contraceptive pill. Blood tests taken on arrival at the hospital are shown.

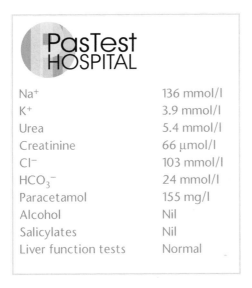

PasTest
HOSPITAL

Na$^+$	136 mmol/l
K$^+$	3.9 mmol/l
Urea	5.4 mmol/l
Creatinine	66 µmol/l
Cl$^-$	103 mmol/l
HCO$_3^-$	24 mmol/l
Paracetamol	155 mg/l
Alcohol	Nil
Salicylates	Nil
Liver function tests	Normal

Would you treat this patient? Detail the logic for your decision.

Answer 4.3

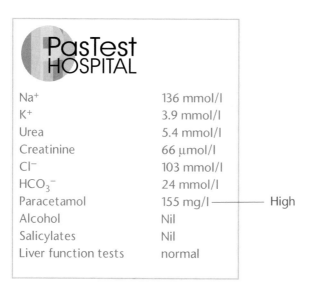

PasTest
HOSPITAL

Na$^+$	136 mmol/l
K$^+$	3.9 mmol/l
Urea	5.4 mmol/l
Creatinine	66 μmol/l
Cl$^-$	103 mmol/l
HCO$_3^-$	24 mmol/l
Paracetamol	155 mg/l ——— High
Alcohol	Nil
Salicylates	Nil
Liver function tests	normal

The three most important pieces of information to ascertain from a paracetamol overdose patient are:

- **How much has been taken?**
- **When was it taken?**
- **Does the patient have any factors to make them 'high risk'?**

Further questions to ascertain the psychiatric state and suicide risk are also clearly important.

In this case:

- **How much?**

16 tablets. Paracetamol tablets are normally 500 mg. Thus total dose = 16 x 500 mg = 8000 mg = 8 g.

- **Timing?**

4 h post-ingestion.

- **Risk?**

No high-risk features from history

The 4 h level in this patient is 155 mg/l.

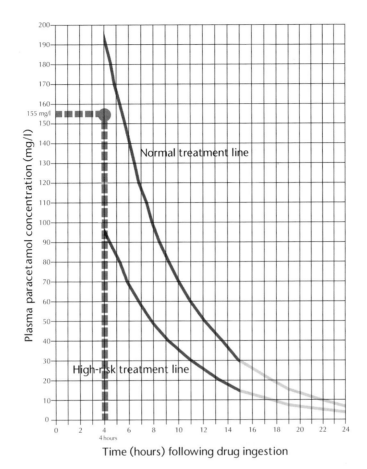

Time (hours) following drug ingestion

Using the graph illustrated earlier, one can interpret a paracetamol level of 155 mg/l at 4 h as not high enough to warrant treatment. Note, however, that if this patient were deemed to be 'high risk', treatment would have been necessary. The cut-off difference between the normal and high-risk groups at 4 h is substantial – 200 mg/l and 100 mg/l.

Case 4.4

A 33-year-old single mother attends A&E with her neighbour who found that she had taken an overdose when she came round to visit. The patient is a difficult historian but does indicate that she took about 30–50 tablets from the cupboard during the midday news. It is now 19:15 hours. The neighbour indicates that the woman has a history of epilepsy and she is on medication for this. Blood tests were taken on arrival.

PasTest HOSPITAL

Na$^+$	139 mmol/l
K$^+$	3.7 mmol/l
Urea	5.1 mmol/l
Creatinine	56 µmol/l
Cl$^-$	106 mmol/l
HCO$_3$$^-$	24 mmol/l
Paracetamol	80 mg/l
Alcohol	25 mmol/l
Salicylates	1.45 mmol/l
Bilirubin	12 µmol/l
AST	78 IU/L
ALT	65 IU/L
GGT	100 IU/L
ALP	67 U/L

State what treatment this woman might need and justify your answer.

Answer 4.4

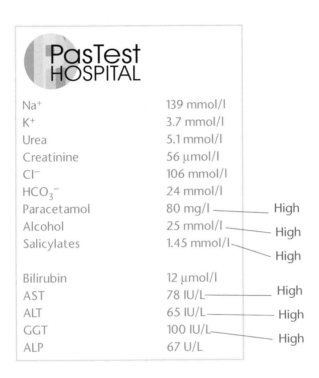

PasTest
HOSPITAL

Na$^+$	139 mmol/l
K$^+$	3.7 mmol/l
Urea	5.1 mmol/l
Creatinine	56 μmol/l
Cl$^-$	106 mmol/l
HCO$_3$$^-$	24 mmol/l
Paracetamol	80 mg/l ———— High
Alcohol	25 mmol/l ———— High
Salicylates	1.45 mmol/l ——— High
Bilirubin	12 μmol/l
AST	78 IU/L ———— High
ALT	65 IU/L ———— High
GGT	100 IU/L ——— High
ALP	67 U/L

This overdose case is more difficult, although perhaps more typical. The patient is only admitting to taking 'tablets', although the quantity, type and timing are more uncertain. At the time of presentation to hospital it is over 7 h since ingestion. To complicate matters further she is also on an unspecified anticonvulsant medication. This patient has taken alcohol with the tablets, has a raised paracetamol level and a mildly raised salicylate level. The patient also has mild impairment of her liver function tests.

On first glance 80 mg/l of paracetamol doesn't appear that remarkable. However, if the exact drug history cannot quickly be ascertained, one must assume that this patient is on hepatic enzyme-inducing antiepileptic medication. When this is transferred to the nomogram, one can see that a level of 80 mg/l is well above the treatment line in high-risk groups. Instigation of an infusion of N-acetylcysteine must commence immediately.

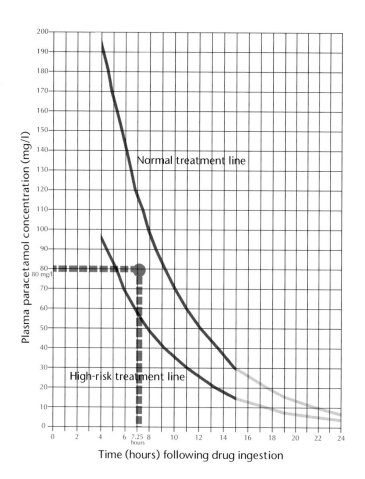

Plasma paracetamol concentration (mg/l)

Normal treatment line

80 mg/l

High-risk treatment line

6 7.25 8
hours

Time (hours) following drug ingestion

Case 4.5

A 41-year-old patient with bipolar disorder presents to A&E indicating that she has taken an overdose of her prescribed lithium. She is subdued and states that she had been feeling low at the time. Her examination is normal and she does not have any direct complaints. Blood tests are shown.

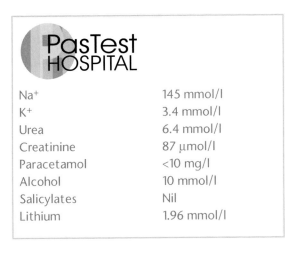

PasTest
HOSPITAL

Na+	145 mmol/l
K+	3.4 mmol/l
Urea	6.4 mmol/l
Creatinine	87 μmol/l
Paracetamol	<10 mg/l
Alcohol	10 mmol/l
Salicylates	Nil
Lithium	1.96 mmol/l

Explain the treatment options in lithium overdose with specific reference to this patient.

Answer 4.5

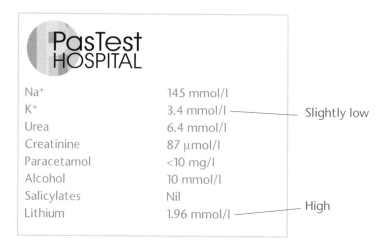

One must be particularly mindful in psychiatric patients of the accuracy of information conveyed and compliance with medication. Lithium is a commonly used drug in bipolar affective disorder, but has one major drawback − overdose. It has a narrow therapeutic ratio. Patients on long-term lithium can become unwell due to toxicity even without deliberate overdose. Overdoses of lithium can be fatal. The normal range is 0.4–1.5 mmol/l with levels above 2.0 mmol/l requiring treatment that may include haemodialysis. Levels between 1.5 and 2.0 mmol/l, as in this case, may require only fluid resuscitation and supportive treatment, along with temporary discontinuation of the drug.

PLEURAL AND PERITONEAL FLUID ANALYSIS

5

PLEURAL AND PERITONEAL FLUID ANALYSIS

In health, only a small volume of fluid surrounds the pleural lining of the lung. In various pathological states, excess fluid can accumulate forming a pleural effusion. When a significant volume has collected it may be detected on clinical examination or on a chest radiograph (see page 265 for further details). Approximately 300 ml of fluid must be present before a pleural effusion is apparent on a chest radiograph. Pleural fluid is not the only fluid that can collect within the pleural cavity. Blood in the pleural space is termed a haemothorax, lymph a chylothorax, and pus an empyema.

Analysis of this fluid may help determine the cause of the effusion. If significant volumes of fluid are removed there can also be symptomatic benefit to the patient. Fluid is collected by performing pleural aspiration ('a pleural tap') which should be performed under imaging guidance.

A number of key parameters are analysed routinely, with many additional tests being possible on request. The first fundamental point to establish is whether the effusion is unilateral or bilateral. Unilateral effusions are more likely to be 'exudates' and bilateral effusions are more likely to be 'transudates', but this is not always the case. The protein concentration of the pleural fluid is a good starting point for fluid analysis.

DON'T FORGET

Unilateral pleural effusions are more likely to be exudates.

For pleural effusions

Exudate ≥30 g/l of protein
Transudate <30 g/l of protein

Reliance on the fluid protein concentration is most useful when there is a clear clinical suspicion of either exudate or transudate, and when the protein concentration of the fluid is either much higher or much lower than 30 g/l. Occasionally, reliance on the protein concentration can result in misclassifying an exudate as a transudate, or vice versa. For this reason, the 'Light's criteria' can be used to make the distinction with greater certainty. This requires knowledge of pleural fluid and serum protein levels, as well as lactate dehydrogenase (LDH) levels.

THE 'LIGHT'S CRITERIA'

A pleural effusion is likely to be an exudate if one or more of the following conditions are met:

- Pleural fluid:serum protein ratio >0.5

- Pleural fluid LDH >200 IU/l (commonly taken as more than two-thirds of the upper limit of normal for blood)

- Pleural fluid:serum LDH ratio >0.6

Light RW, MacGregor MI, Luchsinger PC, et al. Pleural effusions: the diagnostic separation of transudates and exudates. *Ann Intern Med* 1972;**77**:507–13.

COMMON PARAMETERS ANALYSED IN PLEURAL FLUID	REASON FOR ANALYSIS
Total protein	Differentiate exudate and transudate
Lactate dehydrogenase (LDH)	Differentiate exudate and transudate
Microbiology (microscopy, cell count, Gram stain and culture)	Identify an infection
pH	Low in empyema. If pH <7.2, chest drain insertion should be strongly considered
Cytological examination	To identify and characterise malignant cells

ADDITIONAL PARAMETERS ANALYSED IN PLEURAL FLUID	INTERPRETATION
Glucose	Low in rheumatoid disease
Rheumatoid factor	High in rheumatoid disease
Amylase	High in pancreatitis
Ziehl–Neelsen stain and culture	To diagnose tuberculosis
Haematocrit	High in haemothorax

COMMON CAUSES OF A TRANSUDATE PLEURAL EFFUSION

Cardiac failure
Liver failure
Nephrotic syndrome (think 'renal failure' for ease of memory)
Hypoalbuminaemia ('nutritional failure')
Hypothyroidism ('thyroid failure')

Hooper C, Lee YC, Maskell N. Investigation of a unilateral pleural effusion in adults: British Thoracic Society pleural disease guideline 2010. *Thorax* 2010;**65**(suppl 2): ii4–17.

DON'T FORGET
Transudates are usually associated with FAILURE.

COMMON CAUSES OF AN EXUDATE PLEURAL EFFUSION

Cancer
Pneumonia (parapneumonic effusion)
Pulmonary embolus/infarction
Tuberculosis
Connective tissue disease (eg rheumatoid disease)
Acute pancreatitis

DON'T FORGET

An exudate exudes (pumps out) protein so the protein content is normally high.

The colour of the fluid aspirated from a pleural effusion also gives useful information as to the potential cause.

COLOUR OF FLUID	DIAGNOSIS
Straw	Normal
Yellow	Infected
Blood stained	Traumatic, malignancy
Frank blood	Mesothelioma, trauma, other malignancy
Pus	Empyema
Food debris	Oesophageal rupture

Peritoneal fluid analysis

In health, peritoneal fluid is present only in small volumes. In illness it may collect in vast quantities, in which case it should be detected on clinical examination. Smaller volumes may be detected on imaging. An abnormal collection of peritoneal fluid is termed 'ascites'.

Paracentesis (often termed 'peritoneal tap') may be undertaken for diagnostic purposes. Alternatively, large volumes of fluid can be removed to provide symptomatic benefit to the patient.

Analysis of peritoneal fluid has two main purposes:

- To characterise the disease causing ascites

- To detect infection.

Characterising the disease causing ascites

The most common cause of ascites by far is portal hypertension secondary to liver cirrhosis. However, there are a great many other causes. It is important to be able to distinguish between these. In a method analogous to pleural fluid analysis, the causes of ascites can be divided into whether they cause an exudate or a transudate. The total protein content is used to differentiate between the two, with a cut-off level of 25 g/l.

FOR ASCITES
Exudate ≥25 g/l of protein
Transudate <25 g/l of protein

CAUSES OF TRANSUDATE ASCITES

Cirrhosis
Cardiac failure
Hypoalbuminaemia
Nephrotic syndrome

CAUSES OF EXUDATE ASCITES

Intraperitoneal malignancy (primary or secondary)
Intraperitoneal infection including tuberculosis
Pancreatitis
Hypothyroidism
Chylous ascites

Characterising ascites is, however, notoriously unreliable. Accuracy can be improved by comparing the albumin content of the ascitic fluid with its level in the serum. This yields a serum–ascites albumin gradient (SAAG) as shown in the box.

Serum–ascites albumin gradient
SAAG (g/l) = Serum albumin (g/l) – Ascites albumin (g/l)

If the SAAG is ≥11 g/l, one can say that the patient is very likely to have portal hypertension. Bear in mind, however, that a patient may have portal hypertension alongside another cause of ascites. Other causes listed in the 'Transudate' box are possibilities. If the SAAG is <11 g/l, the causes listed in the 'Exudate' box are more likely.

Detecting infection

The detection of infection in ascitic fluid is extremely important. The WCC of the ascites is increased in peritonitis. In most patients with ascites associated with cirrhosis, peritonitis is a primary problem, and is termed 'spontaneous bacterial peritonitis' (SBP). Occasionally another cause of peritonitis, such as a subphrenic abscess or perforated bowel, can be mistaken for SBP.

The diagnosis of SBP can be made when bacteria are identified after culturing ascitic fluid. However, this process takes some time, so the ascites white cell count is usually used to guide treatment. This result should be available within a matter of hours. An ascites neutrophil count ≥250 cells/mm^3 (0.25 x 10^9/l) is in keeping with SBP. If the clinical setting fits with this diagnosis, treatment with an appropriate antibiotic should be commenced.

DON'T FORGET
Ascites neutrophil count of ≥250 cells/mm^3 is in keeping with SBP.

An alternative cause for peritonitis (eg perforated bowel) should be suspected when multiple organisms are seen on Gram staining.

The parameters shown in the box may be analysed. Those marked with an asterisk should be requested only when clinically indicated.

PARAMETER	PURPOSE
WCC (including differential)	To detect infection
Total protein content and albumin	To distinguish exudates and transudates To calculate the serum–ascites albumin gradient
Microscopy including Gram stain	To visualise bacteria
Culture	To identify bacteria
Glucose*	Low in malignant ascites
Cytology*	To detect malignant cells
Amylase*	Raised in ascites associated with pancreatitis

Case 5.1

A 36-year-old man is admitted with shortness of breath and a cough productive of green sputum. He is feverish and complains of left-sided pleuritic chest discomfort. He has led a perfectly healthy life to date. He is a smoker of 10 pack-years. On examination a pleural effusion is noted on the left side to the mid-zone. This finding is confirmed on chest radiography.

The effusion is aspirated at ward level and sent for analysis.

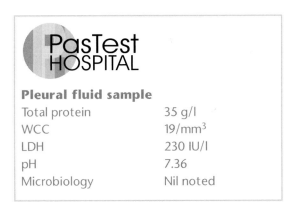

PasTest
HOSPITAL

Pleural fluid sample

Total protein	35 g/l
WCC	19/mm³
LDH	230 IU/l
pH	7.36
Microbiology	Nil noted

Describe the findings and the likely cause of the pleural effusion.

Answer 5.1

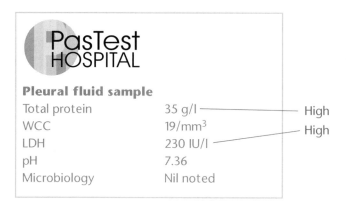

Pleural fluid sample

Total protein	35 g/l	High
WCC	19/mm³	High
LDH	230 IU/l	
pH	7.36	
Microbiology	Nil noted	

This patient has symptoms suggestive of a bacterial pneumonia. He is otherwise healthy and there is little to suspect an underlying sinister or chronic disease. A proportion of bacterial pneumonias will present with a pleural effusion. Pleural fluid is produced in excess in reaction to the local irritation of the pleura from the surrounding infection.

The findings from the simple pleural fluid analysis are in keeping with this clinical suspicion. It is an exudate (total protein >30 g/l) and the lactate dehydrogenase level is high.

This patient has a parapneumonic pleural effusion. Treatment consists of antibiotics for the pneumonia, with the effusion expected to resolve over several weeks. The patient should have a repeat chest radiograph 6 weeks after treatment to ensure resolution of the effusion. If the patient's condition were to deteriorate one would have to consider the development of an empyema (pus collection in the pleural space).

Case 5.2

A 65-year-old retired headmaster presents with progressive shortness of breath and swelling of the feet. Nine years ago he sustained an anterior myocardial infarction and has had subsequent problems with angina requiring coronary artery stenting. He also suffers from hypertension and gout. Following a recent flare of gout his GP prescribed a short course of ibuprofen. Examination reveals pitting oedema to the mid-calves bilaterally and a jugular venous pulse (JVP) raised by 3 cmH$_2$O. The bases of both lungs are dull to percussion. Breath sounds are reduced and vocal resonance is decreased over these areas.

After some initial treatment these examination findings remain and a decision is made to carry out pleural aspiration: 30 ml was aspirated from the right hemithorax and sent for analysis.

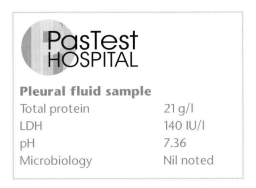

PasTest
HOSPITAL

Pleural fluid sample

Total protein	21 g/l
LDH	140 IU/l
pH	7.36
Microbiology	Nil noted

Describe the findings and likely cause.

Answer 5.2

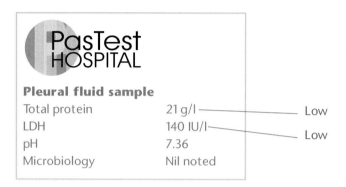

PasTest
HOSPITAL

Pleural fluid sample

Total protein	21 g/l	Low
LDH	140 IU/l	Low
pH	7.36	
Microbiology	Nil noted	

The clinical features of this patient suggest a diagnosis of congestive cardiac failure (CCF). The prescription of a non-steroidal anti-inflammatory drug (NSAID) for acute gout has caused fluid retention, leading to worsening of the underlying cardiac failure. The effusions are bilateral, which suggests that they are likely to be transudative. The pleural fluid sample confirms this suspicion with a total protein content of only 21 g/l and an LDH of 140 IU/l. Of all the causes of transudate pleural effusions, cardiac failure best fits in this case.

Case 5.3

As the medical junior doctor on-call you are asked by your surgical colleagues to see a 45-year-old overweight housewife. She was admitted with abdominal pain 2 days ago and an ultrasound scan of the abdomen showed gallstones with extrahepatic bile duct dilatation. Bowel gas obscured visualisation of the pancreas. Your opinion is sought as the patient is short of breath and complains of left-sided pleuritic chest discomfort. On examination you detect a left-sided pleural effusion which is confirmed on chest radiography. You decide to perform a diagnostic pleural aspiration.

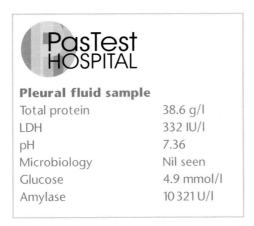

PasTest
HOSPITAL

Pleural fluid sample

Total protein	38.6 g/l
LDH	332 IU/l
pH	7.36
Microbiology	Nil seen
Glucose	4.9 mmol/l
Amylase	10 321 U/l

What is your interpretation of this result?

Answer 5.3

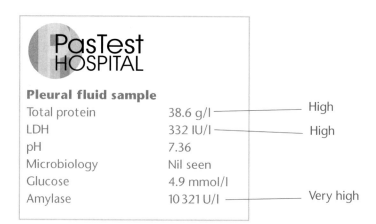

PasTest HOSPITAL

Pleural fluid sample

Total protein	38.6 g/l	High
LDH	332 IU/l	High
pH	7.36	
Microbiology	Nil seen	
Glucose	4.9 mmol/l	
Amylase	10 321 U/l	Very high

Pleural effusions can be found in acute pancreatitis. It is most typical for this to be unilateral; however, bilateral effusions are recognised. The key to diagnosis is the amylase level within the aspirated fluid.

Case 5.4

A 33-year-old secretary presents with malaise, joint discomfort and by her own admission generally feeling 'out of sorts'. She was diagnosed with Graves' disease 3 years ago and has been rendered euthyroid (normal thyroid function). She has also suffered from coeliac disease since her teens. She has no respiratory complaints. As part of her investigative work-up a chest radiograph is taken, which to the medical team's surprise shows a right-sided pleural effusion of moderate size.

Pleural aspiration is performed.

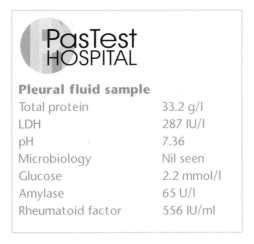

Pleural fluid sample

Total protein	33.2 g/l
LDH	287 IU/l
pH	7.36
Microbiology	Nil seen
Glucose	2.2 mmol/l
Amylase	65 U/l
Rheumatoid factor	556 IU/ml

What is the cause of her effusion?

Answer 5.4

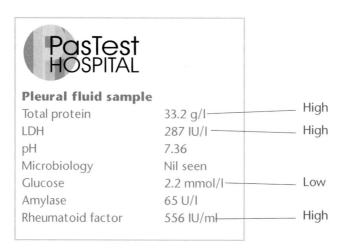

PasTest HOSPITAL

Pleural fluid sample

Total protein	33.2 g/l	High
LDH	287 IU/l	High
pH	7.36	
Microbiology	Nil seen	
Glucose	2.2 mmol/l	Low
Amylase	65 U/l	
Rheumatoid factor	556 IU/ml	High

Pleural effusion is an uncommon but well-documented finding in rheumatoid disease. This is a systemic disease and a number of manifestations occur in the chest. Among these are: pleural effusion, pulmonary nodules, interstitial fibrosis, pleural thickening and bronchiolitis obliterans. This patient has a number of autoimmune diseases so it would not be unreasonable for her to be diagnosed with rheumatoid disease. The pleural effusion is an exudate. The rheumatoid factor level is hugely elevated at 556 IU/ml. In addition the glucose is low at 2.2 mmol/l in the effusion, further supporting the diagnosis.

Case 5.5

A 42-year-old salesman with established alcoholic liver cirrhosis is a known patient to the ward. He has been admitted on multiple previous occasions and continues to drink heavily. On this admission he is a little confused and tremulous. On examination, ascites is present along with small bilateral pleural effusions. His abdomen is mildly tender throughout. Bowel sounds are present.

The on-call doctor performs a diagnostic peritoneal aspiration. One hour later, the laboratory technician phones with the report below.

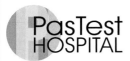

Analysis of peritoneal fluid

WCC	322 cells/mm^3 – predominantly neutrophils
Albumin	16 g/l
Amylase	92 U/l
Microscopy	Gram-negative bacilli seen on Gram stain

His blood albumin level is 29 g/l.

What is the diagnosis, and how should the patient be treated?

Answer 5.5

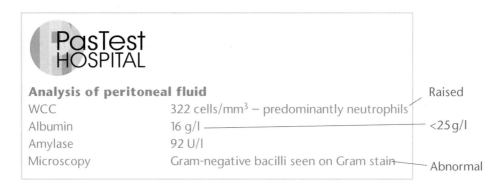

Analysis of peritoneal fluid   Raised

WCC   322 cells/mm^3 – predominantly neutrophils

Albumin   16 g/l ———————————————————— <25g/l

Amylase   92 U/l

Microscopy   Gram-negative bacilli seen on Gram stain ——— Abnormal

His ascites white cell count shows a neutrophilia, with more than 250 cells/mm^3.

The albumin content is less than 25 g/l indicating a transudate.

The SAAG is 13 g/l (29 g/l – 16 g/l). This is in keeping with portal hypertension.

Gram staining shows the most typical finding in SBP – Gram-negative bacilli. In time, one might expect culture to yield *Escherichia coli* or *Klebsiella* species.

This man has spontaneous bacterial peritonitis, on a background of hepatic cirrhosis caused by alcohol. His clinical features are typical with general abdominal discomfort, often accompanied by pyrexia. This infection has also made him mildly encephalopathic, hence the confusion.

In a patient with a history of alcohol dependency, abdominal distension and pain, pancreatitis is a further differential diagnosis. However, this would cause an exudate, and one would expect the amylase level to be raised significantly.

Case 5.6

A frail 88-year-old nursing home resident is brought to hospital because of abdominal pain. Her nurse is also concerned about the progressive increase in her abdominal girth over the past 6 weeks. She has a history of vascular dementia. On examination there is a grossly distended abdomen, with shifting dullness and a fluid thrill. A CT scan of the abdomen and pelvis demonstrated a massive mixed solid–cystic lesion in the pelvis and gross ascites.

Peritoneal aspiration was performed for diagnostic purposes and symptomatic benefit: 9500 ml was drained and sent for analysis. The results are shown.

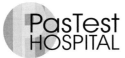

Analysis of peritoneal fluid

WCC	25 cells/mm^3 – mixed leukocytes
Albumin	28 g/l
Microscopy	No organisms seen
Cytology	Tumour cells seen – in keeping with adenocarcinoma

Her blood albumin level is 29 g/l.

Provide a diagnosis and explain your reasoning.

Answer 5.6

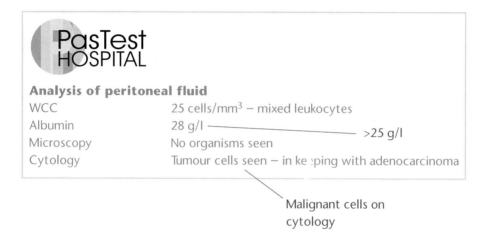

PasTest
HOSPITAL

Analysis of peritoneal fluid

WCC	25 cells/mm³ – mixed leukocytes
Albumin	28 g/l ——————— >25 g/l
Microscopy	No organisms seen
Cytology	Tumour cells seen – in keeping with adenocarcinoma

Malignant cells on
cytology

The WCC is not significantly raised.

The albumin level is greater than 25 g/l, indicating an exudate.

The SAAG is 1 g/l (29 g/l – 28 g/l), indicating a low probability of portal hypertension.

The diagnosis is seen on cytology.

This patient has an advanced intraperitoneal malignancy. The specific primary origin is unknown. The cells present may originate from a primary intraperitoneal malignancy or be due to intraperitoneal metastatic disease. A large volume of ascites in an elderly patient without known liver disease should always arouse the suspicion of malignancy. The CT findings are in keeping with a primary pelvic malignancy of likely ovarian origin.

Case 5.7

A 36-year-old banker attends A&E complaining of recurrent bouts of intense abdominal discomfort. He has been reluctant to present previously for fear of admission. He admits to being a heavy drinker, but his family and colleagues are not aware of his problem. On examination there is distension of the abdomen with ascites present, tenderness in the upper abdomen and a faint upper midline incision.

You are concerned about his level of abdominal pain. He agrees to peritoneal aspiration, but does not wish to be admitted.

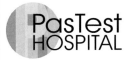

PasTest HOSPITAL

Analysis of peritoneal fluid

WCC	147 cells/mm^3 – predominantly neutrophils
Albumin	29 g/l
Amylase	894 U/l
Microscopy	No organisms seen

The patient's blood albumin level is 32 g/l.

Give a diagnosis and list useful further investigations.

Answer 5.7

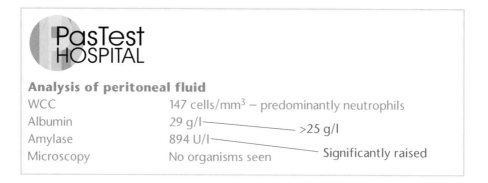

PasTest
HOSPITAL

Analysis of peritoneal fluid

WCC	147 cells/mm³ – predominantly neutrophils	
Albumin	29 g/l	>25 g/l
Amylase	894 U/l	
Microscopy	No organisms seen	Significantly raised

The ascites is an exudate, and there is no evidence of infection.

The SAAG is 3 g/l (32 g/l – 29 g/l), indicating a low probability of portal hypertension.

The amylase is elevated at 894 U/l, in keeping with acute pancreatitis.

Every effort should be made to persuade this man of the need to stay in hospital for further investigation and treatment of his pancreatitis.

MICROBIOLOGY

6

MICROBIOLOGY

Infections account for a wide spectrum of human illness. Bacteria and viruses predominate in clinical medicine in the UK, but one should bear in mind that other organisms (eg fungi, protozoa, helminths and arthropods) can all cause problems. Infections that are rare in clinical practice in the UK should be borne in mind when patients have been travelling or are from endemic regions. In addition, patients who are immunocompromised are prone to infections that are not normally seen in individuals with healthy immune systems.

If treatment is required for an infection, a drug must be chosen that has activity against the pathogen causing the problem. Often, a 'best guess' at treatment is made. For example, an antibiotic called trimethoprim is often given to patients with symptoms of a urinary tract infection because the bacteria that are responsible for most urinary tract infections are likely to be targeted by this drug. In many cases, however, it is appropriate to collect samples from the patient so that an attempt can be made to accurately identify the organism that is causing the infection. It is the results from the analysis of such samples that are considered further here.

To have the best chance of identifying a causative organism, samples should normally be taken from the body site that is affected. Common samples include sputum, urine, faeces, synovial fluid, swabs from mouth, skin or genitals, pus from any site, cerebrospinal fluid and biopsy samples. On occasion, organisms can move from the site of origin into the bloodstream causing septicaemia. Thus, blood is often cultured in addition to material from the likely focus of infection.

Infections with bacteria

Infections with bacteria tend to predominate in undergraduate assessments because they are the infections that most commonly cause serious disease in the UK. Once a sample containing bacteria has been collected, there are two basic methods for identifying the organism. First, the sample can be examined using light microscopy with a stain applied. The stain normally used first is the Gram stain. Organisms that stain blue are termed 'Gram positive' and those that stain pink are termed 'Gram negative'. Bacteria can then be described using their shape. 'Bacilli' are rod shaped whereas 'cocci' are spherical. Thus, very quickly one can have a fair idea of the likely organism contained in a sample. Common organisms characterised by staining characteristics and shape are listed in the box on page 216. 'Aerobes' grow best in oxygen-rich environments, whereas 'anaerobes' grow best in oxygen-poor environments. This will become apparent during culture. Another staining technique, Ziehl–Neelsen staining, can be used to detect mycobacteria (responsible for tuberculosis).

EXAMPLES OF COMMON ORGANISMS

Aerobes	Gram-positive cocci	Staphylococcus aureus Streptococcus pyogenes Streptococcus pneumoniae Enterococcus faecalis
	Gram-positive bacilli	Listeria monocytogenes Bacillus anthracis
	Gram-negative cocci	Moraxella catarrhalis Neisseria meningitidis
	Gram-negative bacilli	Escherichia coli Pseudomonas aeruginosa
Anaerobes	Cocci	Peptococci Peptostreptococci
	Bacilli	Bacteroides fragilis Clostridium difficile

The second method for organism identification is culture. Samples are placed on growth media and given time for the organisms to multiply. After multiplication has taken place, microbiologists use a range of techniques for identifying the particular type of bacteria present. This takes time – several days for most bacteria. The identification of tuberculosis can take weeks, however. The payoff for waiting is that the exact species of organism can usually be identified after culturing. Once a bacterium is cultured, its sensitivity to a batch of suitable common antimicrobial agents is tested. There are three outcomes to this testing: sensitive (S), intermediately sensitive (I) and resistant (R). A typical culture and antibiotic sensitivity report might look like this:

PasTest
HOSPITAL

Urine culture

> 10^5 organisms/ml *Proteus* species

Co-amoxiclav	R
Ampicillin	S
Ciprofloxacin	S
Cefotaxime	S
Nitrofurantoin	I
Tazocin	S
Trimethoprim	R
Cephalexin	S

In this example, the patient's urinary tract infection appears to have been caused by the Gram-negative bacillus *Proteus* species. If treatment is deemed necessary, it would be most appropriate to prescribe one of the drugs shown as sensitive (S), because this would be expected to have the highest likelihood of killing the micro-organism in question.

MINIMAL INHIBITORY CONCENTRATION (MIC) AND MINIMUM BACTERICIDAL CONCENTRATION (MBC) TESTING

Occasionally it is desirable to have more information about an organism's sensitivity to a particular antimicrobial agent rather than a simple yes/no answer. This is commonly the case for infections that are difficult to treat or that require prolonged courses of antibiotics, eg infective endocarditis. In such circumstances detailed testing can be performed to work out the minimum concentration of antibiotic necessary to stop bacterial growth (MIC) and the minimum concentration of antibiotic necessary to kill the bacteria (MBC). These data can then be translated into the most appropriate dose and duration for drug prescription purposes.

Staphylococcus aureus requires special mention for two reasons:

1. If resistant to meticillin, it is deemed meticillin-resistant *Staphylococcus aureus* (MRSA). This is highly important because different antibiotics are required to treat this particular type of bacterium.

2. It is a reasonably common finding to isolate 'coagulase-negative' *Staphylococcus aureus* on blood cultures. Laboratories often test staphylococci for their production of coagulase. Staphylococci that normally colonise skin (such as *S. epidermidis*) do not produce coagulase. The identification of these organisms on blood cultures usually reflects the fact that the skin surface was inadequately sterilised before blood was drawn.

Other methods are available for detecting certain bacteria, but the clinician must actually have the knowledge to suspect a likely organism and request the appropriate test. In patients presenting with pneumonia, for example, urine is often tested for the presence of antigens to *Streptococcus pneumoniae* and *Legionella* species. In patients with diarrhoea, faecal samples are often tested for the presence of *Clostridium difficile* toxin. Genetic testing can also be carried out to look for the presence of bacterial DNA or RNA in a sample. Polymerase chain reaction (PCR) techniques can be used to assist in this process.

Finally, it is possible to perform serological tests to detect antibodies to various organisms in a patient's blood. Immunoglobulin type M (IgM) levels tend to rise early in a disease course, with IgG levels rising later. If IgM is detected to a particular bacterium, it is likely that this is the cause of the illness. The IgG level is more difficult to interpret, however, because the IgG antibody level would be expected to be elevated if a patient has either had a particular illness previously or been immunised against it. It is thus difficult to distinguish between current infection and previous exposure based on a single measure of IgG level. The best use of serological testing is in the measurement of acute and convalescent levels of IgG, ie measure the level during the acute illness and again once the patient has recovered. If there has been a significant rise in the antibody levels to a particular microorganism during the patient's recovery, it is probable that the organism suspected was the likely pathogen. The disadvantage with serological tests is the inevitable time lag in making the diagnosis, and the fact that treatment decisions must therefore be made without confirmation of the pathogen.

Infections with other organisms

The principles for the detection of other microorganisms are similar to those used for bacteria. Light microscopy can be useful in detecting fungi (eg in skin scrapings samples), parasites (eg in faecal samples) and protozoa (eg malaria in blood). Electron microscopy can be used to identify certain viruses. Pathogen antigen testing can be attempted with certain organisms also (eg hepatitis B surface antigen). Genetic testing employing PCR techniques is being increasingly used for the rapid detection of viruses. An example would be the rapid testing of cerebrospinal fluid for herpes simplex virus in patients with suspected encephalitis (viral brain infection). Fungi can be cultured similarly to bacteria, but culture of viruses and other organisms is time-consuming and difficult because they must be grown in cell or tissue preparations. Serological testing is the method most useful in clinical practice for confirming infection with a virus.

It should be apparent that the difficulty with microbiological investigations for a clinician lies with knowing which test to request. Thanks to the efforts of highly skilled laboratory technicians, the interpretation of test results is generally relatively straightforward.

Interpretation of drug levels

Drug treatment of patients with infections sometimes requires the use of drugs with 'narrow therapeutic ratios'. This means that there is a small difference between the dose of a drug required to produce a therapeutic effect and the dose required to cause toxicity. Use too low a dose, and the infection may not be adequately treated. Use too high a dose, and you will put the patient at risk of an adverse drug reaction. Drugs for which levels are commonly tested include aminoglycoside agents (eg gentamicin) and glycopeptides (eg vancomycin). It is possible to measure a peak drug level in the blood (sample taken shortly after drug administration) or a trough level (taken just before the next dose being administered). Target ranges for peak and/or trough levels are listed in drug formularies. Generally, if levels are lower than required, dosing is increased. If levels are too high, the drug is omitted until the level returns to a safe level before a modified dosing regimen is re-started.

Bedside testing for urinary tract infection

Urinary tract infection

Urine samples can be quickly analysed at ward level using a reagent strip that is dipped into the urine. Typical strips allow for the estimation of a range of substances in the urine (see page 9 for urinalysis in haemolysis and page 72 for its use in cholestatic jaundice). Operators wait for a set time period and then compare a colour change with each reagent to a standard set of results. The colour change seen will depend on the amount of a particular substance in the urine. Substances that are useful in the detection of urinary tract infection (UTI) include leukocyte esterase, nitrites, protein and blood. Urinalysis can only at best point towards the diagnosis of UTI – culture is necessary for a definitive diagnosis. The sensitivity and specificity of abnormalities in each of the parameters mentioned have been published with regard to diagnosing a UTI, but a good rule of thumb is to say that, if urinalysis is totally normal, then a UTI is unlikely. If it is abnormal in any way, a UTI is a possibility and culture should be performed if there is clinical suspicion.

Simerville JA, Maxted WC, Pahira JJ. Urinalysis: a comprehensive review. *Am Fam Physician* 2005;**71**:1153–62.

Interpretation of microbiological data is found within Chapter 16.

NEUROLOGICAL INVESTIGATIONS

7

NEUROLOGICAL INVESTIGATIONS

There are three main groups of tests used to investigate neurological disease. Cerebrospinal fluid analysis and neurophysiological investigations are dealt with in this chapter. Imaging is touched upon in Chapter 9. It is the combination of findings from these tests, rather than one in isolation, that frequently enables a diagnosis to be made

Cerebrospinal fluid analysis

Cerebrosinal fluid (CSF) is obtained by performing a lumbar puncture. A wide variety of tests can be performed on CSF as detailed below. This box details the components of a routine CSF analysis.

COMPONENTS OF A ROUTINE CSF ANALYSIS	
Opening pressure	Total protein
Appearance	Glucose
(Gram stain + culture if infection suspected)	Microscopy for cell counts

Bedside tests

Important information on a patient's condition can be gleaned at the bedside during the process of lumbar puncture, even before fluid is sent for analysis.

Opening pressure

Once a needle has been passed and CSF is draining, a manometer can be attached to measure the 'opening pressure'. This is meaningful only if the patient is in the 'standard' lateral decubitus position (lying on their side) at the time of puncture. If lumbar puncture is performed with the patient upright, the opening pressure will be artificially elevated. Normal values for opening pressure are variably quoted between texts, but a pressure of between 8 and 20 cmCSF is probably normal.

CAUSES OF ABNORMAL OPENING PRESSURE	
Abnormally low	**Abnormally high**
CSF leak Recent lumbar puncture	Meningitis Tumour Intracranial haemorrhage Idiopathic intracranial hypertension ('benign intracranial hypertension')

CSF appearance

The gross appearance of CSF can give an early indication of fluid composition. Textbooks list many subtle colour variations of CSF, which are quite difficult to appreciate unless you are experienced in this area. The most abnormal CSF appearances are listed in the box below.

CHARACTERISTIC CSF APPEARANCE	
Appearance	**Characteristic of**
Clear Cloudy or purulent Bloody	Normality Meningitis Traumatic tap or subarachnoid haemorrhage

The inadvertent puncture of a blood vessel during the process of lumbar puncture will result in blood-stained fluid being drained. The operator will not know with any certainty, however, that a blood vessel has been hit, and one must therefore be able to distinguish between CSF that is truly blood stained and CSF that appears blood stained only because of the puncture of a vessel. One simple method for doing this at the bedside involves collecting three separate CSF samples. If the fluid remains blood stained to the same degree in all samples, it is likely that the CSF is truly blood stained. If, however, the fluid becomes less blood stained with time, it is more likely that the lumbar puncture has been a traumatic tap. Laboratory testing of the CSF for the presence of xanthochromia provides another method of distinguishing between these two possibilities and is discussed below.

Laboratory tests

Microscopy

CSF microscopy permits the estimation of cell counting in the fluid. An elevated red cell count is most commonly seen as a result of the lumbar puncture needle puncturing a blood vessel en route to the subarachnoid space. It will also be seen in cases of intracranial haemorrhage. However, a measure of the red cell count in three consecutively collected specimens of CSF can help differentiate between these two possibilities, similar to the bedside test described above.

An elevated white cell count (>5 cells/mm^3) suggests central nervous system infection (ie meningitis or encephalitis), but can also be found in other conditions such as inflammatory diseases and cancer. If puncture of a small blood vessel has occurred during lumbar puncture, the white cell count will also be elevated falsely due to the presence of these cells in the blood. The particular type of white cells present can also be informative. A predominance of neutrophils suggests bacterial meningitis. Lymphocytes predominate in other infective causes of meningitis (eg viral, tuberculosis or fungal).

Microbiological testing

Microscopy after Gram staining (for bacterial infection), Ziehl–Neelsen staining (for tuberculosis), culture and genetic techniques (eg polymerase chain reaction [PCR] techniques to detect bacterial or viral DNA) can all be useful in the analysis of CSF when infection is suspected. Refer to Chapter 6 for further details. It is worth bearing in mind that, as it is imperative that antimicrobial treatment should be administered as soon as possible in patients with suspected bacterial meningitis, lumbar puncture is often (rightly) performed after treatment has been started. This can change the CSF constituents such that 'textbook' patterns may not be seen, and a high index of suspicion is necessary. More specialised microbiological testing can be performed if an unusual organism (eg syphilis, cryptococci, human immunodeficiency virus [HIV]) is suspected.

Protein measurement

Normal CSF contains between 0.15 and 0.45 g/l of protein approximately, but the precise reference range varies depending on the laboratory used. Abnormally elevated CSF protein is a good pointer that some pathological process is active in the central nervous system, but it is impossible to be sure about causality using the protein measure alone. The box on page 226 lists some of the more common conditions that are associated with elevated CSF protein, but this list is by no means exhaustive.

CAUSES OF RAISED CSF PROTEIN	
Meningitis	Neoplastic disease
Brain abscess	Guillain–Barré syndrome
Intracerebral haemorrhage	Multiple sclerosis

Glucose measurement

Interpretation of the CSF glucose concentration in isolation is meaningless – it must be interpreted in relation to the blood glucose concentration. A blood sample for glucose measurement must always be sent at the time of lumbar puncture.

DON'T FORGET
Always interpret CSF glucose results in the context of blood glucose levels.

CSF glucose should be around 40–60% that of the level in blood. An abnormally high glucose level will be seen with simultaneous high blood sugar level (ie in poorly controlled diabetes) and is not a pointer to CSF pathology. An abnormally low CSF glucose level is, however, highly important and is suggestive of, but not limited to, bacterial, fungal or tuberculous infection. Viral infections of the CNS do not characteristically lower the CSF glucose concentration.

Other tests

There are a multitude of specialised tests that can be performed on CSF in certain circumstances. The most commonly requested of these are detailed below.

Xanthochromia

The term 'xanthochromia' describes a yellow discoloration of CSF. This can sometimes be detected by inspecting CSF, but is more reliably quantified in a laboratory using spectrophotometry. A positive test indicates that bilirubin is present in the fluid, and will therefore be found in patients with significant jaundice. Assuming that the patient does not have jaundice, xanthochromia is tested for most commonly in patients who are suspected to have had a subarachnoid haemorrhage (SAH), because blood in the CSF breaks down to form bilirubin. CT scanning of the head should be performed first, with lumbar puncture being performed if SAH is suspected but no evidence of it is seen on the scan. It is routine to wait at least 12 hours after the onset of symptoms to ensure that any blood in the CSF has had time to break down into bilirubin.

The presence of xanthochromia in a sample can also be helpful in distinguishing blood-stained CSF from a traumatic tap in addition to the methods used above. In a traumatic tap, blood will only have entered the CSF at the time of lumbar puncture, and will not have had time to break down into bilirubin. Testing for xanthochromia will therefore be negative in these circumstances.

Oligoclonal bands

The presence of oligoclonal bands in CSF is often tested for in patients who are suspected of having multiple sclerosis (MS). Oligoclonal bands are due to the presence of immunoglobulins in the CSF and are detected when CSF is tested using electrophoresis. Although characteristic of MS, the finding of oligoclonal bands is not diagnostic, because they can be found in a variety of rare neurological diseases.

Cytological examination

Cytological examination of the CSF can be helpful in the diagnosis of neurological malignancy. The specifics of the tests used are beyond the scope of this text, but a cytological report normally incorporates a cytologist's overall impression and is therefore relatively easy to interpret.

Neurophysiological investigations

Neurophysiology is a specialist domain within neurology. Only a brief understanding of the common investigations is necessary for an undergraduate. Likewise, knowledge of the key findings in classic conditions will suffice. It is unlikely that one would be expected to interpret neurophysiological investigations.

The main investigations to be aware of are nerve conduction studies and electromyography. Visually evoked responses and electroencephalography are further aids to diagnosis.

NEUROPHYSIOLOGICAL INVESTIGATIONS
Nerve conduction studies
Electromyography
Visually evoked responses
Electroencephalography

Nerve conduction studies

Nerve conduction studies (NCSs) measure how well individual nerves transmit electrical signals. The nerve of interest is stimulated, usually electrically, with surface electrodes placed on the skin. One electrode stimulates the nerve and the resulting electrical activity is recorded by the other electrodes. The distance between electrodes and the time taken for electrical impulses to travel between electrodes are used to calculate the nerve conduction velocity.

The most common reason for NCSs to be requested is for suspected carpal tunnel syndrome. In this condition, the median nerve is entrapped within the confines of the carpal tunnel.

Electromyography

Surface or needle electrodes are used to detect muscle action potentials following controlled electrical stimulation. The electrical stimulation provokes action potentials within the nerves which in turn stimulate a magnified response in muscles.

Electromyography (EMG) may be modified for some indications. The most important to know is single-fibre EMG and EMG with repetitive stimulation used when myasthenia gravis is clinically suspected.

CASES

Visually evoked responses

In this test, the eye is stimulated in order to evoke a response within the occipital cortex. It is performed by placing a series of electrodes over the scalp in the occipital area while asking the patient to observe a series of visual patterns. The response is recorded via the electrodes. Two indices are noted:

1. The speed of response of the nerve (termed 'P100 latencies')

2. The height of the waveform obtained.

This test is usually performed in patients in whom multiple sclerosis is suspected. In multiple sclerosis, the waveform will be preserved, but the speed of response will be delayed because of optic nerve demyelination.

Electroencephalography

Electroencephalography (EEG) is the recording of electrical activity from the brain using a series of scalp electrodes. Usually, recordings over a period of several minutes are taken. Broadly speaking, EEG can be used to diagnose epilepsy and diffuse brain disease. In epilepsy, it is most valuable if a recording takes place during a seizure since it is not unusual to obtain a normal recording between seizures.

In difficult cases, EEG recording can take place over several hours or days in a supervised room in hospital with video recording. EEG may also be invaluable in diagnosing non-convulsive status epilepticus and distinguishing true seizures from pseudoseizures. In non-convulsive status epilepticus, a patient is having ongoing seizures, despite these not manifesting themselves clinically. Prompt diagnosis by EEG may prevent a permanent neurological deficit.

Classic neurophysiological disease associations

TEST	RESULT	DISEASE
EEG	Spike and wave	Primary generalised epilepsy
EEG	Periodic complexes	Creutzfeldt–Jakob disease
EMG	Short polyphasic motor potentials Sometimes spontaneous fibrillation and high-frequency repetitive discharges	Polymyositis
EMG (single fibre)	Fatiguability following repetitive stimulation	Myasthenia gravis
EMG	Repetitive single motor unit potentials all low amplitude. Short duration polyphasic motor unit potentials	Myotonic dystrophy
EMG	Spontaneous fibrillations	Motor neuron disease
NCS	Delay in conduction of median nerve	Carpal tunnel syndrome (entrapment neuropathy)
Visually evoked responses (VERs)	Delayed P100 latencies, without amplitude loss	Multiple sclerosis

Case 7.1

A 19-year-old university student complains of a headache of 8 h duration accompanied by a dislike for lights. She has vomited twice. She is sweaty to the touch. No rash is apparent. The A&E officer was concerned enough to request a CT scan of the brain which was reported as normal. She proceeds to lumbar puncture. The CSF pressure was normal at the time of lumbar puncture.

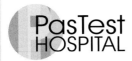

PasTest
HOSPITAL

Appearance	Cloudy. No organisms seen
WCC	228/mm^3 (predominantly neutrophils)
Red cell count	4/mm^3
Glucose	2.1 mmol/l
Total protein	0.96 g/l
Plasma glucose	5.9 mmol/l
Plasma total protein	0.45 g/l

Describe the CSF, and state the most likely diagnosis.

Answer 7.1

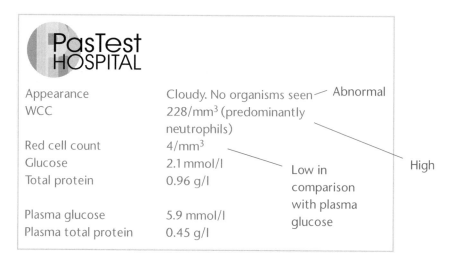

PasTest HOSPITAL

Appearance	Cloudy. No organisms seen	Abnormal
WCC	228/mm³ (predominantly neutrophils)	
Red cell count	4/mm³	
Glucose	2.1 mmol/l	Low in
Total protein	0.96 g/l	comparison
		with plasma
Plasma glucose	5.9 mmol/l	glucose
Plasma total protein	0.45 g/l	

High

Several features in the history should set off alarm bells for bacterial meningitis. The patient is young and in an institutional environment, and has an acute headache with photophobia. In addition, the CSF is cloudy with a raised WCC and a low CSF:plasma glucose ratio.

Three important points can be learned from this case:

1. If the leukocyte count is raised, analysis of the differential leukocyte count will help in distinguishing the cause.

2. A patient may have bacterial meningitis without any organisms being seen on microscopy. Don't be put off by this.

3. In bacterial meningitis, CT of the brain can be normal even when the CSF is highly abnormal.

This patient has bacterial meningitis and requires immediate treatment with intravenous antibiotics.

THE CLASSIC CSF FINDINGS IN BACTERIAL MENINGITIS	
A cloudy appearance Organisms seen in CSF Raised WCC (with >95% neutrophils) Red cell count (RCC) normal	Raised (but only mild–moderate) total protein Significantly reduced CSF glucose Reduced CSF:plasma glucose ratio (to less than two-thirds)

Case 7.2

A 21-year-old soldier complains of a headache for the past 2 days and a dislike of light. He is feverish. He has recently returned from deployment in Germany. Examination did not reveal any focal neurological signs or signs suggestive of raised intracranial pressure. The CSF opening pressure at the time of lumbar puncture was normal (17cmCSF). Lumbar puncture is performed, and the following result obtained.

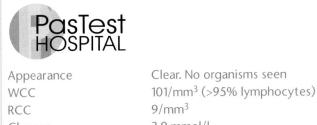

Appearance	Clear. No organisms seen
WCC	101/mm³ (>95% lymphocytes)
RCC	9/mm³
Glucose	3.9 mmol/l
Total protein	1.4 g/l
Plasma glucose	5.8 mmol/l
Plasma total protein	0.45 g/l

Interpret this CSF sample and give a differential diagnosis of the cause.

Answer 7.2

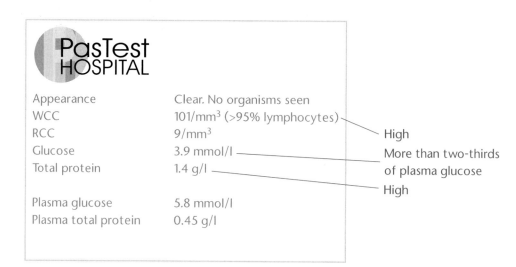

PasTest
HOSPITAL

Appearance	Clear. No organisms seen
WCC	101/mm³ (>95% lymphocytes) — High
RCC	9/mm³
Glucose	3.9 mmol/l — More than two-thirds of plasma glucose
Total protein	1.4 g/l — High
Plasma glucose	5.8 mmol/l
Plasma total protein	0.45 g/l

This history is not dissimilar to Case 7.1. However, the CSF analysis is significantly different. The WCC is raised – although less so than in the example of bacterial meningitis. The differential WCC is also different – lymphocytes being the predominant cell type here. The plasma glucose is a little abnormal, as is the CSF:plasma glucose ratio. Total protein is elevated – but only marginally. In summary many of the parameters are abnormal, but not markedly so.

CAUSES OF LYMPHOCYTE-PREDOMINANT LEUKOCYTOSIS IN CSF

Viral meningitis	Tuberculous meningitis
Mumps meningoencephalitis	Partially treated bacterial meningitis

The most common cause for these findings is viral meningitis – the virus itself may never be identified. Polymerase chain reaction analysis of CSF can be performed to test for a number of viruses, including herpes simplex. The treatment and outcome of viral meningitis are markedly different to those of partially treated bacterial meningitis, and if any diagnostic doubt exists treatment should continue for bacterial meningitis. The reason for partial treatment may have been the commencement of an antibiotic by a GP.

Case 7.3

A 39-year-old man is admitted to the neurology ward following a short illness. He is unable to move his legs. He was previously well, although he did have a short bout of diarrhoea a week ago after his return from holiday in Turkey.

Lumbar puncture was performed. The CSF opening pressure at the time of lumbar puncture was 18 cmCSF.

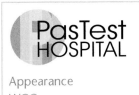

PasTest
HOSPITAL

Appearance	Clear. No organisms seen
WCC	5/mm^3
RCC	2/mm^3
Glucose	3.6 mmol/l
Total protein	2.1 g/l
Plasma glucose	4.7 mmol/l
Plasma total protein	0.45 g/l

1. **What are the significant findings and what condition could cause this appearance?**

2. **What other test might help in coming to a diagnosis?**

Answer 7.3

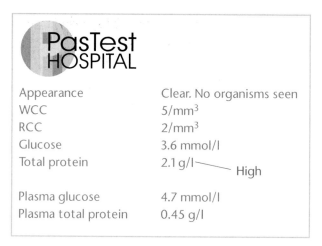

PasTest
HOSPITAL

Appearance	Clear. No organisms seen
WCC	5/mm³
RCC	2/mm³
Glucose	3.6 mmol/l
Total protein	2.1 g/l ⎯⎯ High
Plasma glucose	4.7 mmol/l
Plasma total protein	0.45 g/l

1. The history is short and the symptoms significant. However, the only significant abnormality on the CSF sample is the elevated level of protein within the CSF. The plasma total protein is normal. The CSF protein is raised to a greater degree than one would usually expect for a viral or bacterial meningitis/encephalitis. Note that the WCC and the CSF:plasma glucose ratio are also not in keeping with an infective pathology. The differential diagnosis is therefore of a high CSF protein.

    When interpreted in the context of the history of leg weakness after an episode of infectious diarrhoea, the diagnosis is most likely to be Guillain–Barré syndrome (an acute inflammatory polyneuropathy).

2. Nerve conduction studies (NCS) would help diagnosis (see Neurophysiological investigations on page 228 for further details).

Case 7.4

A 29-year-old bank clerk has become known to local neurologists over the past year following several presentations to both the hospital and the outpatient clinic with a variable constellation of neurological symptoms. Initially a complaint of numbness over the lateral aspect of the left leg was mentioned. This resolved. Of late, she has had an episode of loss of vision in the right eye lasting 4 weeks. Examination reveals global hyperreflexia and a mild cerebellar gait.

The patient attends the ward for a series of tests including lumbar puncture. The CSF opening pressure was 17cmCSF.

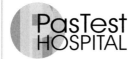

PasTest
HOSPITAL

Appearance	Clear. No organisms seen
WCC	$2/mm^3$
RCC	$1/mm^3$
Glucose	3.9 mmol/l
Total protein	0.46 g/l
Oligoclonal bands	Present
ACE level	Normal

A blood sample was taken at the same time:

Plasma glucose	5.1 mmol/l
Plasma total protein	0.46 g/l
Oligoclonal bands	Absent

What is the likely diagnosis?

Answer 7.4

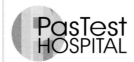
PasTest
HOSPITAL

Appearance	Clear. No organisms seen
WCC	2/mm³
RCC	1/mm³
Glucose	3.9 mmol/l
Total protein	0.46 g/l
Oligoclonal bands	Present
ACE level	Normal

Appearance   Clear. No organisms seen
WCC $2/mm^3$
RCC $1/mm^3$
Glucose   3.9 mmol/l
Total protein   0.46 g/l
Oligoclonal bands Present
ACE level   Normal —————— Abnormal

A blood sample was taken at the same time:
Plasma glucose   5.1 mmol/l
Plasma total protein 0.46 g/l

Oligoclonal bands   Absent

This CSF sample shows essentially normal values for all the common indices. Additional analyses have been performed, including oligoclonal bands which are present.

These bands represent immunoglobulin G (IgG). The presence of this has been noted in a number of conditions – it is therefore of poor specificity in isolation. However, it is found in over 80% of patients with multiple sclerosis (MS). MS is the most common cause for its presence on CSF analysis. It is a supportive feature rather than a diagnostic feature of the disease, since MS is a clinical diagnosis defined as 'two episodes of neurological deficit disseminated in time and place'.

CAUSES OF OLIGOCLONAL BANDS IN CSF

Multiple sclerosis
Subacute sclerosing panencephalitis
Guillain–Barré syndrome
Neurosyphilis
Lyme disease
Neurosarcoidosis

IMMUNOLOGY

8

IMMUNOLOGY

Interpretation of autoantibodies is often difficult. This is because of the degree of overlap in the presence of antibodies between various disease states. For example, rheumatoid factor can be found in well over a dozen diseases. Furthermore, certain autoantibodies may be found in healthy people, and the absence of an autoantibody may not rule out a particular disease. Therefore, always bear in mind that the presence of an autoantibody does not necessarily mean that a patient has a particular disease.

> **DON'T FORGET**
> A disease may be present without the typical autoantibody profile.

For the purpose of undergraduate examinations, the classic autoantibody associations will be tested. These are listed in the box below. Those tested commonly in examinations are in bold type.

DISEASE	AUTOANTIBODIES
Addison's disease	Anti-21-hydroxylase
Anti-phospholipid syndrome	**Anti-cardiolipin** **Lupus anticoagulant antibodies**
Autoimmune haemolytic anaemia	**Red blood cell autoantibodies** (this disease can be classified into warm and cold, depending on the temperature at which the antibodies best attach to red cells)
Autoimmune hepatitis	**Anti-nuclear** **Anti-smooth muscle** **Anti-liver/kidney microsomal-I** Myeloperoxidase anti-nuclear cytoplasmic antibody (MPO-ANCA), also called perinuclear ANCA (pANCA)
Churg–Strauss syndrome	**MPO-ANCA**
Coeliac disease	**Anti-endomysial** **Anti-tissue transglutaminase** **Anti-reticulin** **Anti-gliadin**

Diffuse cutaneous scleroderma	Rheumatoid factor Anti-nuclear **Anti-ScL-70** **Polymerase 1, 2 and 3**
Goodpasture syndrome	**Anti-glomerular basement membrane**
Graves' disease	**Anti-TSH receptor** Anti-peroxidase
Hashimoto's thyroiditis	**TSH-receptor-blocking antibodies** Anti-peroxidase
Lambert–Eaton myasthenic syndrome	Anti-P/Q-type voltage-gated calcium channels
Limited cutaneous scleroderma	Rheumatoid factor Anti-nuclear **Anti-centromere**
Mixed connective tissue disease (overlap syndrome)	Anti-U1-RNP
Myasthenia gravis	Anti-nuclear **Anti-acetylcholine receptor antibodies**
Paraneoplastic conditions	Anti-YO Anti-Hu Anti-Ri Anti-MA Anti-CV2/CRMP5 Anti-amphiphysin
Pernicious anaemia	**Anti-parietal cell** **Anti-intrinsic factor**
Polyarteritis nodosa	**MPO-ANCA**

Polymyositis/dermatomyositis	Anti-nuclear Rheumatoid factor **Anti-Jo-1**
Primary biliary cirrhosis	**Anti-mitochondrial** (more particularly against pyruvate dehydrogenase complex type E2- and/or E3-binding protein)
Rheumatoid disease	**Rheumatoid factor** Anti-nuclear
Sjögren syndrome	Rheumatoid factor Anti-nuclear **Anti-Ro (SS-A)** **Anti-La (SS-B)**
Systemic lupus erythematosus	**Double-stranded DNA** Rheumatoid factor Anti-nuclear Anti-Ro (SS-A) Anti-Sm Anti-U1-RNP Anti-cardiolipin
Wegener syndrome	**Proteinase 3 anti-nuclear cytoplasmic antibody** (PR3-ANCA), also called cytoplasmic ANCA (cANCA)

IMAGING 9

With Dr Barry Kelly
Consultant Radiologist
Royal Victoria Hospital, Belfast
and Reader in Radiology,
The Queens University of Belfast

IMAGING

The interpretation of imaging investigations is a comprehensive topic that forms a specialty in its own right. Its influence and remit in contemporary medicine are vast forming huge amounts of 'digital data' for interpretation. It is essential that medical students and trainee doctors have a sound basic understanding of plain radiographs (X-rays), in particular chest and abdominal radiographs. Likewise an appreciation and insight into the more advanced imaging investigations at their disposal is increasingly important, in particular the ever popular and influential computed tomography (CT). A good professional relationship with the radiology department, including thoughtful and selective referral, can hugely aid patient care.

This chapter does not aim to be a concise undergraduate textbook on radiology. Nor will it be an exhaustive description of characteristic radiological findings in common diseases or a gallery of images. It is a guide to approaching the interpretation of common X-rays and the basics of CT of the head. In the clinical cases featured the emphasis will be on inpatient films – these are X-rays that one might be expected to interpret during work on general medical and surgical wards or the accident and emergency department. Films are presented in a symptom-based manner to best reflect everyday practice and to provide instruction on how interpretation may immediately assist your diagnostic pathway and therefore your management decisions. No film will be viewed in isolation without clinical information. As with all the data interpretation considered in this book, investigations should be assessed in the light of the clinical scenario and laboratory results. This should also be the gold standard to aspire to in clinical practice.

Imaging studies may feature in both written and clinical examinations, offering the chance to assess a broad knowledge base.

DON'T FORGET

Always interpret X-ray findings in a clinical context.
Compare the images with old films if available.

Interpreting the chest X-ray

The chest X-ray (CXR) is the single most requested imaging investigation and is also the most likely film to feature in daily practice or an undergraduate exam. It is the perfect prompt for questioning other aspects of a patient's condition and to explore management strategies. To be able to comment confidently on the film's findings, and have an understanding of how to approach interpretation, an appreciation of normality is required. Don't forget that a CXR is a two-dimensional representation of a three-dimensional structure.

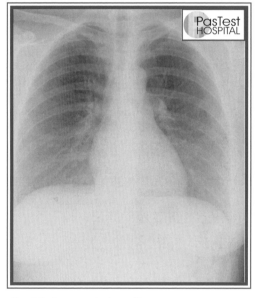

Fig 9.1: A normal chest X-ray.

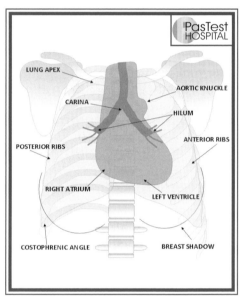

Fig 9.2: Normal anatomy on CXR.

One may think of a CXR as a picture that contains five 'shades' on a black-and-white scale. These shades represent four different natural 'tissues' and one for artefacts.

These are:

1. Bone is WHITE

2. Gas is BLACK.

3. Soft tissue is GREY

4. Fat is DARKER GREY.

5. Most man-made things on the film are BRIGHT WHITE.

Film specifics and technical factors

Before proceeding to interpret a CXR, always comment on film specifics and technical factors as shown in the boxes below.

FILM SPECIFICS (DETAILS)

Name of patient
Age and date of birth
Location of patient
Date taken
Film number (if applicable)

FILM TECHNICAL FACTORS

Type of projection (see box below)
Markings regarding any special techniques used (eg taken in expiration)
Rotation
Inspiration
Penetration

TYPES OF PROJECTION

Posteroanterior (PA): the X-ray tube is behind the patient and film against the chest. The GOLD standard projection
Anteroposterior (AP): the X-ray tube is in front of the patient and film against the back
Supine: the patient is lying on his or her back
Erect: the patient is upright
Semi-erect: the patient is partially upright
Mobile: the X-ray has been taken with a mobile X-ray unit. VERY SICK patients ONLY (on the ITU/HDU/CCU usually)

These descriptions may be combined. For example, an acutely unwell patient who has a CXR taken on an intensive therapy unit (ITU) may have a mobile, semi-erect AP film.

You might think of this part of the interpretation, like the safety announcement on an airplane, as one you have heard many times: necessary to acknowledge, but tedious and of little consequence. However, this could not be further from the truth. Changes in these parameters can give the impression of abnormalities in the structures visualised. For example, a widened mediastinum, on an AP chest X-ray may provoke the impression of a thoracic dissection or a pneumothorax may be overlooked if one does not appreciate that the chest X-ray is supine rather than erect.

Assess the film in detail

A structured systematic approach is needed for thorough interpretation, just as one would approach a clinical system examination in a methodical manner.

It is good practice to mention a clear-cut abnormality at the outset. A reasonable way to say this would be, 'The technical quality of the film is satisfactory. The most striking abnormality on initial assessment is ...'.

The examiner will then expect the candidate to demonstrate an organised approach to looking at the rest of the film. Do not stop when one abnormality has been noted (termed 'the satisfaction of search') – there may be more to see.

DON'T FORGET

Keep looking – multiple findings may give the definitive diagnosis.

The structures below need to be assessed in the interpretation of the CXR. It is fair to assume that, if one major abnormality is clearly 'spotted' at the beginning, this structure or system should be commented on first.

Structures to assess on CXR

- Heart and major vessels
- Lungs and pleura
- Mediastinum (including hila)
- Bones and soft tissues.

Be particularly careful not to miss the following REVIEW areas. They should be specifically checked as abnormalities in these areas may be easily overlooked.

Review areas

- Costophrenic angles (1)
- Apices (2)
- Behind the heart (3)
- Below the diaphragms (4)
- Breast shadows (in females) (5).

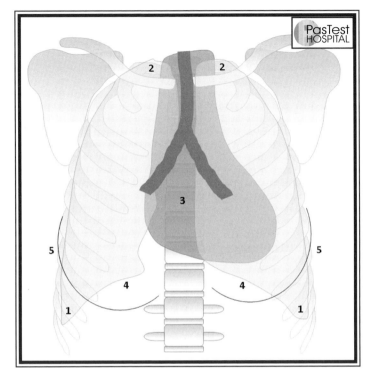

Fig 9.3: Review areas on a chest X-ray assessment.

Heart and major vessels

Assess:

- Size of the heart
- Size of individual chambers of the heart
- Size of pulmonary vessels
- Evidence of stents, clips, wires, valves, pacemakers
- Outline of aorta, inferior (IVC) and superior (SVC) vena cava.

DON'T FORGET

Do not comment on heart size on an AP chest X-ray because it is magnified.

Lungs

Assess:

- Size
- Intrapulmonary pathology
- Bronchovascular lung markings.

Pleura

Assess:

- Thickness or calcification
- Fluid or air in the pleural space.

Mediastinum (including hila)

Assess:

- Width of the mediastinum
- Contour of the mediastinum
- Size and density of the hila
- Level and symmetry of the hila.

Bones and soft tissues

Assess:

- Diffuse or focal bony abnormalities
- Surgical emphysema
- Breast presence/absence and symmetry.

Interpreting the abdominal X-ray

Abdominal X-ray

The abdominal X-ray (AXR) has more limited value in diagnosis than a CXR. Its chief value is in the diagnosis of bowel obstruction and renal tract calculi, although other pathology may be identified. Even in these cases, the abdominal X-ray is often just a 'stepping stone' to further imaging with ultrasonography or CT. Indiscriminate requesting of the abdominal X-ray is discouraged.

The radiation exposure of an AXR compared with a CXR is also considerably higher. One AXR is equivalent to 35 CXRs.

As with a CXR, an appreciation of normality is vital in order to make a correct interpretation.

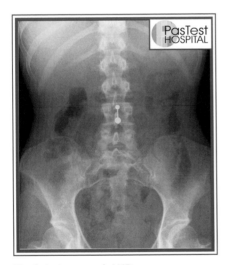

Fig 9.4: A normal AXR

Fig 9.5: Normal anatomy on AXR

Film specifics and technical factors

The initial assessment of an AXR is similar to for a CXR.

FILM SPECIFICS	FILM TECHNICAL FACTORS
Name of patient Age of patient Location of patient Date taken Film number (if applicable)	Type of projection (supine is standard) Markings of any special techniques used Adequate anatomical coverage

Assess the film in detail

A simple guide to interpretation is shown below. Working through these headings, one covers 'black bits', 'white bits', 'grey bits' and 'bright white bits' in turn. Alternatively one may take an anatomical approach to interpretation.

'Black bits'
Intraluminal gas

Intraluminal gas can be normal. Extraluminal gas is abnormal. However, intraluminal gas can be abnormal if it is in the wrong place or if too much is seen.

The maximum normal diameter of the large bowel is 5.5 cm. Small bowel should be no more than 3.5 cm in diameter. The natural presence of gas within the bowel allows assessment of calibre, although the amount varies between individuals. The caecum is not considered to be dilated unless wider than 8.0 cm in diameter.

Large and small bowel may be distinguished by looking at bowel wall markings.

DON'T FORGET

The haustra of the large bowel extend only a third of the way across the diameter of the large bowel from each side. The valvulae conniventes of the small bowel traverse the whole diameter.

It is usual to see small volumes of gas throughout the gastrointestinal (GI) tract and the absence in one region may in itself represent pathology. For example, if gas is seen to the level of the splenic flexure and nothing is apparent distal to this, a site of the obstruction at this site − a 'cut-off' point − is assumed.

Extraluminal gas

When a bowel or any other gas-containing structure perforates, its contained gas becomes extraluminal. Extraluminal gas is never normal, but it may be seen following intra-abdominal surgery or laparoscopy.

CAUSES OF EXTRALUMINAL GAS

Post-abdominal surgery/laparoscopy
Perforation of viscus (eg bowel, stomach)
Abscess/Collection

DON'T FORGET

An erect CXR (not AXR) is the best projection to diagnose a pneumoperitoneum (gas in the peritoneal cavity).

'White bits'
Calcification

Calcified structures are often seen on an AXR. The main question is: 'Does their presence have any important implications?' Calcification can be broadly divided into three types:

1. Calcification that is an abnormal structure, eg gallstones, renal calculi, calcified splenic artery aneurysm.

2. Calcification that is within a normal structure, but represents pathology, eg pancreatic ductal calcification.

3. Calcification that is within a normal structure, but is not clinically significant, eg lymph node calcification or a calcified pelvic phlebolith.

Bones are normal 'white' structures. On the AXR they comprise mainly those of the thoracolumbar spine and pelvis. Findings are often incidental.

'Grey bits'
Soft tissues

Soft tissues represent most of the contents of the abdomen and feature prominently in the AXR. However, these tissues are poorly visualised and delineated when compared with other imaging techniques such as ultrasonography, CT or MRI.

The outlines of the kidneys, spleen, liver and bladder (if filled) can be seen in addition to psoas muscle shadows. An abdominal X-ray, however, should not be requested to specifically look at these structures.

'Bright white bits'
Foreign bodies

Foreign bodies represent an interesting final observation. These may have been purposely placed in or on the body, for example, an aortic stent, an inferior vena cava filter or abdominal drains. Sterilisation clips and an intrauterine device are common findings in women. Other objects that may be seen include ingested and rectal foreign bodies, as well as items in the path of the X-ray beam, such as belt buckles, dress buttons and umbilical jewellery.

Other imaging modalities

There is a range of other imaging modalities in regular use – the majority of which do not feature significantly in undergraduate exams. Knowledge of their importance in diagnosis should be sufficient, in particular which investigation should be requested for different common clinical scenarios.

IONISING RADIATION TECHNIQUES

Contrast/fluoroscopic studies (mostly barium)   Positron emission tomography (PET)
Computed tomography (CT)   Nuclear (radionuclide) imaging

NON-IONISING RADIATION TECHNIQUES

Ultrasonography
Magnetic resonance imaging (MRI)

Computed tomography (CT) and MRI play a diverse and pivotal role in contemporary clinical care. These cross-sectional imaging modalities have a hugely influential position in the diagnostic process.

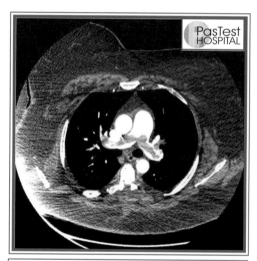
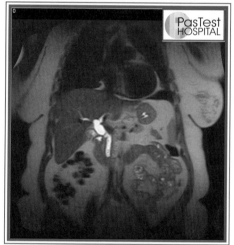
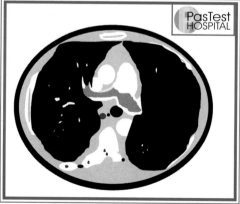
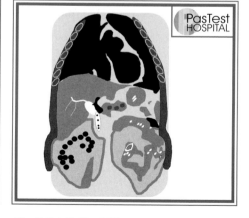

Fig 9.6: CT Pulmonary angiography: saddle pulmonary embolus.

Fig 9.7: MRCP: CBD stones

CT of the head

In the last decade the use of computed tomography (CT) has exploded, with clinicians increasingly becoming familiar with its value and undertaking self-review of images within their specialty areas. This is particularly true for CT of the head. With this there is a growing expectation of familiarity and knowledge of key pathologies.

The most commonly requested CT scan, all hours of the day and night, is a head CT. Quick and inexpensive to acquire, and fast to report, an ever-growing number of clinicians view CT of the head independently. For this reason an introduction to CT of the head is included and key pathologies are featured in the clinical cases.

Specific NICE (National Institute for Health and Clinical Excellence) guidelines have been written with respect to the indications for head CT after trauma. These include:

- Glasgow Coma Scale (GCS) <13 when first assessed or GCS <15 2 hours after injury
- Suspected open or depressed skull fracture
- Signs of base of skull fracture
- Post-traumatic seizure
- Focal neurological deficit
- More than one episode of vomiting (SIGN [Scottish Intercollegiate Guidelines Network] guidance suggests two distinct episodes of vomiting)
- Coagulopathy + any amnesia or loss of consciousness since injury
- More than 30 minutes of amnesia of events before impact.

DON'T FORGET

If there is concern over intracranial haemorrhage, the scan must be performed unenhanced. Acute blood and contrast look the same!

Approach to assessment of a head CT

A brief outline of how to approach reviewing a head CT study is outlined below, starting with an understanding of the major anatomical structures.

The normal appearances of key structures in the supra- and infratentorial brain are shown in Figs 9.8–9.12.

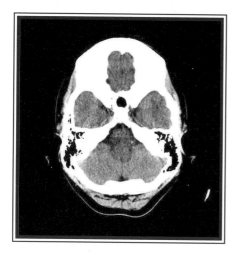
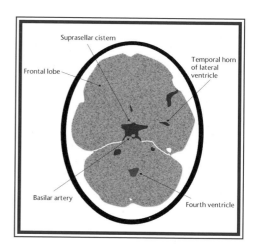

Fig 9.8

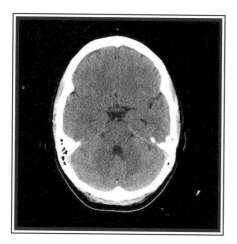

Fig 9.9

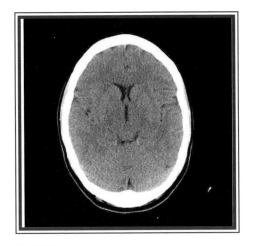

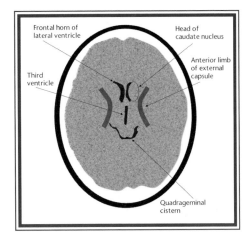

Frontal horn of
lateral ventricle

Head of
caudate nucleus

Anterior limb
of external
capsule

Third
ventricle

Quadrageminal
cistern

Fig 9.10

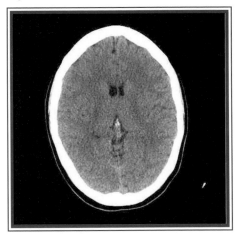

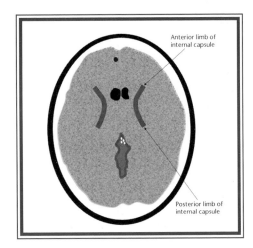

Anterior limb of
internal capsule

Posterior limb of
internal capsule

Fig 9.11

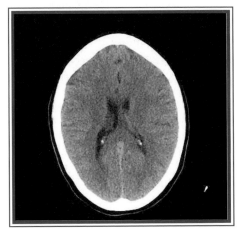

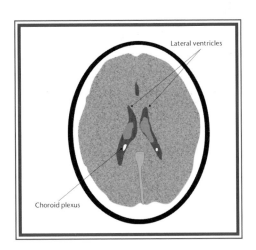

Lateral ventricles

Choroid plexus

Fig 9.12

Head CT: key basic facts

CT demonstrates a wide-ranging grey scale, referred to as attenuation. In the brain this is often stated to be hypo-, iso- or hyperdense in relation to the brain normal parenchyma:

- CSF in the brain will appear black
- The bone of the skull will appear white
- Grey and white matter within the brain have different attenuations; the densely packed nerve cell bodies of the grey matter have a higher attenuation than the nerve axons of the white matter, meaning that surprisingly white matter is darker than grey matter on CT
- Blood contains protein, making it dense, and areas of acute haemorrhage appear high attenuation (white) on a CT scan
- Areas of dead or damaged brain tissue (encephalomalacia or ischaemic brain) will become less dense, meaning that they will appear darker than the surrounding brain (low attenuation)
- Intravenous contrast on CT highlights blood vessels or vascular areas of the brain. It is also useful for identifying areas of high cell turnover, such as tumours and infection. Aneurysms, tumours and abscesses all become brighter after contrast administration.

Assessment of the CT head

- Is the ventricular system the appropriate size?
- Is there any acute blood present? If so, is it intraparenchymal, subarachnoid or an extra-axial collection?
- Is there any evidence of ischaemia? If so is it focal or territorial in nature?
- Is there normal differentiation between the grey and white matter of the brain?
- Is there space around the cord at the level of the foramen magnum?
- Are the sulci effaced or the ventricles displaced suggesting mass effect?
- Check the bony skull (on bone window settings) to look for a fracture or other bony abnormality.

Check the review areas to finish:

- Anything in the ventricular system, eg blood in the occipital horns?
- Are the visualised orbits normal?
- Is there any abnormality in the mastoid air cells or paranasal sinuses?

Scenarios presenting with shortness of breath

Case 9.1

This 23-year-old university student presents to A&E acutely short of breath.

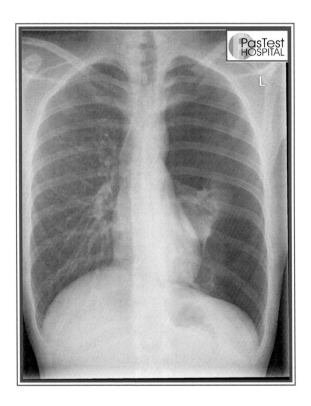

1. **Describe your findings on the chest X-ray.**
2. **List five conditions that predispose to this condition.**

Answer 9.1

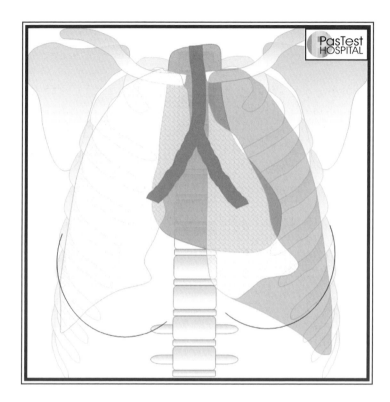

1. The left hemithorax is translucent with absent pulmonary markings. The collapsed left lung is apparent centrally. No evidence of mediastinal shift.

    The appearances are consistent with a large left-sided pneumothorax.

2. Numerous chronic pulmonary diseases predispose to pneumothoraces. These include: chronic obstructive pulmonary disease (COPD), asthma, pulmonary fibrosis and cystic fibrosis. Other important causes of pneumothorax include: trauma, congenital pulmonary blebs and iatrogenic reasons (eg central venous line insertion, mechanical ventilation).

Case 9.2

This 46-year-old retired firefighter has become increasingly short of breath over the past 6 months. He complains of a dry cough. Pulmonary function tests and CXR were requested.

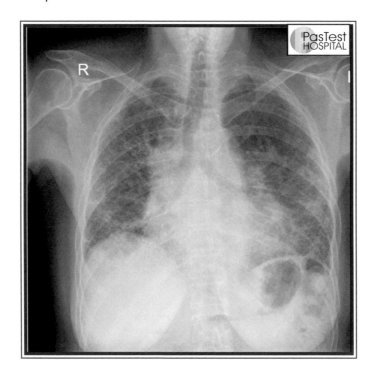

1. **How would you describe the lungs on this CXR?**

2. **What are the possible causes for these findings?**

3. **What are his pulmonary function tests likely to demonstrate?**

Answer 9.2

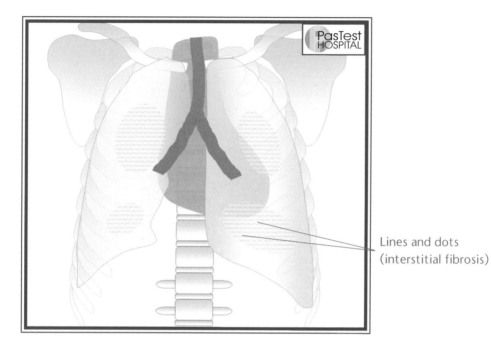

Lines and dots
(interstitial fibrosis)

1. Diffuse reticulonodular ('lines and dots') shadowing is evident in both lungs. This has lower zone predominance.

   The appearances of this CXR are of pulmonary (interstitial) fibrosis.

2. The causes may be divided according to whether the fibrosis predominantly affects the upper or lower zones.

MEMORY AID	
Upper lobe fibrosis (mnemonic = BREAST)	**Lower lobe fibrosis**
Berylliosis (uncommon)	Cryptogenic fibrosing alveolitis
Radiation fibrosis	Drug induced (eg amiodarone, metho-trexate)
Extrinsic allergic alveolitis	Asbestosis
Ankylosing spondylitis	Connective tissue diseases
Sarcoidosis	(eg rheumatoid diseases)
Tuberculosis	

3. Spirometry would demonstrate a restrictive pattern (see page 429 for further details).

Case 9.3

This 55-year-old man attended his local hospital feeling increasingly short of breath over the past week. He has lost 1 stone in weight recently. He is a smoker of 60 pack-years. His CXR is shown.

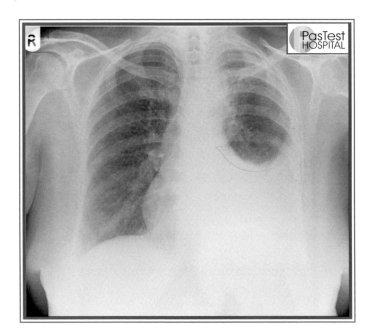

1.   **Describe the appearances on the CXR.**

2.   **List the causes of this finding, and state the most likely cause in this patient.**

3.   **What other simple test may assist in forming a diagnosis?**

Answer 9.3

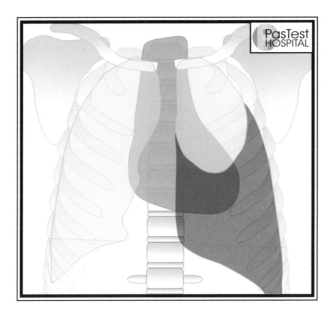

1. There is an area of increased radio-opacity in the lower left hemithorax. The
    edge can be seen to taper at the lateral aspect of the chest, forming a
    meniscus. There is no shift of mediastinal structures. This is a moderately
    sized left-sided pleural effusion.

2. For unilateral pleural effusions, the causes are mostly exudates. These include:

  - malignant tumours (both primary and metastatic disease)

  - parapneumonic

  - pulmonary embolus or infarction

  - rheumatoid disease.

  A malignant effusion would be most likely in this patient because of his weight loss and smoking history.

3. A diagnostic pleural aspiration could be performed. This will help distinguish whether the effusion is an exudate or transudate based on the protein content (see page 191 for details).

  In this case, malignant cells may be identified when the pleural fluid is examined cytologically.

Case 9.4

This 45-year-old smoker of 30 pack-years attends his GP with increasing shortness of breath over the past 2 weeks.

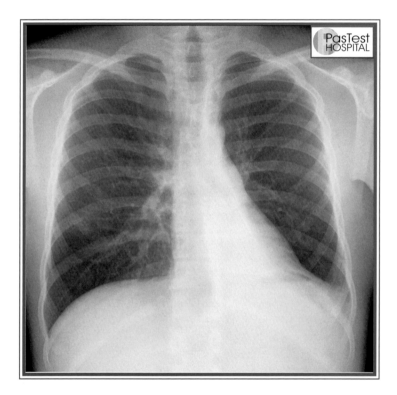

1. **Describe the abnormality on this chest X-ray.**

2. **What is your concern regarding these appearances and what would you recommend?**

Answer 9.4

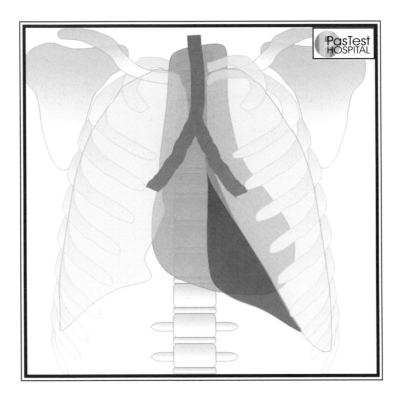

1. A triangular density is present in the left retrocardiac position, which is separate from the left heart border. The medial aspect is difficult to delineate, but the abnormality has a 'sail-like' appearance. The left hilum is inferiorly displaced and there is volume loss within the left hemithorax.

   The appearances are consistent with a 'tight' left lower lobe collapse.

2. The nature of further investigation depends on the clinical scenario. The three most common causes of a left lower lobe collapse are:

   (a) a central hilar or endobronchial mass

   (b) an endobronchial foreign body

   (c) an endobronchial mucus plug.

   In children a foreign body is most likely and, in a postoperative or ITU patient, a mucus plug; both can be dealt with by bronchoscopy. In adults, especially smokers, left lower lobe collapse must always be viewed with suspicion for an underlying tumour. Bronchoscopy and CT of the chest are indicated, after clinical assessment by a respiratory team.

Case 9.5

This 21-year-old patient, well known to the local hospital, attends A&E with acute-on-chronic shortness of breath.

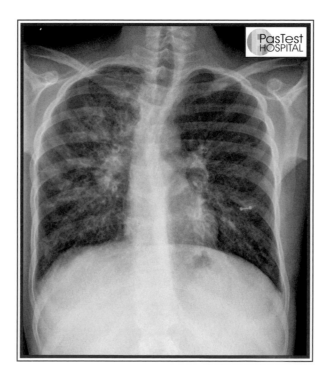

1. **Describe the appearances on this chest X-ray.**

2. **Give a short summary of the underlying condition.**

Answer 9.5

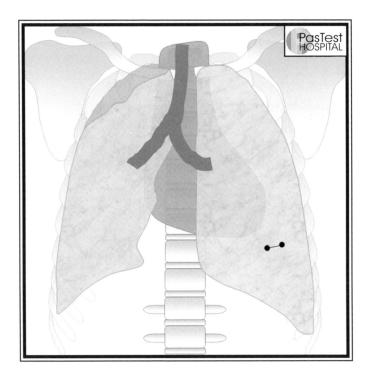

1. Throughout both lungs there are increased interstitial markings, most pronounced in the upper lobes, consistent with fibrosis. At the right lung apex, the lung edge is apparent with no lung markings peripheral to this, consistent with a small apical pneumothorax.

   Given the patient's young age this would be compatible with a pneumothorax on a background of cystic fibrosis.

2. Cystic fibrosis is the most common lethal inherited disease in white individuals. It is an autosomal recessive disorder, for which most carriers of the gene are asymptomatic. It is caused by defects in the *CFTR* gene, which encodes for a protein that functions as a chloride channel, and also regulates the flow of other ions across the apical surface of epithelial cells. It is a disease of exocrine gland function that involves multiple organ systems, albeit most commonly associated with pulmonary manifestations. Pancreatic insufficiency is also a common element of the disease. The median survival is now 36 years of age.

Scenarios presenting with chest pain

Case 9.6

This 62-year-old patient presented to A&E with chest pain and shortness of breath.

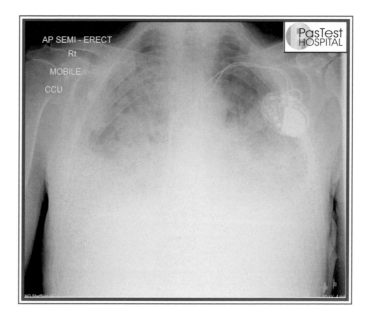

1. **Describe the appearance on this chest X-ray.**

2. **What conditions may cause these appearances with a normal-sized heart?**

Answer 9.6

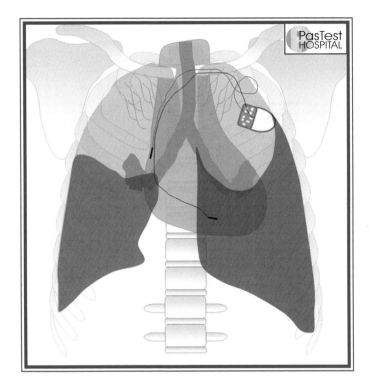

1. This AP erect film demonstrates evidence of bilateral perihilar consolidation ('bat's wings'). The remainders of both lungs are plethoric. The AP projection indicates an ill patient; however, it does limit the assessment of cardiac size.

   The appearances are in keeping with acute pulmonary oedema.

2. The most common cause of pulmonary oedema is cardiac failure, which is typically associated with cardiomegaly. However, pulmonary oedema can occur in a number of situations where the heart is normal in size. These include:

   (a) in acute renal failure – so-called 'flash' pulmonary oedema

   (b) non-cardiogenic pulmonary oedema in adult respiratory distress syndrome (ARDS)

   (c) after aggressive fluid resuscitation

   (d) with a massive acute myocardial infarction/valve rupture

   (e) in association with a subarachnoid haemorrhage.

Case 9.7

This 34-year-old woman attends A&E with chest pain. She is known to the departmental staff from previous admissions.

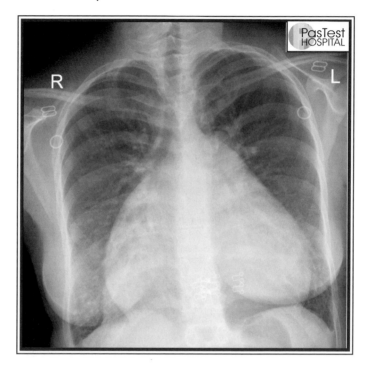

1. **Describe the appearances on this chest X-ray, especially the cardiac outline.**

2. **What else might you consider doing to establish the exact cause of these appearances?**

Answer 9.7

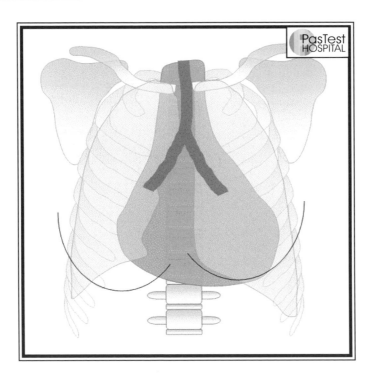

1. The heart is severely enlarged with a globular configuration, suggesting a diffuse cardiac abnormality rather than individual chamber enlargement. There is no evidence of cardiac failure.

   The differential diagnosis for these appearances includes congenital cardiac disease, cardiomyopathy and a pericardial effusion.

2. Important aspects that may help establish the exact cause include:

   (a) a full clinical history, including childhood illness and a family history of cardiac disease

   (b) a review of previous radiological investigations, eg old films may indicate that the cardiomegaly is longstanding and therefore unlikely to be due to a pericardial effusion

   (c) an echocardiogram.

Case 9.8

This 80-year-old woman is brought to A&E by her daughter due to a short history of chest pain.

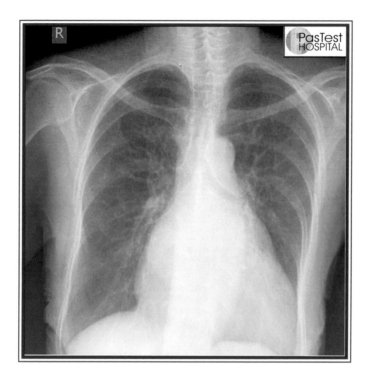

1. Outline the features on the chest X-ray that suggest mitral valve disease.

2. If this patient presented with cardiac failure due to her underlying condition, what signs might be present on a chest X-ray?

Answer 9.8

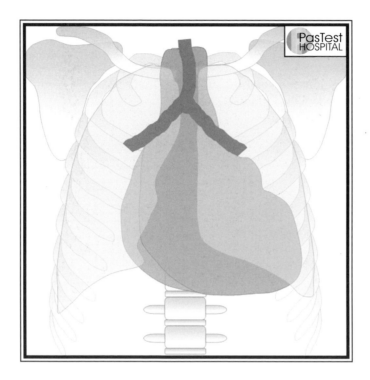

1. The heart is moderately enlarged, with prominence of the left atrial appendage. A double right heart border is evident, indicating enlargement of the left atrium. The subcarinal angle is normal; however, the other features all point towards a diagnosis of left atrial enlargement (a 'mitral heart').

2. The following are all features of cardiac failure on chest X-ray:

   (a) cardiomegaly

   (b) pleural effusions

   (c) perihilar consolidation ('bat's wings')

   (d) upper lobe venous distension

   (e) interlobular septal lines ('Kerley B lines').

Scenarios presenting with weight loss

Case 9.9

This 67-year-old man was admitted with shortness of breath and weight loss. A large lung mass was seen on his CXR. Other investigations confirmed that the lesion was a bronchial carcinoma at the left lung apex.

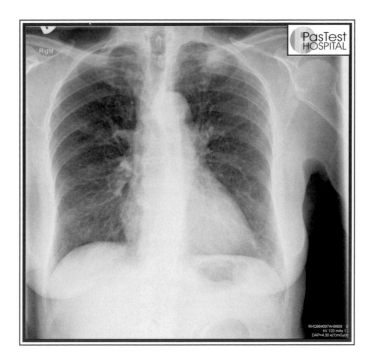

1. **What other findings might be seen on CXR in a patient with bronchial carcinoma?**

2. **What else could cause the appearance of a mass like this on a CXR?**

3. **What other imaging investigation would be helpful?**

Answer 9.9

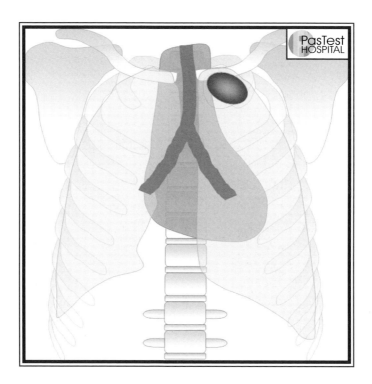

1. A lung mass on a CXR in a smoker over 50 years of age should be regarded as a bronchial carcinoma until proven otherwise. Other features that may be seen on CXR with bronchial carcinoma include:

   - pleural effusion
   - lung collapse (due to endobronchial tumour)
   - pulmonary metastases
   - bony metastases (and pathological fracture)
   - secondary pneumonia
   - lymphangitis carcinomatosis
   - enlarged lymph nodes (hilar and paratracheal).

2. Causes of a lung mass on CXR include:

    - bronchial carcinoma

    - pulmonary metastasis

    - round pneumonia

    - lung hamartoma

    - encysted pleural effusion

    - rheumatoid nodule

    - lung abscess (usually cavitating).

3. Computed tomography of the chest would image the mass in greater detail. It will also help in the assessment of lymphadenopathy and provide evidence of local or metastatic spread

Case 9.10

This 52-year-old man attends his GP complaining of non-intentional weight loss of 8 kg.

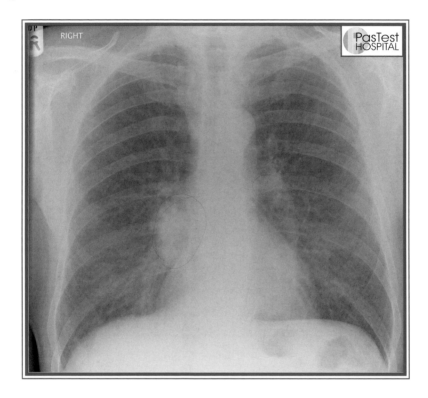

1. **Describe the appearances on the chest X-ray.**

2. **Provide a short differential diagnosis.**

Answer 9.10

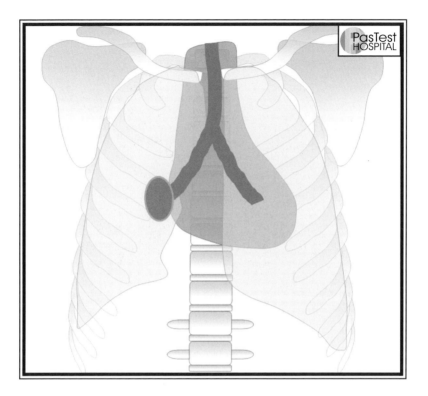

1. The inferior aspect of the right hilum is dense and enlarged. The left hilum and paratracheal regions are normal. The lungs are clear. Further investigation advised.

2. The differential diagnosis for unilateral hilar enlargement includes:

    (a) bronchial carcinoma

    (b) tuberculosis

    (c) lymphoma

    (d) metastatic mediastinal lymph node disease

    (e) atypical sarcoidosis

    (f) vascular anomaly.

Case 9.11

This 34-year-old man is admitted with weight loss, shortness of breath and fever.

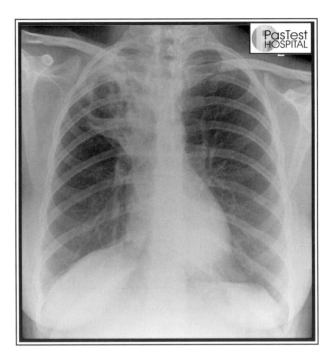

1. **Describe the findings on this CXR.**

2. **What are the potential causes of such an appearance?**

Answer 9.11

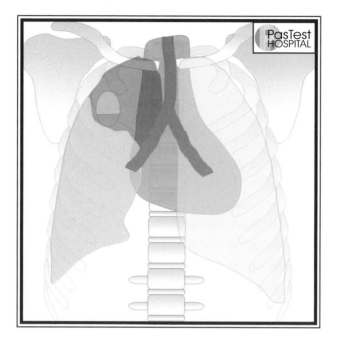

1. There is dense consolidation in the right upper lobe with an area of cavitation within. There is an air–fluid level within the cavity.

2. The differential diagnosis for a cavitating lung lesion is:

    •   bronchial carcinoma (especially squamous cell carcinoma)

    •   pulmonary metastasis

    •   tuberculosis

    •   cavitating pneumonia

    •   lung abscess

    •   vasculitic disease (eg Wegener's granulomatosis)

    •   lung infarction

    •   rheumatoid nodule.

Case 9.12

This 67-year-old ex-coal miner presents with a history of weight loss over the past month, now accompanied by shortness of breath.

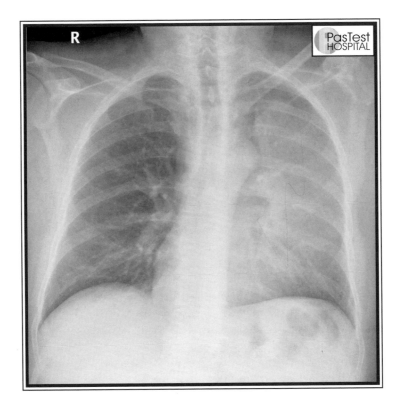

1. **Describe the appearances on the chest X-ray.**
2. **What further investigations are required and why?**

Answer 9.12

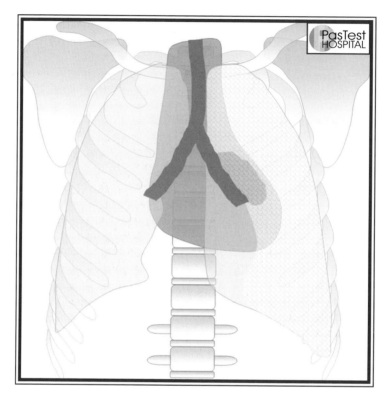

1. The left hemithorax is opacified in a 'veil-like' manner. There is the impression of a dense and enlarged left hilum. The right lung is clear.

   The appearances are in keeping with a left upper lobe collapse, with a strong suspicion of an underlying hilar mass.

2. The chest X-ray appearances are highly suspicious for a central (hilar) bronchial carcinoma, which has resulted in a left upper lobe collapse due to obstruction of the left upper lobe bronchus. This merits urgent referral to the lung cancer multidisciplinary team (MDT) meeting for work-up and discussion. This will entail CT of the chest and upper abdomen and bronchoscopy. With a central tumour, bronchoscopic biopsy is likely to be performed to confirm the histology and so plan for treatment.

Scenarios presenting feeling generally unwell

Case 9.13

A 32-year-old man attends A&E complaining of shortness of breath and the development of a rash on his shins.

A CXR was requested.

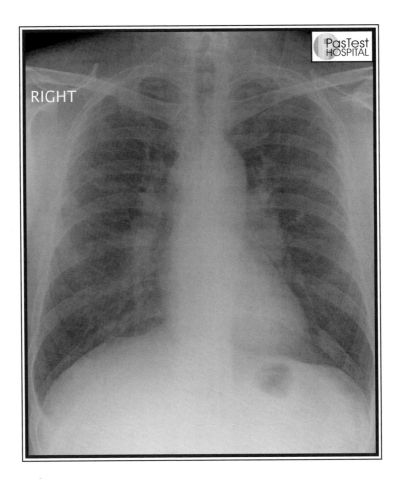

1. **Outline any abnormal findings seen on this film.**

2. **Give a differential diagnosis for this appearance.**

Answer 9.13

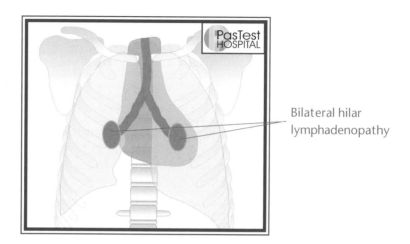

Bilateral hilar lymphadenopathy

1. The mediastinal contour is abnormal. There is bilateral hilar enlargement. When bilateral hilar enlargement is observed the three important potential diagnoses are sarcoidosis, lymphoma (enlarged nodes) and pulmonary hypertension (enlarged pulmonary vessels). You should therefore pay special attention to the lungs to assess for the presence of other signs that might point to one of these diagnoses.

DISEASE	SUPPORTING FEATURES
Sarcoidosis	Interstitial fibrotic change
Lymphoma	Enlargement of other nodes (para-tracheal)
Pulmonary hypertension	Peripheral pruning Chronic lung disease (cause of secondary pulmonary hypertension)

2. Causes of bilateral hilar enlargement include:

- sarcoidosis
- lymphoma
- pulmonary hypertension (primary and secondary)
- metastatic nodal disease.

Case 9.14

This 30-year-old man presents with fatigue, for which a chest X-ray is among numerous investigations.

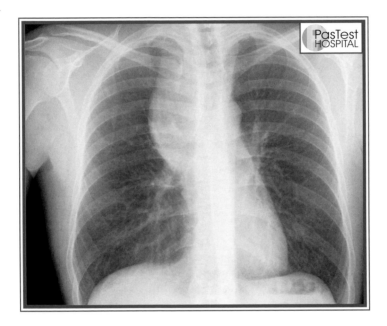

1. **Describe the appearances on this chest X-ray.**

2. **Give a short differential diagnosis and how you might establish the exact diagnosis.**

Answer 9.14

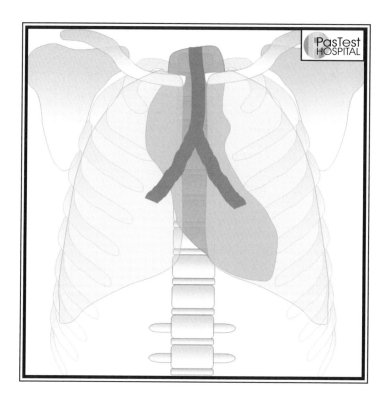

1. Large, predominantly right-sided, anterior mediastinal mass. This is causing displacement of the trachea to the left. The heart and lungs are normal in appearance.

2. The main differential diagnoses for an anterior mediastinal mass are: thyroid enlargement, thymoma, teratoma and lymphoma. CT of the chest will assist in identifying the extent of the mass and may also point towards a diagnosis, such as internal calcification in the case of a teratoma. Histological confirmation can be ascertained by CT-guided biopsy.

Case 9.15

This 61-year-old woman complains of non-specific symptoms, including malaise and anorexia.

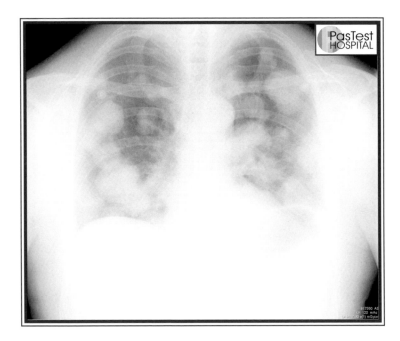

1. **Succinctly describe the appearances on this film and the likely diagnosis.**

2. **Which primary tumour types are most likely to result in these appearances?**

Answer 9.15

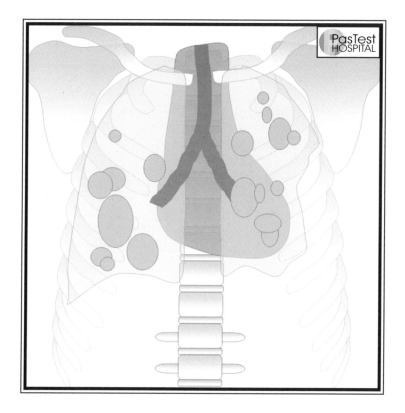

1. Multiple masses in both lungs of variable size, measuring up to 4 cm, consistent with pulmonary metastases. The appearances are those of 'cannon-ball' metastases and identification of the primary tumour is recommended, with CT of the chest, abdomen and pelvis.

2. The most likely primary tumour to cause cannon-ball metastases is renal cell carcinoma. Others include testicular malignancy and choriocarcinoma.

Scenarios presenting with fever

Case 9.16

This 39-year-old woman attends A&E with a high fever, following a recent holiday overseas.

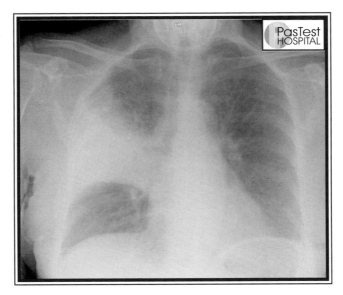

1. **Describe the appearances on the chest X-ray.**

2. **What follow-up imaging is necessary, how long after treatment should this be performed and why is it performed?**

Answer 9.16

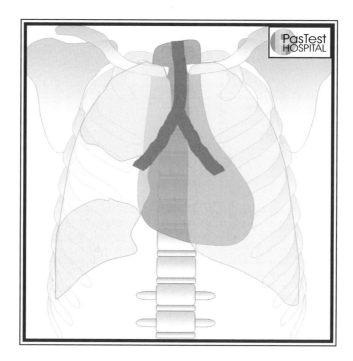

1. Dense consolidation is evident in the right upper and mid-zones, clearly delineated inferiorly by the horizontal fissure. This, combined with the right heart border remaining distinct, implies that the consolidation is in the right upper lobe The left hilum cannot be clearly visualised in its entirety. The right lung is clear.

    The appearances are in keeping with right upper lobe pneumonia.

2. A follow-up chest X-ray is indicated with a dense lobar pneumonia, especially a case like this, where the hilum cannot be properly assessed. A lobar pneumonia may be the presentation of something more sinister underlying it, such as a central bronchial carcinoma, which has resulted in a distal 'obstructive' pneumonia. A follow-up film should be performed 6 weeks after antibiotic treatment. For every decade of life after 60 years of age, an additional week should be added. Radiological resolution may lag behind clinical resolution. The follow-up film enables assessment for resolution of the pneumonia for any underlying mass.

Scenarios presenting with incidental findings

Case 9.17

This 55-year-old retiree has a chest X-ray as part of a medical insurance assessment.

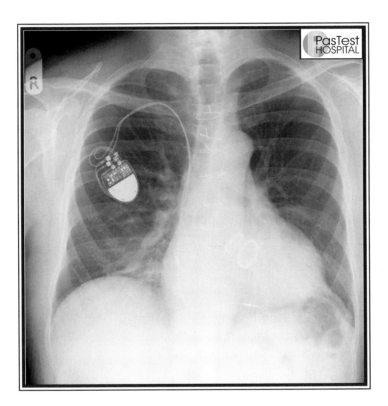

1. **Report the chest X-ray including what previous surgery has been performed.**

2. **List five indications for the surgery performed.**

Answer 9.17

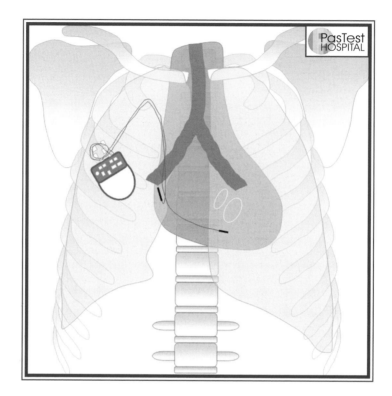

1. Dual lead pacemaker. Median sternotomy, aortic and mitral valve replacements. The heart is mildly enlarged, but there is no evidence of cardiac failure. The lungs are clear.

2. Cardiac valve replacement may be with a tissue or metallic valve. Only the latter will be visible on chest X-ray. Most commonly a single valve is replaced. The most common valve replacements are those of the 'left side of the heart' − the mitral and aortic valves. Indications for valve replacement include:

    (i) endocarditis

    (ii) rheumatic heart disease (usually mitral valve)

    (iii) congenital valve disease (eg a biscupid aortic valve)

    (iv) severe acquired valve incompetence or stenosis

    (v) acute valvular rupture.

Case 9.18

This 57-year-old woman is attending a follow-up clinic after previous surgery.

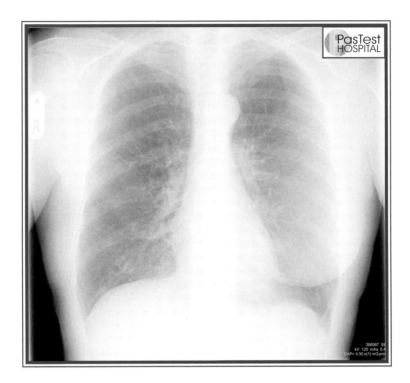

1.   **Describe the appearances on the chest X-ray.**
2.   **Name the other review areas when examining a chest X-ray.**

Answer 9.18

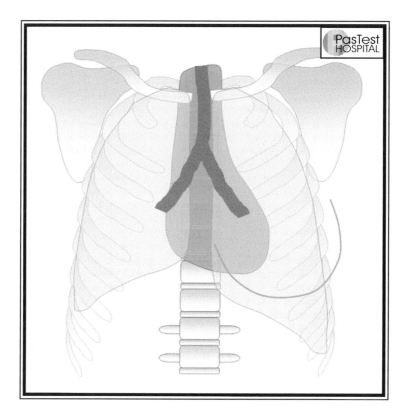

1. The right breast shadow is absent in keeping with a mastectomy. No evidence of recurrent disease in the lungs. Normal bony skeleton.

2. There are five key areas to review on chest X-ray:

   (i) costophrenic angles

   (ii) apices

   (iii) behind the heart

   (iv) below the diaphragms

   (v) breast shadows (in females)

Scenarios presenting with a distended abdomen

Case 9.19

This 63-year-old man attends A&E complaining of a short history of abdominal distension.

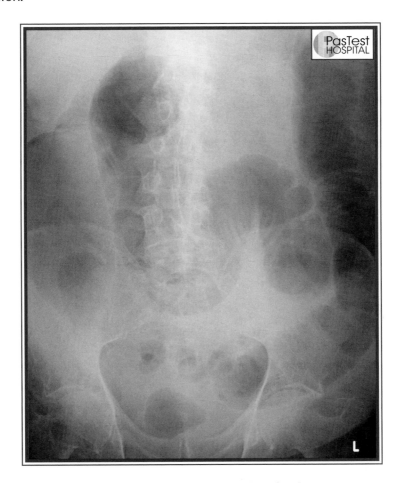

1. Describe the appearance on this abdominal X-ray.

2. What investigation should be performed next and how will it be useful?

Answer 9.19

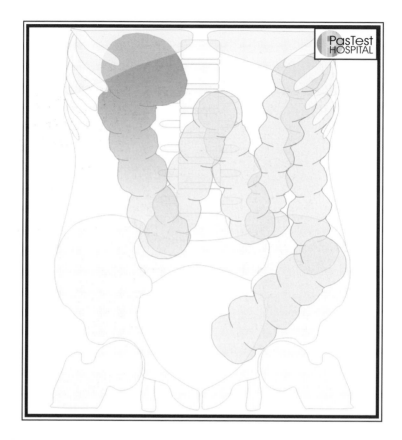

1. The large bowel is gas filled and dilated up to 6 cm in diameter down to the left side of the pelvis, where there is an abrupt cut-off. The rectum is non-distended and the small bowel collapsed. The appearances are consistent with a large bowel obstruction at the level of the sigmoid colon.

2. A CT of the abdomen is indicated to investigate further, before probable surgical intervention. This will enable the following:

    (a) confirmation of the site of obstruction

    (b) establishment of the cause of obstruction; a sigmoid tumour is most likely, although other causes include a diverticular stricture or hernia

    (c) identification of whether a perforation has occurred

    (d) in the case of the cause being a tumour, identification of any local, regional or distal metastatic disease.

Case 9.20

A 55-year-old man was admitted with acute abdominal pain and a CXR was performed.

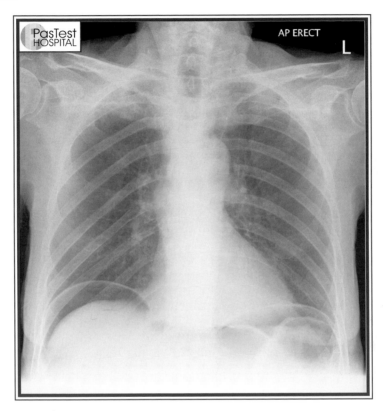

1. **What abnormality is seen on this film?**
2. **What projection has been used?**
3. **List some causes of this finding.**

Answer 9.20

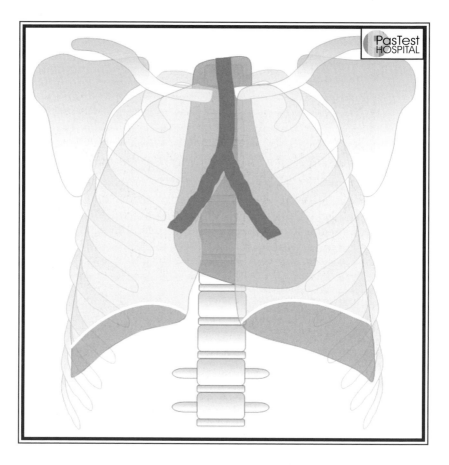

1. A radiolucent linear abnormality is noted inferior to the diaphragm bilaterally.

   Remember that gas on a plain X-ray is black so this must be gas in the abdomen.

   It is outside the bowel lumen – an abnormal finding. This is called a pneumoperitoneum.

2. This is an ERECT CXR. An erect film is invariably requested to assess for free gas within the abdomen (pneumoperitoneum).

3. The causes of pneumoperitoneum are listed on page 254 (see table 'Causes of extraluminal gas').

Case 9.21

This 69-year-old woman was admitted to the surgical ward with malodorous vomiting and a distended abdomen.

An AXR was taken while she was in A&E.

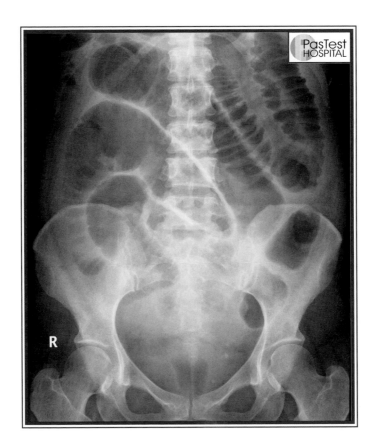

1. **Describe the findings on the AXR.**
2. **What are the causes of this abnormality?**

Answer 9.21

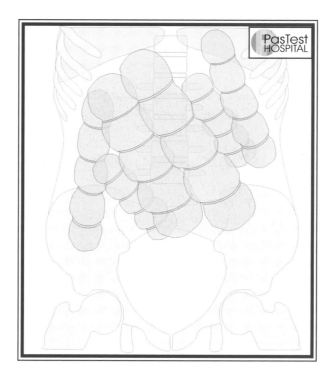

1. Multiple dilated small bowel loops. The bowel measures 4 cm in diameter and is located in the centre of the film. Multiple loops suggest that the obstruction lies in the distal small bowel. These findings are in keeping with a diagnosis of small bowel obstruction.

FEATURES OF SMALL BOWEL OBSTRUCTION

Bowel lies in centre of the film
Markings seen across the bowel wall (valvulae conniventes)
Several loops (more loops the lower the obstruction)

2. Causes of small bowel obstruction include (most common first):

- adhesions

- hernia

- extraluminal causes more common than intraluminal (obstructing mass)

- intussuception.

Case 9.22

This 77-year-old nursing home resident is brought to hospital because her carers are concerned about an enlarged abdomen over the last 24 hours.

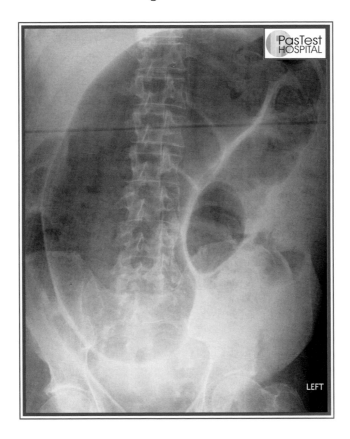

1. **Describe the appearances on the AXR.**

2. **What are the treatment options for this condition?**

Answer 9.22

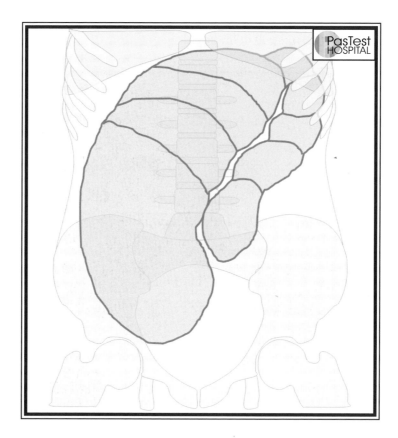

1. A large distended featureless loop of bowel arises from the pelvis into the mid/upper abdomen, with a 'coffee-bean' configuration. Proximal to this there is distended large bowel consistent with obstruction. The small bowel is collapsed. Appearances are consistent with a sigmoid volvulus.

2. The usual treatment for sigmoid volvulus is insertion of a flatus tube. A plain film is usually sufficient for diagnosis and a management decision. On occasion the volvulus might result in a section of ischaemic bowel requiring surgical resection. Sigmoid volvulus is commonly recurrent, which in itself may merit surgery. Of the three types of volvulus of the gastrointestinal tract, sigmoid is the most common followed by caecal and gastric.

Case 9.23

This 38-year-old woman attends A&E with abdominal distension and discomfort lasting the previous 12 hours.

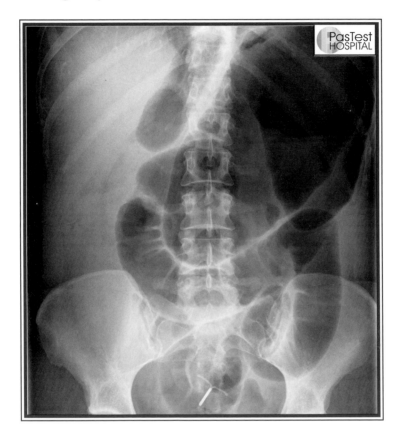

1. **Describe the findings on the AXR and provide a diagnosis.**
2. **Which group of patients typically get this condition?**

Answer 9.23

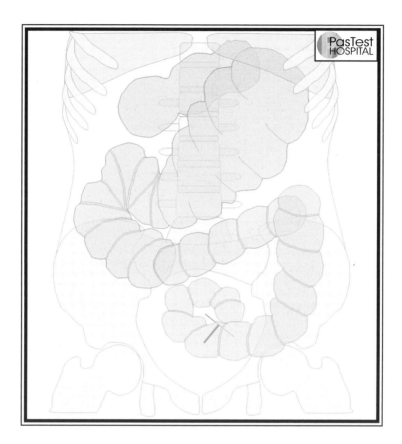

1. A large, distended, gas-filled, featureless viscus is sited in the right upper abdomen, which is separate from the collapsed stomach. The caecum is not apparent in the right iliac fossa. The small bowel is dilated. The appearances are consistent with a caecal volvulus with a resultant small bowel obstruction

2. Caecal volvulus typically occurs in young/middle-aged women with 'virgin' abdomens in comparison to sigmoid volvuli, which tend to cluster in the elderly population. Treatment is with surgery, requiring a caecopexy.

Scenarios presenting with abdominal pain

Case 9.24

This 35-year-old man is a regular attendee at the hospital with severe upper abdominal pain.

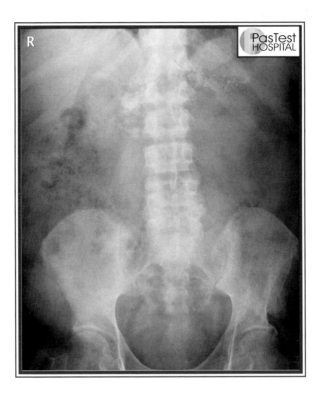

1. **Give a brief report of your findings on this AXR.**

2. **List the potential complications after acute pancreatitis.**

Answer 9.24

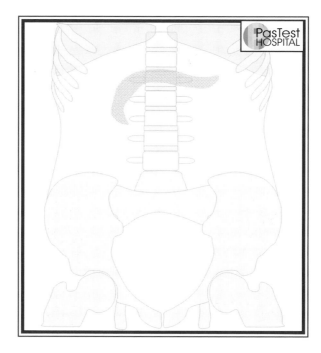

1. Extensive punctate calcification is evident in the upper abdomen, extending across the midline, conforming to the shape of the pancreas, in keeping with chronic pancreatitis.

2. Numerous complications may follow acute pancreatitis, which can be identified on imaging, in particular CT. Complications may be acute, subacute or chronic in nature, including the following:

    (a) pancreatic necrosis

    (b) pancreatic haemorrhage

    (c) pancreatic or peripancreatic abscess

    (d) pancreatic pseudocyst

    (e) pseudoaneurysm formation

    (f) thrombosis of adjacent vessels, eg the superior mesenteric vein

    (g) pancreatic calcification, which occurs in the chronic phase of pancreatitis and may involve the parenchyma or ductal components of the pancreas.

Case 9.25

This 43-year-old man complains of left-sided flank pain.

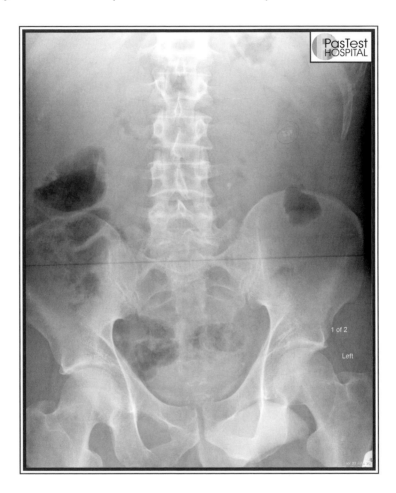

1. **Describe any abnormalities present on this AXR.**

2. **Which other imaging modality is best for imaging renal stone disease?**

Answer 9.25

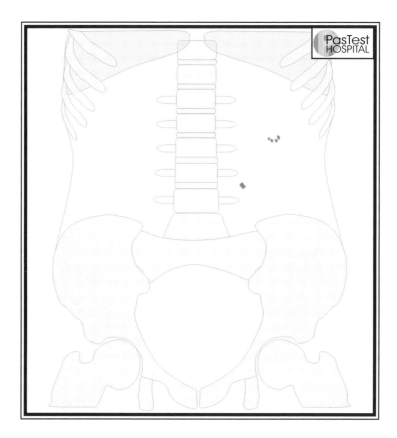

1. Multiple calcific densities project over the lower pole of the left kidney in keeping with renal calculi. An additional similar density projects between the left L3 and L4 transverse process, in keeping with a calculus within the left mid-ureter.

2. CT KUB (kidneys, ureters and bladder) is the gold standard imaging investigation for the assessment of renal calculi, with over 99% sensitivity for calculi as small as 1 mm. This is performed without contrast with 1-mm (thin) slice acquisition. Renal calculi and the level of obstruction are identified. In addition perinephric/periureteric inflammatory change and fluid are visualised. Complications, such as hydronephrosis or pyonephrosis, can be seen. Pyonephrosis due to renal stone disease is a urological emergency and is an indication for percutaneous nephrostomy insertion.

Scenarios presenting with an abdominal mass

Case 9.26

This 25-year-old man presented with upper abdominal discomfort. An AXR was performed because the admitting doctor was concerned about bowel obstruction.

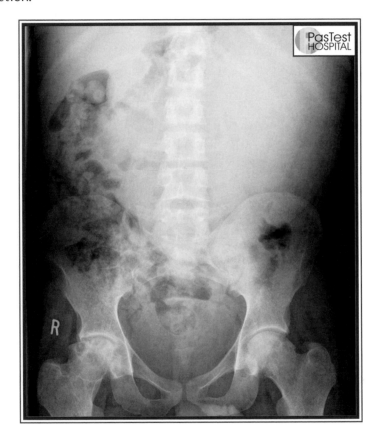

1. **Describe the appearances on the abdominal radiograph.**

2. **List some potential causes.**

Answer 9.26

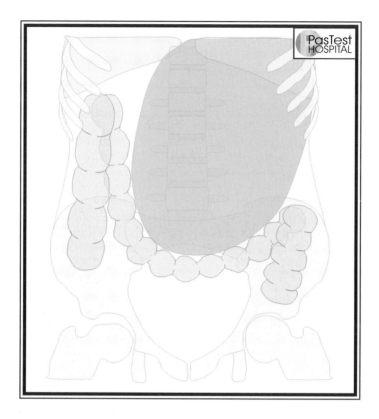

1. A large soft-tissue mass is present in the left upper quadrant extending inferomedially into the lower abdomen and upper pelvis. This is displacing both large and small bowel, consistent with being located within the peritoneal cavity. The findings are consistent with splenomegaly.

2. Potential causes of splenomegaly include: sickle cell disease, myelofibrosis and lymphoma.

    Note the bilateral hip abnormalities (much more pronounced on the right) of sclerosis and collapse consistent with avascular necrosis. The unifying diagnosis is sickle cell disease. Later in the disease process the spleen may become small due to infarction.

Case 9.27

This 75-year-old man complains of an ongoing aching pain in the centre abdomen.

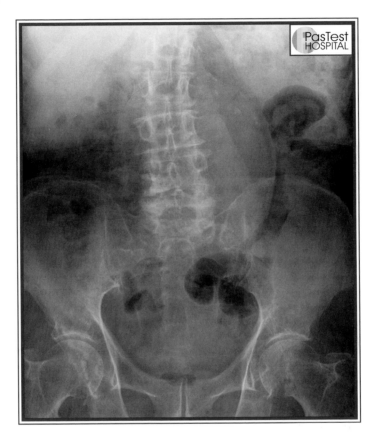

1. **Describe your findings on this AXR**

2. **What additional imaging investigation is recommended?**

Answer 9.27

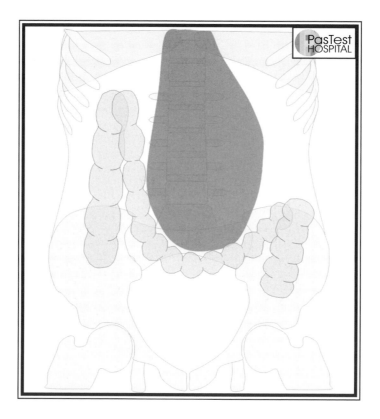

1. A large, left, paraspinal, soft tissue abnormality is present in the mid-abdomen with a curvilinear lateral aspect, which contains a rim of calcification. The psoas shadow is separate from this. Appearances are consistent with a large abdominal aortic aneurysm.

2. Although both ultrasonography and CT can be used to assess the aorta, in this instance CT is the best choice. Ultrasonography is used for surveillance of aneurysm size. This aneurysm is large enough to warrant elective surgery and therefore full assessment with CT is merited. CT is the investigation of choice in the acute setting to assess for rupture.

Case 9.28

This 37-year-old woman complains of lower abdominal pain and early bladder fullness.

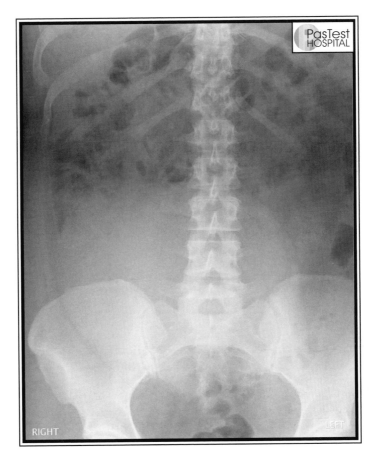

1. **Describe the abnormality present on the AXR.**

2. **Give a differential diagnosis and suggest an additional imaging technique to assess further.**

Answer 9.28

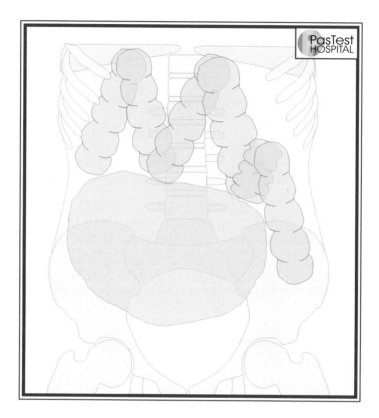

1. A large soft-tissue mass arises from the pelvis extending to the level of the umbilicus. This is well defined superiorly and is displacing the bowel into the upper abdomen. Appearances are in keeping with a pelvic mass, most likely gynaecological in origin.

2. The differential diagnosis for these appearances includes: ovarian cyst, dermoid cyst, pelvic abscess/collection and an enlarged fibroid uterus. In the first instance assessment with ultrasonography is recommended. Depending on this further cross-sectional imaging may also be required.

Scenarios presenting with headache

Case 9.29

This 37-year-old woman attended A&E complaining of a severe sudden headache.

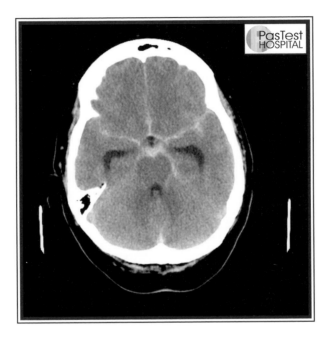

1. **Describe the appearances on the head CT.**
2. **What other imaging investigation(s) would be helpful in the patient's management plan?**

Answer 9.29

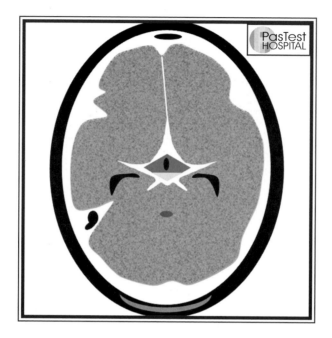

1. Extensive high-attenuation material consistent with acute blood is present within the suprasellar cistern and sulci of the brain in keeping with subarachnoid haemorrhage. The temporal horns of the lateral ventricles are dilated in keeping with early hydrocephalus.

2. Spontaneous subarachnoid haemorrhage is commonly associated with an underlying vascular abnormality, most commonly a cerebral ('berry') aneurysm. Imaging is focused on trying to identify an aneurysm, which will permit definitive treatment, such as a coil embolisation or less commonly now surgical clipping. This usually involves CT angiography of the circle of Willis, although catheter angiography may be performed alone or in addition to CT, especially if endoluminal treatment is to be performed.

Case 9.30

This 39-year-old man was brought to A&E by his wife, because he has developed a progressively worsening headache over the past 2 weeks, particularly severe first thing in the morning.

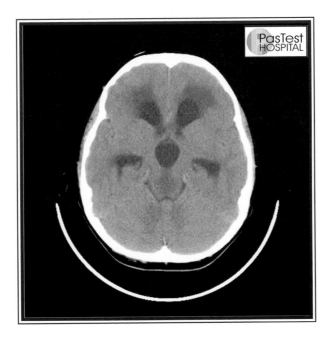

1. **Describe the appearances on the head CT.**

2. **List potential causes for these appearances.**

Answer 9.30

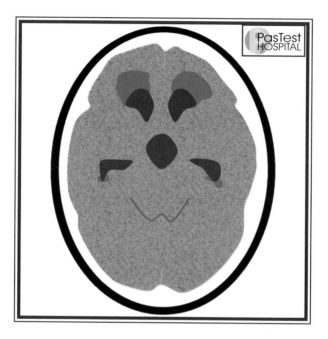

1. The ventricular system of the brain is dilated, in particular on the single image provided, note that the lateral ventricles (frontal and temporal horns) are dilated as is the third ventricle, which is also uncharacteristically round. Periventricular low attenuation is evident around the frontal horns, in keeping with transependymal oedema, which typically occurs in acute hydrocephalus (the CSF leaks across the ependymal lining of the ventricle due to high pressure within).

2. Hydrocephalus may be obstructive or non-obstructive. It may involve individual ventricles or the whole ventricular system. Causes include:

    (a) an obstructive malignant mass, such as a tumour; potential tumours include an ependymoma

    (b) an obstructive non-malignant mass, such as a third ventricular colloid cyst

    (c) obstruction due to intraventricular debris, such as blood post-subarachnoid haemorrhage.

Case 9.31

This 69-year-old man developed a severe headache while attending a local football match.

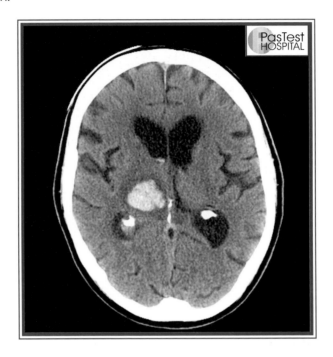

1. **Describe the appearances on the head CT.**
2. **What is the most likely cause for these appearances?**

Answer 9.31

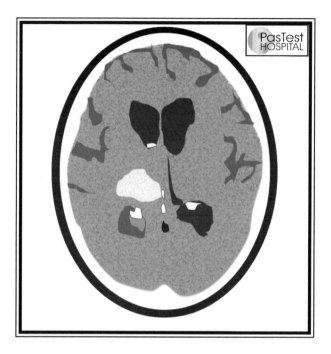

1. A moderate-sized, well-defined, high-attenuation focus is present in the right thalamus, in keeping with a thalamic haemorrhage. This is an intraparenchymal haematoma, and there is a little reactive surrounding oedema.

2. Thalamic haemorrhage is typically due to hypertension. This would be classed as a haemorrhagic stroke, which accounts for 15% of all strokes, most being due to infarction. Other typical locations for hypertensive haemorrhage include the basal ganglia and dentate nucleus of the cerebellum.

   With large intraparenchymal haemorrhages there may be intraventricular extension. A small proportion of infarcts may undergo haemorrhagic transformation.

Scenarios presenting with confusion

Case 9.32

This 55-year-old woman was brought to A&E by her relatives who state that she has been confused over the past 24 hours. She had a mastectomy for breast cancer 2 years ago.

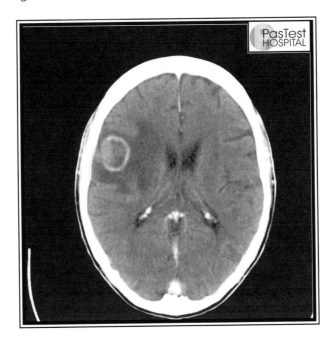

1. Describe the appearances on the CT head.

2. If this was the patient's first presentation, what is the potential differential diagnosis?

Answer 9.32

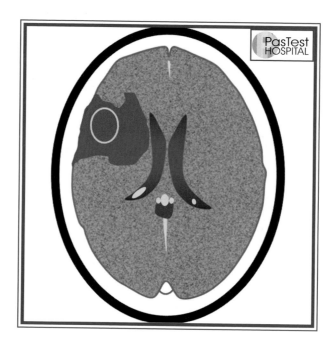

1. This CT has been performed following contrast administration. An approximately 3-cm rim-enhancing mass lies within the right frontoparietal region, with significant surrounding perilesional oedema. This is causing a mass effect, as demonstrated by sulcal effacement and mild displacement of the body of the right lateral ventricle. In the context of the clinical history a cerebral metastasis is the most likely diagnosis.

2. The differential diagnosis for a single rim-enhancing intraparenchymal mass includes:

   (a) cerebral metastasis

   (b) primary brain malignancy

   (c) cerebral abscess

   (d) tumefactive multiple sclerosis (mass like in appearance).

Case 9.33

This 24-year-old intravenous drug user is accompanied to A&E by his friend who states that he has been 'really muddled' over the last 3 days and has a fever.

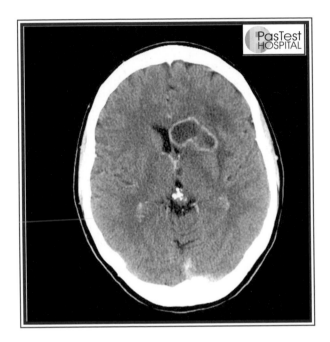

1. Describe the appearances on the head CT.

2. Name some other complications that commonly occur in those using intravenous drugs.

Answer 9.33

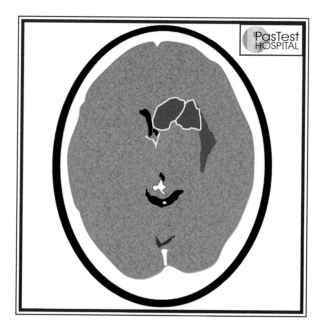

1. This scan has been performed following contrast administration. Adjacent to the frontal horn of the left lateral ventricle is an avidly rim-enhancing lesion, with a low attenuation centre. There is a moderate amount of perilesional oedema. Although there is a wide differential for a rim-enhancing solitary cerebral lesion (see Case 9.32), correlation with the clinical history makes a cerebral abscess by far the most likely cause.

2. Although not necessarily unique to those taking intravenous drugs, there are a number of conditions that occur much more commonly in this patient subgroup, including:

   (a) infective endocarditis

   (b) cerebral abscesses

   (c) groin pseudoaneurysms, which may also become infected

   (d) septic pulmonary emboli.

Scenarios presenting with reduced GCS score

Case 9.34

This 18 year old was involved in a skiing accident 2 hours previously. His GCS on arrival at A&E is 9/15.

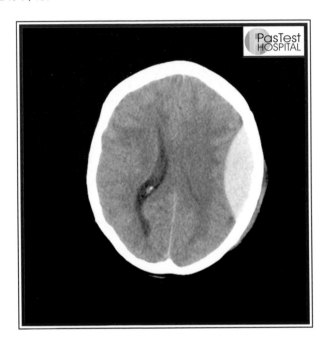

1. Describe the appearances on the head CT.

2. What is normally associated with this finding on CT and which vessel is typically damaged?

Answer 9.34

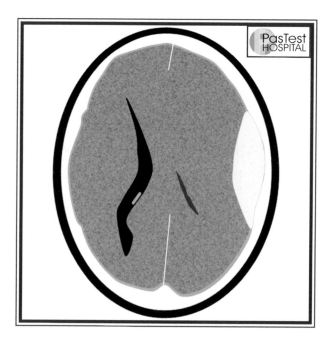

1. A high-attenuation, lens-shaped (biconvex), extra-axial abnormality is present in the left parietal region, which is causing a mass effect in the form of sulcal effacement, along with both compression and displacement of the left lateral ventricle.

   The appearances are consistent with an acute extradural haematoma.

2. Ninety-five per cent of extradural haematomas are associated with a skull fracture. The middle meningeal artery is usually the vessel damaged and is responsible for the haematoma. This differs from subdural haematomas, which are usually due to tears of the bridging veins.

Case 9.35

This 77-year-old widow is found at home by her neighbour. On arrival at A&E her GCS is 12/15.

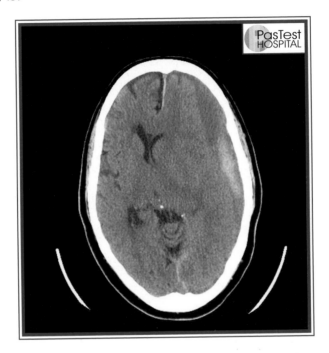

1. Describe the appearances on the head CT.

2. There is no history of severe head trauma. How might this haematoma have arisen?

Answer 9.35

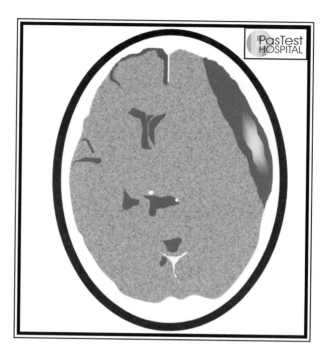

1. Blood of variable age is present within the left subdural space, in keeping with a moderate-sized subdural haematoma. Most of the haematoma content is isodense, with the brain parenchyma indicating subacute blood with some high-attenuation material within, consistent with more acute blood. The haematoma is causing significant mass effect, with displacement of the frontal horn of the left lateral ventricle and subfalcine herniation.

2. Subdural haematomas are not uncommonly found after relatively low-impact head trauma. Often, if questioned directly, patients might recall a slight blow to the head or a fall before presentation – which is often considered too trivial to be mentioned. This history may not be given, however, due to the presence of confusion.

Case 9.36

This 35 year old was found on the street late at night. She was intubated at the scene for a GCS of 3/15.

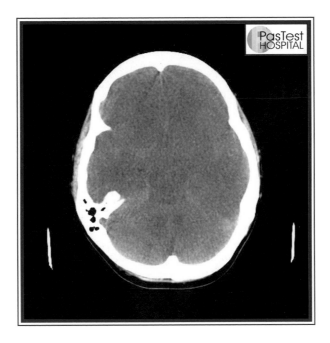

1. **Describe the appearances on the head CT.**

2. **What is the likely cause?**

Answer 9.36

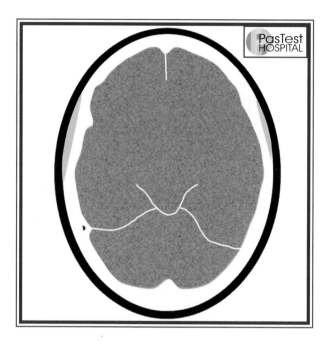

1. Throughout the visualised brain (on the single slice provided) there is diffuse loss of grey–white material differentiation of the brain parenchyma. In addition to this the basal cisterns are completely effaced. The sulci of the brain are also non-apparent.

2. The appearances of the CT are consistent with cerebral anoxia. When the brain is deprived of sufficient oxygenation for a prolonged period of time, eg during a cardiac arrest in the community with a long period of lost cardiac output, anoxia occurs. This results in the loss of grey–white matter differentiation and cytotoxic oedema.

Scenario presenting with neurological deficit

Case 9.37

This 66-year-old man gives a 3-hour history of right-sided weakness. Examination confirms a right hemiparesis.

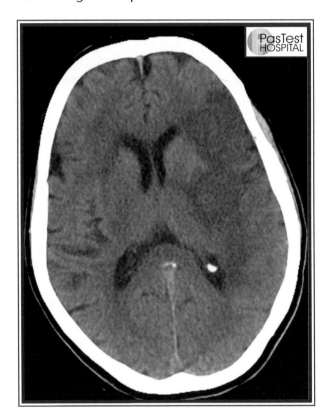

1. **Describe the appearances on the head CT.**

2. **Explain the concept of 'time is brain' in the modern management of stroke.**

Answer 9.37

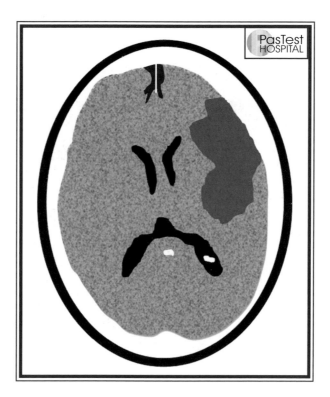

1. Extensive low attenuation is present throughout the left temporoparietal region with sparing of the head of caudate and lentiform nucleus (basal ganglia). These appearances are consistent with a left middle cerebral artery (MCA) territory infarction. No evidence of haemorrhagic transformation. No visible intra-arterial thrombus.

2. 'Time is brain' refers to the urgency with which acute stroke should be treated, where appropriate, with intravenous thrombolysis. Those patients who present to hospital within a specified time window with the clinical diagnosis of stroke, and who fill a number of pre-agreed criteria, should receive intravenous thrombolysis. The concept is that ischaemic, but not yet dead, brain (ischaemic penumbra) is reperfused and saved, resulting in a reduction in neurological deficit. At present the time window that is adopted in many centres is 4.5 hours from the onset of symptoms. The patient must receive a CT of the head before treatment to exclude intracranial haemorrhage.

Case 9.38

This 78-year-old woman has developed progressive right-sided weakness in recent days.

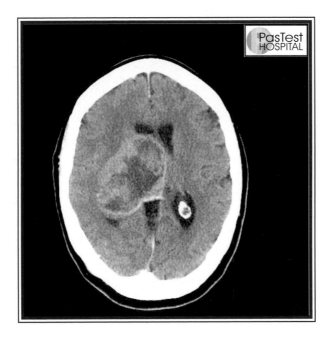

1. **Describe the appearances on the head CT.**

2. **Name three primary brain tumours that occur in the supra- and infratentorial brain.**

Answer 9.38

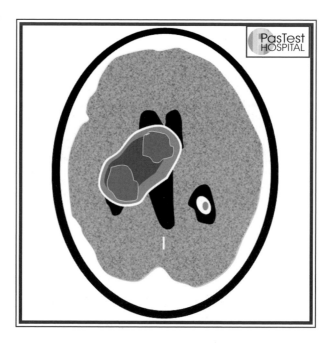

1. This post-contrast scan outlines a large heterogeneous enhancing mass in the right cerebral hemisphere bulging into and compressing the right lateral ventricle. The most likely cause for these appearances is a glioma. At present there is no evidence of hydrocephalus.

2. In adults, primary brain tumours are more common in the supratentorial than the infratentorial brain. The reverse is true in children. Potential supratentorial tumours include: glioblastoma multiforme, astrocytoma, meningioma, oligodendroglioma, neurofibroma and craniopharyngioma. Infratentorial (or posterior fossa) tumours include: ependymoma, pilocytic astrocytoma, brain-stem glioma, cerebellar haemangioblastoma and medulloblastoma, some of which are essentially unique to children.

Case 9.39

This 62-year-old man developed a left-sided visual deficit 3 months previously. On this occasion CT was performed after head trauma.

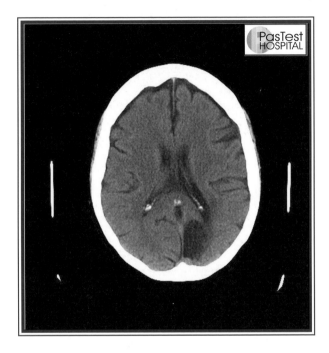

1. **Describe the appearances on this CT of the brain.**
2. **List a few factors that predispose to stroke.**

Case 9.39

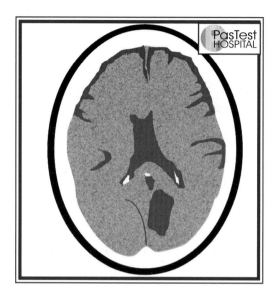

1. There is a focal area of low attenuation in the left occipital lobe. The appearances are consistent with an established posterior cerebral artery stroke involving the left occipital lobe. No acute findings to suggest an injury following trauma.

2. There are a number of factors that predispose to stroke. These include:

   • hypertension

   • atrial fibrillation

   • cardiovascular disease elsewhere ('arteriopath' status)

   • diabetes mellitus

   • smoking

   • hyperlipidaemia

   • family history of cardiovascular disease

   • atheromatous plaques in the carotid or vertebrobasilar arteries

   • infective endocarditis – resulting in septic emboli

   • vasculitis

   • dissection of the carotid or vertebrobasilar arteries (especially in stroke of young people)

   • procoagulant states, such as polycythaemia.

CARDIOLOGY

10

CARDIOLOGY

Electrocardiography

The electrocardiogram (ECG) is one of the most important commonly requested tests in medical practice.

Components of an ECG tracing

A standard ECG comprises 12 individual tracings (called leads). An ECG machine produces these tracings by comparing electrical signals from 10 sensors. Six are placed on the chest and one on each of the four limbs. By convention, the tracings are given standard names, with each representing an electrical signal from a particular part of the heart. V1, V2, V3, V4, V5 and V6 'look at' the heart in a horizontal plane. Each of these tracings represents the electrical signal detected at one of the chest sensors; aVL, aVF, aVR, I, II and III look at the heart in a vertical plane.

LEAD	LOOKS AT
V1, V2, V3 and V4	Anterior surface (right ventricle and septum)
V5, V6, aVL and I	Lateral surface (left ventricle)
II, III and aVF	Inferior surface
aVR	Right atrium

In a patient having an acute myocardial infarction, it is therefore possible to determine which part of the heart is affected by assessing which leads show changes.

If any individual lead is examined in detail, various peaks and troughs will be noted. These represent electrical activity at various times in the cardiac cycle. It is sometimes difficult to see every detail on each tracing. Names are attached to particular parts of the tracing as follows.

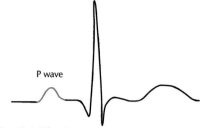

P wave

Fig 10.1: The P wave.

The first bump in a tracing is called a 'P wave'. This represents the electrical activity associated with depolarisation of the atria. There is a further electrical signal associated with atrial repolarisation, but this cannot usually be seen on an ECG, since the small electrical signal is overshadowed by the much more powerful ventricular activity.

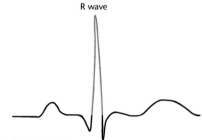

Q wave

Fig 10.2: The Q wave.

Following along from the P wave, a downward dip in the tracing is known as a Q wave. This may or may not be present.

R wave

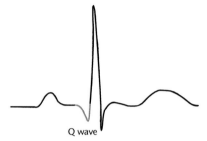

Fig 10.3: The R wave.

The first upward peak after the P wave is known as an R wave.

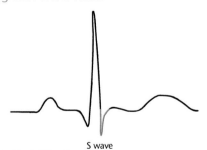

S wave

Fig 10.4: The S wave.

Any dip below the baseline following an R wave is called an S wave.

The Q, R and S waves are known collectively as the QRS complex. This represents ventricular depolarisation.

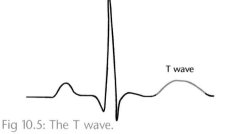

T wave

Fig 10.5: The T wave.

Following the QRS complex, an upward deflection in the tracing is known as a T wave. This represents ventricular repolarisation. T waves are followed by P waves, and the cycle is complete.

Interpreting an ECG

The following aspects should be addressed when interpreting an ECG:

Heart rate	QRS complexes
Heart rhythm	ST segment
Cardiac axis	Q–T interval
P waves	T waves

Heart rate

ECGs are printed on squared paper. This paper usually runs through the ECG machine at a standard rate (25 mm/s). If, for some reason, the machine is set to run at a different speed, interpretation is more difficult.

DON'T FORGET

Always check that the paper speed is at 25 mm per second.

At this speed, on a horizontal axis, each small square represents 0.04 second, and each large square (which is five small squares wide) represents 0.2 second.

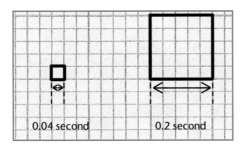

Fig 10.6: Standard squared paper used when recording ECGs.

The ventricular rate is calculated by looking at the distance between consecutive QRS complexes. Usually the distance between R waves is analysed.

When there are a number of large squares between each R wave, the ventricular rate is most easily calculated by counting the number of large squares between each R wave and dividing this number into 300.

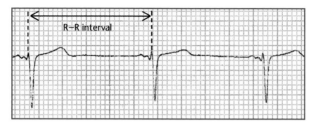

Fig 10.7: Measuring the R–R interval.

In the ECG shown, there are approximately five large squares between each R wave. The ventricular rate is therefore 300 ÷ 5 = 60 beats/min.

When the ventricular rhythm is more rapid, counting large squares can prove difficult. In such instances, the number of small squares between consecutive R waves is counted, and this number divided into 1500.

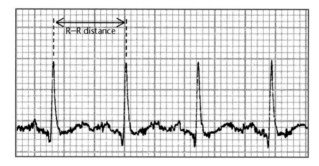

Fig 10.8: Measuring the R–R interval with a faster heart rate.

In the example, there are 12 small squares between each R wave. The ventricular rate is therefore 1500 ÷ 12 = 125 beats/min.

Ventricular rate (beats per minute) = 300 ÷ number of large squares between R waves
OR
Ventricular rate (beats per minute) = 1500 ÷ number of small squares between R waves
Both approaches give the same answer, but the second approach tends to be easier if the heart rate is rapid.

A heart rate of less than 60 beats/min is termed **bradycardia**. A rate of greater than 100 beats/min is **tachycardia**.

If the heart rhythm is irregular, calculate the rate using the number of squares between several R waves. Divide the answer to obtain an average R–R interval.

For example, if there are 40 large squares between the first and the eleventh R wave, the average R–R interval is 4 large squares and the heart rate is approximately $300 \div 4 = 75$ beats/min.

Heart rhythm

There are several heart rhythms that you will be expected to recognise. To assess rhythm, look for P waves and their relationship to QRS complexes. Remember that normally one P wave should be followed by one QRS complex. Good leads for assessing P waves are leads II, V1 and V2.

Sinus rhythm

Sinus rhythm describes a normal heart rhythm in which electrical signals begin in the sinus node. A P wave should precede each QRS complex, and be at a normal, fixed interval from it. The P–R interval is used to measure the interval between P waves and QRS complexes. It is measured by counting the number of squares between the start of the P wave and the start of the QRS complex. This distance should be between three and five small squares.

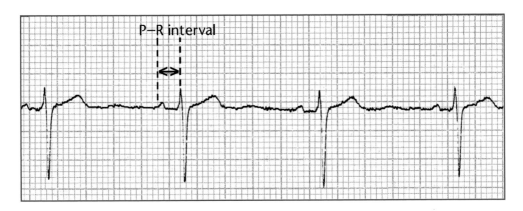

Fig 10.9: Normal sinus rhythm illustrating the P–R interval.

- Sinus tachycardia describes sinus rhythm at a rate of over 100 beats/min.

- Sinus bradycardia describes sinus rhythm at less than 60 beats/min.

- Sinus arrhythmia is the term used to describe the normal variation in heart rate with respiration. Normally, the heart rate increases on inspiration.

In sinus arrhythmia, the heart rate **IN**creases on **IN**spiration.

SINUS RHYTHM CHECKS

To diagnose sinus rhythm, all of the following criteria should be met:
1. P wave preceding every QRS complex
2. P–R interval is normal
3. P–R interval is constant

Atrial fibrillation

This is the term used to describe erratic electrical activity in the atria. In this condition, no P waves are seen, and the ECG baseline commonly shows irregularity. QRS complexes occur irregularly.

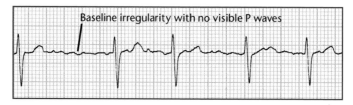

Baseline irregularity with no visible P waves

Fig 10.10: Atrial fibrillation.

This tracing fails sinus rhythm check 1, as no P waves are visible.

Atrial flutter

This condition is similar to atrial fibrillation in many ways. However, the ECG shows the presence of F waves (flutter waves). The baseline of the ECG therefore adopts a 'saw-toothed' appearance. Atrial flutter may occur with a fixed degree of atrioventricular block, eg three-to-one block. This means that, for every three flutter waves, there would be one QRS complex. Alternatively, the rhythm may have variable block, where the number of flutter waves preceding each QRS complex varies from beat to beat.

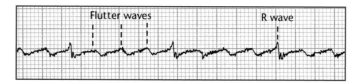

Flutter waves   R wave

Fig 10.11: Atrial flutter.

This tracing fails sinus rhythm check 1, as no P waves are visible. You should be able to instantly recognise atrial flutter on account of its distinctive appearance.

Heart block

Heart block describes a problem with conduction between the atria and ventricles. There are various types.

First-degree heart block

In first-degree heart block, a P wave precedes each QRS complex, but the P–R interval is prolonged (more than five small squares). The P–R interval remains constant from beat to beat.

In simple terms, imagine first-degree heart block as a condition in which the wiring of the heart is still intact, but is a little slow. It therefore takes longer than normal for electrical signals to travel from the atria to the ventricles.

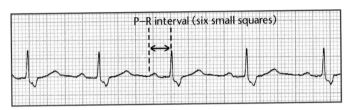

Fig 10.12: First-degree heart block.

You will appreciate that this example is not sinus rhythm because, although there is a P wave before every QRS complex (check 1), the P–R interval is prolonged (six small squares).

Second-degree heart block

Second-degree heart block describes the spectrum of conduction problems that are more severe than first-degree, but less severe than third-degree, heart block.

There are three main types:

1. Mobitz type I (Wenckebach phenomenon)
   This rhythm runs in cycles, and will be identified if the tests for sinus rhythm are checked. The first P–R interval in a cycle is often normal. With each successive heart beat, the P–R interval lengthens. Eventually, there will be a P wave with no following QRS complex. The cycle then begins again.

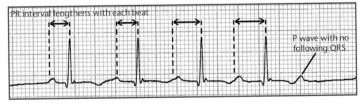

Fig 10.13: Mobitz type I heart block.

2. Mobitz type II
    Again, you will diagnose this rhythm if you check the requirements for
    sinus rhythm. In this rhythm, the P—R interval is constant. Its duration
    may be normal or prolonged. However, periodically there will be no
    conduction between the atria and ventricles, and there will be a P wave
    with no associated QRS complex.

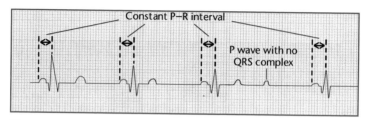

Fig 10.14: Mobitz type II heart block.

3. Fixed degrees of atrioventricular block
    These rhythms are described as two-to-one, three-to-one, four-to-one
    block, etc. In two-to-one block, for example, two P waves are found for
    every QRS complex.

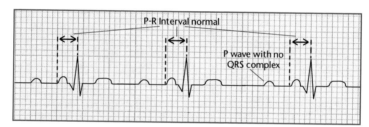

Fig 10.15: Two-to-one atrioventricular block.

Third-degree heart block

In this condition, there is no functioning electrical connection between the
atria and ventricles. You may like to think of this as a state in which the 'wires'
between atria and ventricles have been 'cut'. P waves and QRS complexes will
be seen, but these will have no constant relationship to each other. If you
suspect this rhythm, take a sheet of paper and lay it alongside the ECG in
question. Mark on the paper the position of the P waves. Next, move your paper
so that the first mark you have made lines up with the first QRS complex. You
will see that the P waves and QRS complexes are completely dissociated. The
QRS complex arises because of intrinsic pacemaker activity below the
atrioventricular node.

Note that QRS complexes can be normal in width or wide (see below).

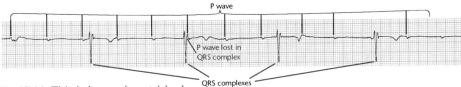

Fig 10.16: Third-degree heart block.

Cardiac axis

The cardiac axis is an arbitrary concept used to describe the average direction of electrical activity in the heart. Normally, the average flow of electrical energy is from the upper right heart border towards the apex. In various disease states, the cardiac axis can shift.

There are several methods for assessing axis, but students often find this a difficult exercise. One method relies on looking at leads I, II and III, and determining whether the QRS complexes are predominantly upgoing or downgoing. QRS complexes in a particular lead are upgoing if average electrical flow (axis) is towards that lead, and downgoing if it is away from the lead (see Fig 10.17).

A good rule of thumb is to assess the QRS complexes in leads I and II and, if both are predominantly upgoing, the axis is normal as shown in Fig 10.19. In right axis deviation, the axis shifts clockwise and, as a result lead I becomes downgoing because average electrical flow is away from it. In left axis deviation, the axis shifts anti-clockwise, and as a result, leads II and III become downgoing. Figure 10.18 illustrates the standard convention for quantifying the cardiac axis. Figure 10.19 illustrates all three scenarios.

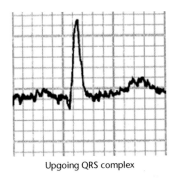

Upgoing QRS complex

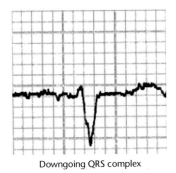

Downgoing QRS complex

Fig 10.17: Upgoing and downgoing QRS complexes.

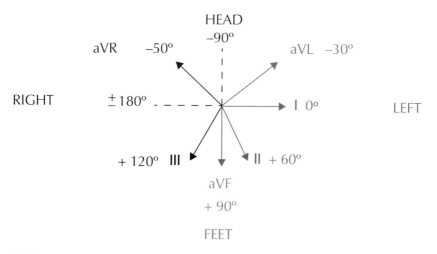

Fig 10.18

AXIS	LEAD I	LEAD II	LEAD III
Normal	Upgoing	Upgoing	Upgoing (or downgoing)
Right axis deviation	Downgoing	Upgoing	Upgoing
Left axis deviation	Upgoing	Downgoing	Downgoing

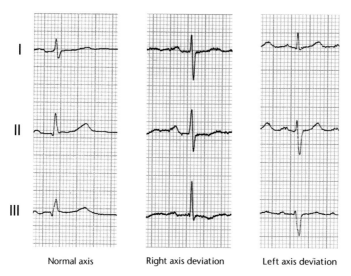

Fig 10.19: Leads I, II and III showing a normal axis, right axis deviation and left axis deviation.

P waves

Look at leads II, V1 and V2 for the best views of P waves. Assess their size and shape. P waves should not exceed the maximum dimensions shown in Fig 10.20. Always make sure that an ECG has been correctly calibrated before commenting on the heights of peaks. The standard calibration is 10 mm = 1 mV.

DON'T FORGET

Always check that an ECG is calibrated to 10 mm = 1 mV.

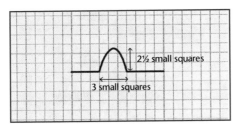

Fig 10.20: Normal P-wave dimensions.

- P pulmonale describes tall, peaked P waves. These occur in conditions when the right atrium becomes enlarged.
- P mitrale describes wide P waves that are often bifid. This may be seen in patients with mitral stenosis.

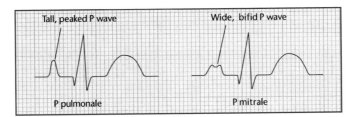

Fig 10.21: P pulmonale and P mitrale.

MEMORY AID

In P **P**ulmonale, the P waves are **P**eaked.
In P **M**itrale, the P waves are bifid and look like the letter **M**.

QRS complexes

Q waves

Look at the location and size of Q waves. The maximum dimensions of Q waves should not exceed those shown in Fig 10.22.

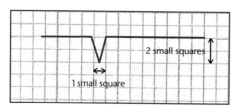

Fig 10.22: Q-wave maximum dimensions.

Because of the direction taken by electrical signals in the heart, small Q waves may normally be seen in leads looking at the lateral aspect of the heart (V5, V6, aVL and I). Large Q waves or Q waves in other locations are abnormal, and indicate the presence of scar tissue in the heart (eg after a myocardial infarction).

Height of R and S waves

Much information can be gleaned by looking at the height of R and S waves. The most common abnormality detected is left ventricular hypertrophy. There are many ECG criteria for predicting whether hypertrophy is present. One method involves finding the sum of the height of the S wave in V1 (in mm) and the height of the R wave in V6 (in mm). If greater than 35 mm, it is probable that left ventricular hypertrophy is present. An echocardiogram is necessary to confirm hypertrophy.

There are several causes of very small complexes, the most common being pericardial effusions, pericarditis and emphysematous lungs.

QRS duration

A normal QRS complex should be less than three small squares wide.

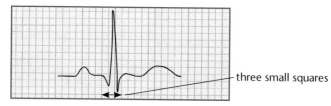

Fig 10.23: Normal maximum QRS complex duration.

Wide complexes indicate abnormal conduction through the ventricles. Normally, electrical signals are carried through the ventricular muscle in specialised conducting tissue – the bundle of His and its left and right branches. Problems in this conducting tissue result in electrical impulses being carried more slowly through non-specialised cardiac tissue. This results in widening of the QRS complex. You should be able to recognise the typical ECG features of both problems in both the left and right bundle branches (named left and right bundle-branch block). Problems with QRS duration and other ECG abnormalities can be seen in tricyclic antidepressant toxicity – see page 173 for details.

In right bundle-branch block (RBBB), two upward deflections (ie two R waves) are seen in the QRS complex in V1. This is known as an RSR pattern. A deep S wave is normally seen in V6.

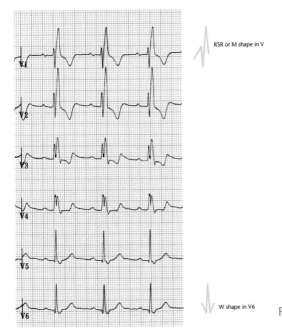

RSR or M shape in V

W shape in V6

Fig 10.24: Right bundle-branch block.

In left bundle-branch block (LBBB), the ECG is typically highly bizarre in appearance. An RSR pattern may be seen in V6. Conduction is so disordered in LBBB that many of the normal morphological features of an ECG are not distinguishable. After establishing heart rate, rhythm, axis and that LBBB is present, analysis of the ECG should stop. Confusion often arises in practice when students attempt to comment on what appear to be highly abnormal ST segments and T waves. It is important to be able to identify LBBB, because, if it develops in a patient, it can be a sign of myocardial infarction.

Do not attempt to comment on the ST segment when LBBB is present.

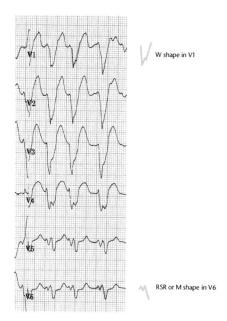

W shape in V1

RSR or M shape in V6

Fig 10.25: Left bundle-branch block.

Remember the name William Morrow, to remind you that:
In LBBB, there is a W shape to the QRS complex in V1 and an M shape to the complex in V6
In RBBB, there is an M shape to the QRS complex in V1 and a W shape to the complex in V6

	V1						V6
LBBB	W	I	L	L	I	A	M
RBBB	M	O	R	R		O	W

ST segment

The ST segment is that part of a tracing that lies between the QRS complex and the T wave.

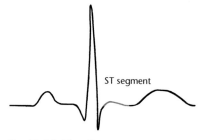

ST segment

Fig 10.26: The ST segment.

Normally, the ST segment should be horizontal and isoelectric (ie lying on the baseline of the tracing). Abnormalities include elevation and depression.

The ST segment may be elevated. The most common causes for this are myocardial infarction (where ST elevation occurs in the heart leads 'looking at' damaged parts of the heart) and pericarditis (where ST elevation occurs in most or all ECG leads). The ST elevation associated with myocardial infarction is typically convex upwards, whereas it is concave (saddle-shaped) in pericarditis.

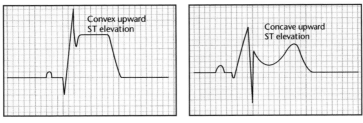

Fig 10.27: Convex and concave ST elevation (exaggerated for clarity).

ACUTE MYOCARDIAL INFARCTION REQUIRING URGENT REPERFUSION .

1. ST segment elevation (convex upwards) in keeping with acute myocardial infarction,

or

2. New LBBB: in a patient with typical chest pain

ST elevation that persists over weeks and months after a myocardial infarction commonly signifies the presence of a ventricular aneurysm.

Horizontal ST depression can represent cardiac ischaemia, and may be seen during episodes of angina pectoris. ST depression may also indicate a non-ST elevation myocardial infarction (NSTEMI), which can be distinguished from ischaemia only by measuring biochemical markers of cardiomyocyte damage (see page 366 for details).

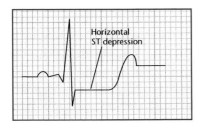

Fig 10.28: Horizontal ST depression.

When ST depression in lateral chest leads is seen alongside features in keeping with left ventricular hypertrophy, this is called a strain pattern, and is a feature of marked left ventricular hypertrophy. It can be difficult to differentiate from changes associated with ischaemia.

Down-sloping ST depression (often called 'reverse tick' ST depression) is seen in patients on digoxin.

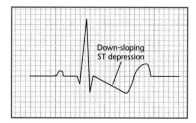

Fig 10.29: Down-sloping ST depression.

Q–T interval

The Q–T interval is the distance from the start of the QRS complex to the end of the T wave. Long Q–T intervals predispose to cardiac dysrhythmias. The Q–T interval varies with heart rate, but should in general not be more than two large squares in duration.

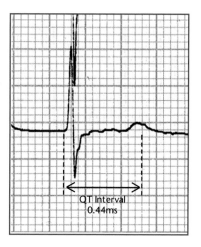

Fig 10.30: Prolonged Q–T interval.

To make matters a little more complicated, the Q–T interval increases as the heart rate slows. Thus bradycardia can be associated with an apparently long Q–T interval. To correct for this, the Bazett correction is applied to the Q–T interval to take the heart rate into account. The corrected Q–T interval (Q–Tc) is calculated as follows:

$$Q\text{–}Tc = \frac{Q\text{–}T}{\sqrt{R\text{–}R}}$$

where R–R is the number of seconds between consecutive R waves.

This value should generally be less than 0.45 second.

T wave

The final stage in ECG interpretation should be to look at the T waves. T waves may be upright or inverted (upside down). They are generally less than two-thirds of the height of their neighbouring R wave, and should not be more than two large squares tall.

Inverted T waves are normally seen in leads aVR and III. They may also be seen in lead V1 ± V2, but not V2 alone. T-wave inversion in other leads may be of little consequence, but is often a sign of cardiac ischaemia, or of NSTEMI.

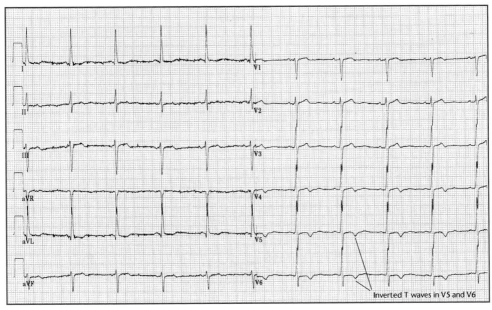

Inverted T waves in V5 and V6

Fig 10.31: 12-lead ECG with T-wave inversion in the lateral chest leads.

T-wave changes often accompany changes in the serum potassium level. Typical findings are shown in the table.

HYPERKALAEMIA	HYPOKALAEMIA
Tall, tented T waves	Flat, broad T waves
Loss of P waves	ST depression
QRS complex broadening	Long Q–T interval
Sine-wave-shaped ECG	Ventricular dysrhythmias
Cardiac arrest rhythms	

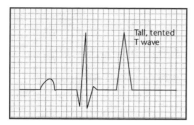

Fig 10.32: T waves in hyperkalaemia.

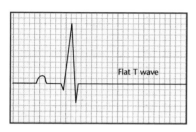

Fig 10.33: T waves in hypokalaemia.

Summary

When interpreting an ECG, always use the following headings:

Heart rate	QRS complexes
Heart rhythm	ST segment
Cardiac axis	Q–T interval
P waves	T waves

Cardiac arrest rhythms

When a patient has a cardiac arrest, the heart stops pumping blood around the body. The electrical activity in the heart does not always stop immediately, however, and the immediate advanced management of patients with cardiac arrest is largely determined by exactly what is happening to the heart rhythm. It is imperative that you are able to identify each of the following rhythms.

'Shockable' rhythms

If one of these rhythms is identified, the priority in treatment is to deliver electricity to the heart using a defibrillator.

Ventricular fibrillation (VF)

This is identified by the erratic nature of the electrical activity. It is random and unpredictable. It is sometimes classified as being fine or coarse depending on whether the electrical activity is of small (fine) or large (coarse) amplitude.

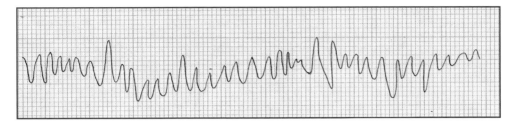

Fig 10.34

Ventricular tachycardia (VT)

This is a broad QRS complex tachycardia that has a very distinctive appearance on an ECG monitor. It is not always associated with cardiac arrest, but is always a significant arrhythmia.

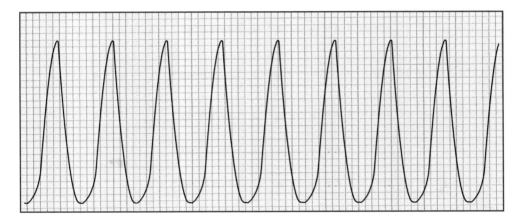

Fig 10.35

'Non-shockable' rhythms

Defibrillation will not be helpful to patients with one of these rhythms. Cardiopulmonary resuscitation should be administered and attempts made to reverse the cause of the cardiac arrest.

Pulseless electrical activity (PEA) (also known as electromechanical dissociation or EMD)

The heart rhythm is indistinguishable from a heart rhythm normally compatible with life.

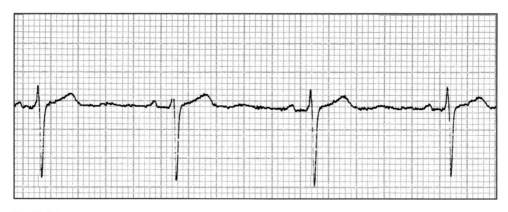

Fig 10.36

Asystole

There is no identifiable cardiac electrical activity. It is important to adjust the gain on the ECG monitor to ensure that 'fine' ventricular fibrillation is not missed.

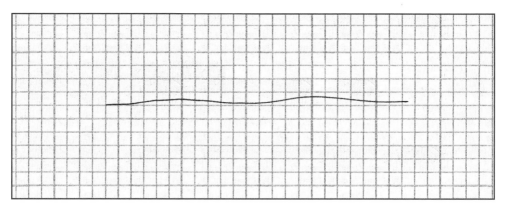

Fig 10.37

P-wave asystole

In this rhythm, only P waves are seen. There is no ventricular activity. This rhythm may respond to cardiac pacing.

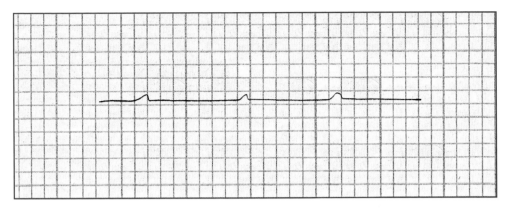

Fig 10.38

Cardiac imaging

Echocardiography

It is unlikely that you will be required to have detailed knowledge of echocardiography at undergraduate level. However, it is important that you are familiar with echocardiographic reports and understand how to interpret them.

You may find it helpful to use the following headings when reading echocardiographic reports. Common abnormalities and points to bear in mind are also listed.

COMPONENT OF REPORT	COMMENT
Size of heart chambers (atria and ventricles)	The normal maximum diameter of the left atrium is 4.5 cm. Enlargement of the left atrium is particularly significant in patients with atrial fibrillation. The normal maximum diameter of the left ventricle in diastole is 5.5 cm – this will be increased in abnormally enlarged left ventricles, eg with dilated cardiomyopathy
Ventricular septal thickness	This should be less than 1.2 cm. A thickened septum should raise suspicions of hypertrophic obstructive cardiomyopathy (HOCM)
Left ventricular function	Hypokinesis refers to walls that contract poorly. Akinesis refers to walls that do not appear to contract at all. The left ventricular ejection fraction is normally around 65%
Details about each valve	Stenotic or regurgitant valves will often be described in terms of severity as trace, mild, moderate or severe. Often pressure gradients across valves and valve areas are documented. For the aortic valve, severe stenosis is present if there is a pressure gradient of more than 50 mmHg across the valve, or if the valve area is less than 1 cm^2

COMPONENT OF REPORT	COMMENT
Vegetations or tumours	Bear in mind that a small vegetation may be missed with transthoracic echocardiography. Transoesophageal echocardiography is more reliable
Estimated pulmonary artery pressure	A pressure >35 mmHg suggests pulmonary hypertension. Note that this is an estimated pressure reading only
Pericardial effusion	Present or absent

Other imaging modalities

Increasingly, computed tomography (CT) and magnetic resonance imaging (MRI) of the heart are being performed in patients with suspected cardiac disease. CT assessment of the coronary arteries, including an assessment of calcification (calcium scoring), is likely to be used increasingly in the non-invasive assessment of patients with chest pain. MRI of the heart can provide detailed information on many aspects of cardiac structure and function. Interpretation of such images is in the territory of a specialist cardiologist and is certainly beyond the scope of this book. Thankfully the written reports from such imaging investigations are usually self-explanatory.

Dynamic tests in cardiology

Dynamic heart testing is commonly used to investigate chest pain and known ischaemic heart disease. In the resting state, a patient with significant coronary artery atherosclerosis may have a normal ECG. However, when the heart is put under stress by increasing its rate, its energy requirements increase. If sufficient blood cannot be supplied to the myocardium under such circumstances, the tissue becomes ischaemic and the ECG will change.

Features that would be in keeping with ischaemic heart disease include horizontal or down-sloping ST segment depression or elevation, particularly if these are associated with angina or a reduction in blood pressure.

Other dynamic tests are used to assess cardiac function in particular patient groups. In patients who are unable to exercise, pharmacological agents (eg dobutamine) can be administered to increase the heart rate and put the heart under stress. Cardiac function can then be assessed by performing echocardiography or by nuclear imaging techniques which look at the uptake of isotopes by cardiac muscle. By so doing, areas of the heart that pump defectively or have inadequate blood supply can be identified.

Cardiac biomarkers

Testing for the presence of the cardiac contractile protein troponin (type I or T) is currently the test most commonly performed to assess for myocardial cell damage. Troponin is normally involved in cardiac muscle cell contraction, and is released systemically when cardiac muscle cells are damaged. Troponin may be elevated after 2 hours, and can stay elevated for up to 7 days. Levels are generally measured 12 hours after the onset of symptoms. A fairly recent development in this area is in the use of 'high-sensitivity' troponin, which rises more quickly than standard troponin. Unfortunately, elevated troponin levels are not specific to myocardial infarction, and may be found in conditions such as those listed in the box:

CAUSES OF RAISED TROPONIN	
• Myocardial infarction	• Renal failure
• Heart failure	• Severe sepsis
• Myocarditis	• Supraventricular tachycardia
• Pulmonary embolism	

Aside from troponin measurement, a range of enzymes rises in concentration after heart damage. These vary in the time taken to peak and to be cleared from the blood after a cardiac event. Differences in the tests are shown in the table below.

TEST	TIME TO PEAK (h)	DURATION OF ELEVATED BLOOD LEVEL AFTER CARDIAC EVENT
Creatine kinase (CK)	24	48
AST	30	60
Lactate dehydrogenase (LDH)	72	240

Creatine kinase is also released from damaged skeletal muscle. Its level will therefore rise in several instances other than myocardial damage, such as trauma, polymyositis/dermatomyositis (when muscle is inflamed) and rhabdomyolysis (when muscle breaks down). To aid differentiation between these conditions, isoenzymes (different types) of CK can be measured. The isoenzyme released mainly from cardiac muscle is called CK-MB, and a high level of this enzyme should raise suspicions of cardiac damage.

B-type natriuretic peptide (BNP)

In heart failure, heart chambers are stretched more than normal. In such circumstances, substances are released that cause increased sodium excretion (natriuresis) in an attempt to improve the situation for the failing heart. One such substance is BNP. BNP, and its inactive cleavage fragment (N-terminal pro-BNP), tend to be elevated in patients with heart failure to such an extent that, if the level of these hormones is normal, then heart failure is an unlikely diagnosis. The extremely low likelihood of heart failure in a patient who has the combination of a normal ECG and a normal BNP or N-terminal pro-BNP level makes this approach a very effective screening test for this condition.

Case 10.1

A 50-year-old manager presents to the accident and emergency department complaining of chest pain. He is very worried that he may be having a heart attack, since his brother had one last year. He has no other risk factors for cardiac disease. On further questioning, he describes doing heavy work in his garden on the previous day. Examination reveals an anxious man with tenderness on either side of the sternum. An ECG is performed.

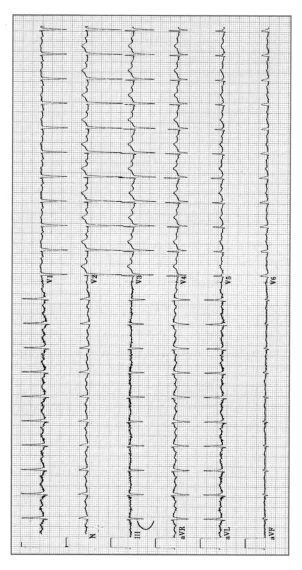

What is your interpretation?

Answer 10.1

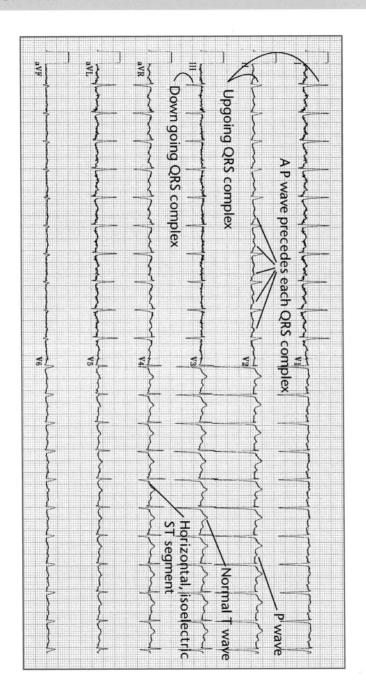

Heart rate

There are 12 small squares between consecutive R waves. The ventricular rate is therefore 1500 ÷ 12 = 125 beats/min.

Heart rhythm

A P wave precedes each QRS complex. The P–R interval is normal (four small squares) and does not vary from beat to beat. The rhythm is sinus rhythm.

Cardiac axis

Leads I and II are upgoing. Lead III is downgoing. The axis is normal.

P waves

P waves are of normal size and shape.

QRS complexes

There are no abnormal Q waves. The R and S waves are of normal height. The QRS complex is of normal duration (two small squares).

ST segment

The ST segment is horizontal and isoelectric.

Q–T interval

The Q–T interval is normal (1.5 large squares).

T waves

T waves are normal in size and shape.

Conclusion – sinus tachycardia. The most likely cause of this is anxiety. Sinus tachycardia is the most common ECG finding in patients with a pulmonary embolism, so this diagnosis should be considered. However, in this case, history and examination point to the true cause of this man's chest pain – muscular strain.

Case 10.2

A 70-year-old woman with a history of a myocardial infarction presents with palpitations that are of recent onset. Her ECG is shown.

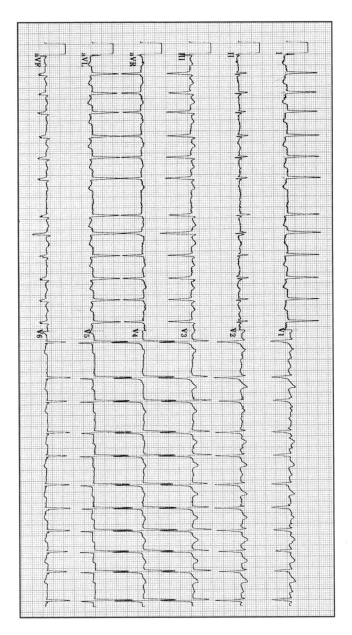

How would you interpret it?

Answer 10.2

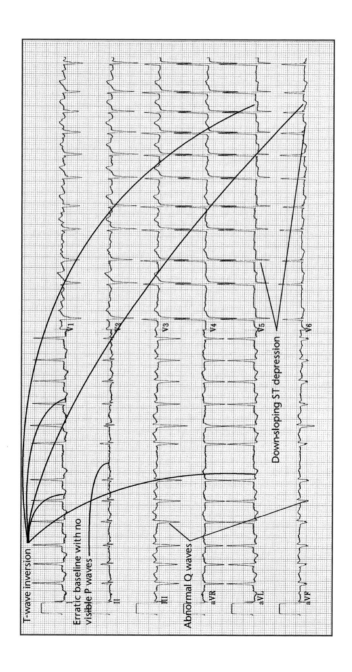

T-wave inversion

Erratic baseline with no visible P waves

Abnormal Q waves

Downsloping ST depression

V1
V2
V3
V4
V5
V6

II
III
aVR
aVL
aVF

Heart rate

There are nine small squares between the first two consecutive R waves in lead I. The ventricular rate is therefore 1500 ÷ 9 = 167 beats/min. However, since the rhythm is clearly irregular, a more accurate assessment of heart rate can be made by measuring the distance between the first and eleventh R waves and dividing this distance by 10 to find the average R–R interval.

By this method, there are approximately 20.5 large squares between the first and eleventh R waves. The average R–R interval is therefore 2.05 large squares. The heart rate is 300 ÷ 2.05 = 146 beats/min.

Heart rhythm

No P waves are visible. The baseline is erratic. QRS complexes occur irregularly. The rhythm is atrial fibrillation.

Cardiac axis

Leads I and II are upgoing. Lead III is downgoing. The axis is normal.

P waves

No P waves are visible.

QRS complexes

There are abnormal Q waves in leads III and aVF, indicating a previous inferior myocardial infarction. The R and S waves are of normal height. The QRS complex is of normal duration (two small squares).

ST segment

The ST segment is horizontal and isoelectric in leads II, III, aVR, aVF, V1, V2 and V3. There is slight downsloping ST depression in the other leads, most marked in I and V6.

Q–T interval

The Q–T interval is normal (seven small squares).

T waves

T waves are normal in size. There is T-wave inversion in leads I, aVL, V5 and V6.

Conclusion – atrial fibrillation with a ventricular rate of 146 beats/min. Inferior Q waves. There is downsloping ST elevation and T-wave inversion in the leads looking at the lateral aspect of the heart. The patient may be on digoxin, but the T-wave changes probably indicate ischaemia. This may be related to the rapid heart rate, and may disappear if the rate is slowed. This woman's palpitations are due to a sudden onset of atrial fibrillation.

Case 10.3

A 74-year-old man is admitted complaining of dizziness. He has had several myocardial infarctions in the past. Clinical examination reveals a pulse rate of 30 beats/min, and a blood pressure of 62/46 mmHg. An ECG is performed.

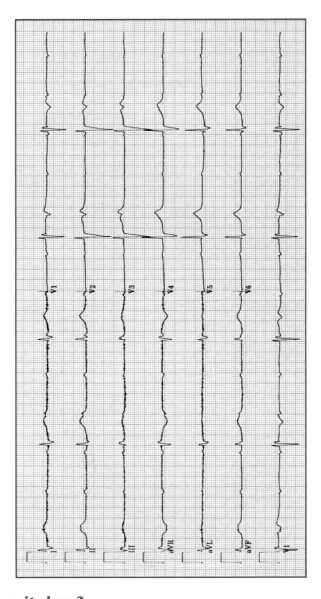

What does it show?

Answer 10.3

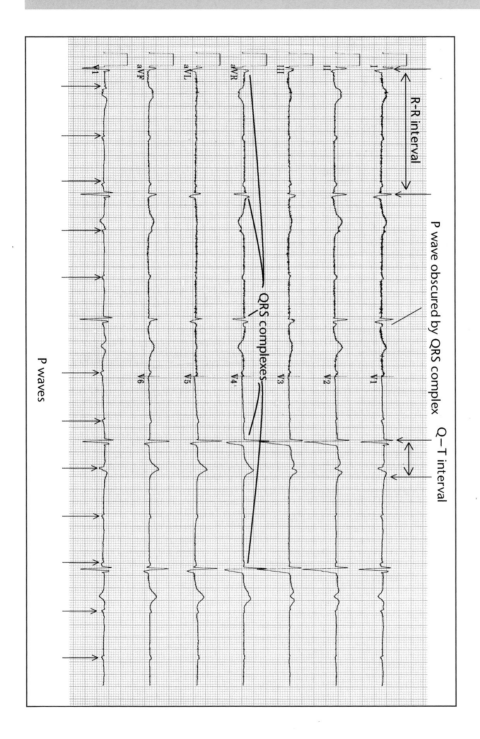

Heart rate

There are 10 big squares between consecutive R waves. The ventricular rate is therefore 300 ÷ 10 = 30 beats/min.

Heart rhythm

P waves are seen, but these show no consistent relationship with the QRS complexes. The P waves and QRS complexes are completely dissociated. The rhythm is third-degree heart block.

Cardiac axis

Leads I, II and III are all upgoing. The axis is normal.

P waves

P waves are of normal size and shape. One P wave is difficult to see because it is obscured by a simultaneous QRS complex.

QRS complexes

There are no abnormal Q waves. The QRS complexes are narrow (two small squares). This indicates that the electrical signal to the ventricles is originating in specialised conducting tissue. The R and S waves are of normal height.

ST segment

The ST segment is horizontal and isoelectric.

Q–T interval

The Q–T interval is prolonged (three large squares). The Bazett correction is therefore required. Three large squares= 3 x 0.2 second = 0.6 second. The R–R interval is 10 large squares = 10 x 0.2 second = 2 seconds. The Q–Tc is therefore:

$$\frac{0.6}{\sqrt{2}} = 0.42 \text{ second}$$

T waves

T waves are normal in size and shape.

Conclusion – third-degree heart block with a ventricular rate of 30 beats/min. This rhythm is resulting in symptomatic hypotension. Consideration should be given to an emergency pacing procedure, followed by the placement of a permanent pacemaker.

The patient eventually had a permanent pacemaker inserted. An ECG was performed to check its function, and is shown below. Note the presence of pacing spikes, which indicate that the pacemaker is discharging. When a pacemaker stimulates the ventricles directly, the QRS complexes will be wide and bizarre. It is impossible to interpret anything else from the ECG in such circumstances, other than that an artificial pacemaker is present.

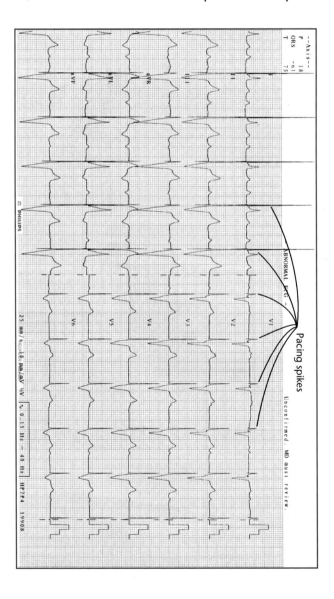

Case 10.4

A 52-year-old male shop assistant presents as an emergency to his general practitioner complaining of central chest pain. This has been present for 30 minutes. He is sweaty and short of breath, and complains of nausea. His risk factors for ischaemic heart disease include smoking and hypertension.

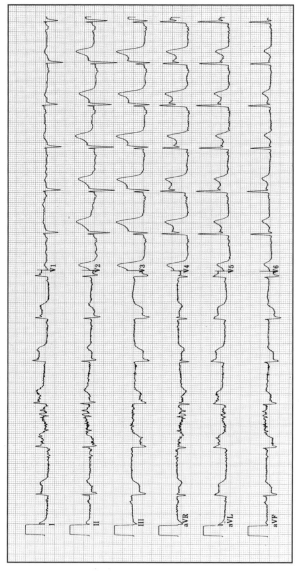

His ECG is shown. How would you interpret it?

Answer 10.4

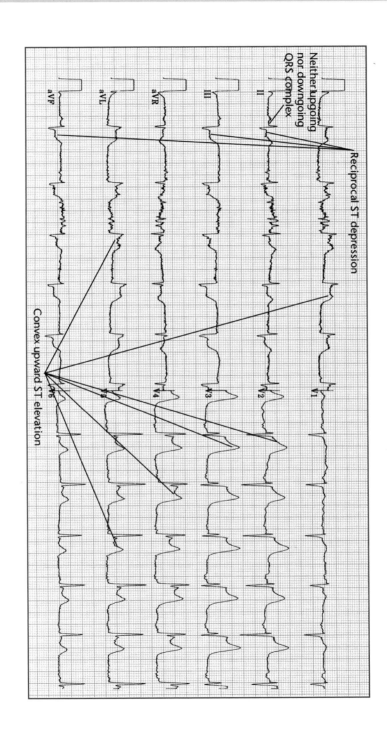

Neither upgoing nor downgoing QRS complex

Reciprocal ST depression

Convex upward ST elevation

Heart rate

There are 4.2 big squares between consecutive R waves. The ventricular rate is therefore 300 ÷ 4.2 = 71 beats/min.

Heart rhythm

A P wave precedes each QRS complex. The P–R interval is normal (four small squares) and does not vary from beat to beat. The rhythm is sinus rhythm.

Cardiac axis

Lead I is upgoing. Lead III is downgoing. Lead II is neither upgoing nor downgoing. The axis is approaching that of left axis deviation.

P waves

P waves are of normal size and shape.

QRS complexes

There are no abnormal Q waves. The R and S waves are of normal height. The QRS complex is of normal duration (two small squares).

ST segment

The ST segment is elevated, in a convex shape, in leads I, aVL, V2, V3, V4 and V5. The ST segment is depressed and horizontal in leads II, III, aVR and aVF. When ST depression accompanies ST elevation, it is known as reciprocal ST depression.

Q–T interval

The Q–T interval is normal (1.5 large squares).

T waves

The T waves appear large, but are difficult to interpret on account of the ST segment changes.

Conclusion – anterolateral ST elevation myocardial infarction or STEMI (ie affecting the anterior and lateral surfaces of the heart). Reciprocal ST depression in some of the limb leads.

Case 10.5

An 80-year-old female nursing home resident presents with acute confusion. No other history is available. On examination, she is tachypnoeic, with oxygen saturations of 83% on 85% oxygen. She is peripherally cyanosed. Blood pressure is 74/32 mmHg. On auscultating her lungs, she has medium inspiratory crepitations to her midzones.

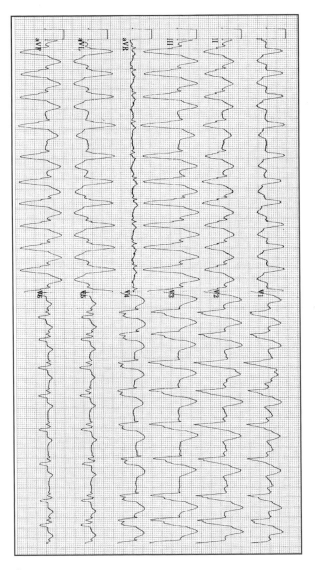

Interpret the ECG

Answer 10.5

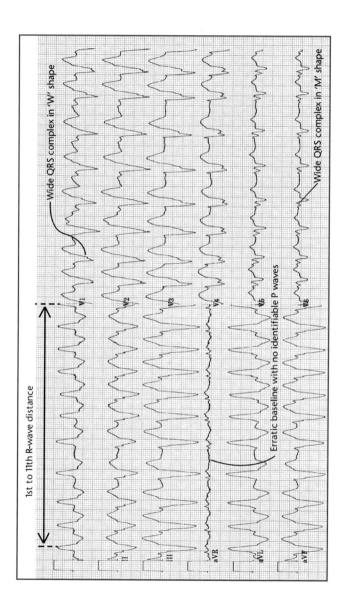

Heart rate

There are 11 small squares between the first two consecutive R waves in lead I. The ventricular rate is therefore 1500 ÷ 11 = 136 beats/min. However, since the rhythm is irregular, a more accurate assessment of heart rate can be made by measuring the distance between the first and eleventh R waves and dividing this distance by 10 to find the average R–R interval.

By this method, there are 24 large squares between the first and eleventh R waves. The average R–R interval is therefore 2.4 large squares. The heart rate is 300 ÷ 2.4 = 125 beats/min.

Heart rhythm

No P waves are visible. The baseline is erratic. QRS complexes occur irregularly. The rhythm is atrial fibrillation.

Cardiac axis

Lead I is upgoing. Leads II and III are downgoing. There is left axis deviation.

P waves

No P waves are visible.

QRS complexes

The QRS complexes are abnormally wide. The complex in V1 has a 'W' shape, and that in V6 is 'M' shaped. This is left bundle-branch block.

ST segment

The ST segment is difficult to visualise.

Q–T interval

The Q–T interval is difficult to measure.

T waves

T waves appear grossly abnormal in size and shape.

Conclusion – atrial fibrillation at 125 beats/min with left bundle-branch block. When this pattern is present, it is impossible to make any further comments about an ECG (ie ST segment changes or T-wave abnormalities). Left bundle-branch block that is of new onset would be in keeping with an acute myocardial infarction. Old ECGs should be reviewed to determine whether this ECG finding is new.

Case 10.6

You are called to a cardiac arrest. Nursing staff have attached ECG electrodes, and the following rhythm is noted on the monitor. What is the rhythm?

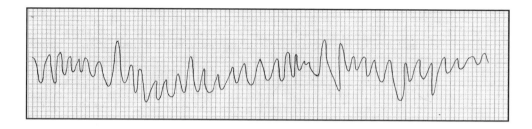

Answer 10.6

It is entirely possible to approach the interpretation of this rhythm as with all the ECGs above. However, for practical purposes, this rhythm should be instantly recognised as ventricular fibrillation (VF) by its erratic nature, and appropriate treatment given. This involves cardiac defibrillation.

After delivering three shocks, the rhythm on the monitor changes to that shown below. A pulse is still not present. What is the rhythm now?

Again, this strip can be analysed in detail, but it should be instantly recognised by its shape as ventricular tachycardia (VT). The ECG shows a tachycardia with wide QRS complexes. This rhythm can be associated with a cardiac output, so it would be imperative to check for the presence of a pulse. Cardiac arrest associated with VT is treated with defibrillation.

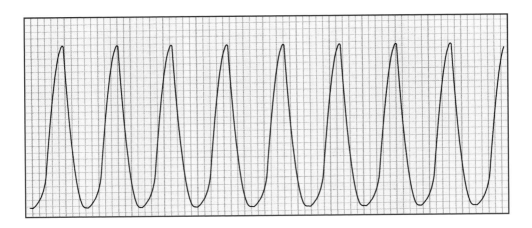

Case 10.7

A 67-year-old woman is reviewed in the cardiology clinic 2 months after a myocardial infarction. She complains of shortness of breath on walking 100 metres on the flat, which she did not have before her heart attack. On further questioning, she reports having to sleep on five pillows to prevent shortness of breath. An echocardiogram is requested.

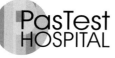

PasTest
HOSPITAL

Aortic root diameter is 3.3 cm
Morphologically normal aortic valve. No restriction of aortic valve leaflet opening. Aortic regurgitation (trace)
Left ventricular cavity size and wall thickness are normal. Left ventricular diastolic cavity diameter is 5.1 cm. Septal diastolic thickness is 1.1 cm
Posterior wall thickness is 1.1 cm. Severely hypokinetic anterior wall. Left ventricular ejection fraction is 25%
Morphologically normal mitral valve. Mitral regurgitation (trace)
Normal left atrial dimensions
Estimated pulmonary artery systolic pressure is 22 mmHg
Normal right ventricular cavity dimension. Right ventricular systolic function is normal. Normal tricuspid valve
Normal inferior vena cava and hepatic vein size indicating normal venous pressures
Technically fair study. Other cardiac valves and chambers appear normal. No pericardial effusion. No evidence of bacterial endocarditis on this study

How would you explain this woman's symptoms?

Answer 10.7

The important points to take away from the echocardiographic report are as follows:

Size of heart chambers (atria and ventricles)	Normal
Ventricular septal thickness	Normal
Left ventricular function	Severe left ventricular wall hypo-kinesis. Markedly reduced left ventricular ejection fraction
Details about each valve	Only a trace of aortic and mitral regurgitation
Vegetations or tumours	None seen
Estimated pulmonary artery pressure	Normal
Pericardial effusion	None

This woman has symptoms (dyspnoea and orthopnoea) of left ventricular failure. Her echocardiogram demonstrates the poor residual function of her left ventricle following her myocardial infarction.

Case 10.8

You assess a patient after a short-lived episode of central chest pain. His medical history includes chronic kidney disease, not requiring dialysis at present. A 12-lead ECG is normal. Blood is sampled 12 hours after the onset of pain.

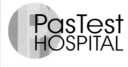

Na+	143 mmol/l
K+	4.6 mmol/l
Urea	13.8 mmol/l
Creatinine	355 µmol/l
eGFR	25 ml/min per 1.73 m²
Troponin T	0.56 µg/l

Has the patient suffered a myocardial infarction?

Answer 10.8

It is difficult to be sure whether or not the patient has had a myocardial infarction (MI) based on the information given. The chest pain was short-lived, and the ECG normal which points away from MI. Although the troponin T level is quite markedly raised over normal, there is an alternative explanation for this other than MI, namely renal failure. A reasonable course of action in this case would be to repeat an ECG and repeat the troponin T level after several more hours. If the patient has really had an MI, one would expect the ECG to change and/or the troponin level to change.

Case 10.9

You assess an elderly man who complains of shortness of breath on exertion. He has fine crepitations on auscultation of both lung bases, and you suspect cardiac failure as a possible diagnosis. On review of his blood tests, you note that a colleague requested the following test 1 month ago.

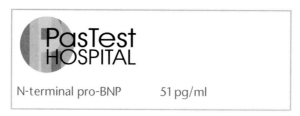

PasTest
HOSPITAL

N-terminal pro-BNP   51 pg/ml

Should you order an echocardiogram?

Answer 10.9

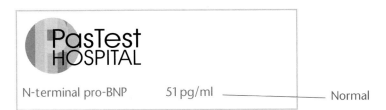

N-terminal pro-BNP	51 pg/ml	Normal

The finding of a normal N-terminal pro-BNP level in this man makes the diagnosis of cardiac failure extremely unlikely. Another cause for his breathlessness and crepitations should be found. A chest X-ray would seem like a useful first test.

Case 10.10

A 55-year-old man who smokes and has a strong family history of coronary heart disease presents 14 h after a 30-min episode of central crushing chest pain. He was afraid to come to hospital at the time. He is currently pain free, and his ECG was normal. The A&E officer requests the following test:

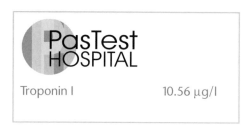

Troponin I	10.56 µg/l

Where should this patient be managed?

Answer 10.10

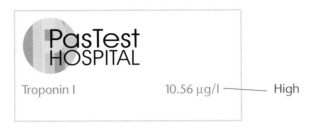

PasTest
HOSPITAL

Troponin I   10.56 µg/l ———— High

This patient has a significantly elevated troponin I indicating a significant amount of cardiac damage. The clinical information is consistent with myocardial infarction. The patient is at significant risk of cardiac arrhythmias and should be managed in a coronary care unit.

PATHOLOGY

11

PATHOLOGY

This chapter lists typical pathological findings for a range of disease states. It is not by any means comprehensive, but includes most of the classic abnormalities that are commonly tested in general medical examinations. Further reading will be required when preparing for pathology examinations.

DISEASE	TYPICAL PATHOLOGICAL CHANGES
Gastroenterology	
Barrett's oesophagus	Lower oesophageal epithelium undergoes metaplasia to become gastric or intestinal-type epithelium
Coeliac disease	Total or subtotal villous atrophy in the small bowel Crypt hyperplasia with inflammatory cells in the mucosa
Crohn's disease	Can affect any part of the gastrointestinal tract *Macroscopically*: skip lesions (ie lengths of normal bowel between diseased segments); cobblestone appearance with fissured ulcers *Microscopically*: thickened wall with transmural inflammation; granulomas
Ulcerative colitis	Affects large bowel only Affects mucosa and submucosa only Crypt abscesses and superficial ulcers
Chronic cholecystitis	Chronic inflammatory changes Rokitansky–Aschoff sinuses
Hepatology	
Acute viral hepatitis	Swelling of hepatocytes with spotty necrosis Councilman bodies

DISEASE	TYPICAL PATHOLOGICAL CHANGES
Alcoholic hepatitis	Fatty accumulation in cytoplasmic vacuoles, necrosis, Mallory hyaline material
Chronic active hepatitis	Piecemeal necrosis
Autoimmune hepatitis	Interface hepatitis, portal plasma cell infiltration
Haemochromatosis	Excessive hepatic iron (shows up blue on Perl's stain)
Primary biliary cirrhosis	Portal hepatitis and granulomatous destruction of bile ducts. Later, periportal hepatitis and bile duct proliferation
Liver cirrhosis	*Macroscopically*: macronodular or micronodular *Microscopically*: fibrous tissue (shows up red on von Gieson stain)

Respiratory

Diffuse alveolar damage (DAD) which can lead to adult respiratory distress syndrome (ARDS)	Alveolar hyaline membranes and thickened alveolar walls
Previous asbestos exposure	Asbestos bodies in lung
Pulmonary fibrosis	Proliferation of type II pneumocytes with thickening of the alveolar walls

Nephrology

Malignant hypertension	Renal arteriole fibrinoid necrosis
Diabetic glomerulosclerosis	Kimmelstiel–Wilson nodules, thickened capillary basement membranes with hyalinisation of arterioles

DISEASE	TYPICAL PATHOLOGICAL CHANGES
Haematology	
Hodgkin's disease	Reed–Sternberg cells Abnormal lymph node architecture Nodular sclerosing type has fibrous tissue
Myelofibrosis	Bone marrow fibrosis secondary to fibroblast proliferation
Multiple myeloma	Plasma cell proliferation in bone marrow
Rheumatology	
Temporal arteritis	Temporal artery biopsy may be normal Alternatively, plasma cells, lymphocytes and multinucleate giant cells can be present
Polymyositis	Muscle fibre necrosis Lymphocyte infiltration
Endocrinology	
Pituitary tumours	Acromegaly is associated with acidophil macroadenomas (somatotroph adenomas) Hyperprolactinaemia is associated with chromophobe adenomas ACTH excess is associated with basophil microadenomas (corticotroph adenomas)
Neurology	
Alzheimer's disease	*Macroscopically*: thinning of gyri *Microscopically*: neurofibrillary tangles; plaques
Parkinson's disease and dementia with Lewy bodies	Lewy bodies (inclusions inside neurons)
Obstetrics and gynaecology	
Ovarian endometriosis	*Macroscopically*: chocolate cyst

GENETICS

12

GENETICS

Family trees

In clinical practice, family trees are often recorded when there is a suspicion that a disease may have a familial element.

To the untrained eye, interpretation of family trees can seem like a daunting process, and many students resort to guessing what the inheritance pattern might be. However, if a few simple rules are borne in mind, interpretation can be made fairly simple. Being able to work out the expected inheritance patterns for the common mendelian disorders from first principles is a good way to check that your answer is correct.

Work through the various inheritance patterns for the common mendelian disorders below, and attempt to reproduce the information for yourself. This will be much easier to remember than if you simply learn off a list of rules.

The two main classes of conditions that are inherited in a mendelian manner are:

- autosomal conditions (affecting the autosomes, ie chromosomes 1 to 22)
- sex chromosomal conditions (affecting the sex chromosomes, ie X and Y).

> Genotype refers to the genetic code.
> Phenotype refers to the actual manifestation of the genetic code.

Autosomal conditions

Autosomal dominant inheritance

There are usually two copies of each chromosome in each cell, each carrying copies of the same genes. In autosomal dominant conditions, inheritance of one faulty gene is sufficient to give rise to the disorder. Thus one chromosome in the pair will be normal; the other will carry the faulty gene.

In the following diagram, the letter 'a' is used to denote a normal chromosome. The capital letter 'A' represents a chromosome with an abnormal gene. Thus an individual with two 'a' chromosomes will be normal. Someone with one 'a' chromosome and one 'A' chromosome will have the disorder, since only one faulty gene is needed for the condition to be manifest. If both parents are affected, it would also be possible for offspring to have two 'A' chromosomes.

Since 50% of the offspring's genetic code comes from one parent and 50% from the other, there is a 50% chance that either chromosome will be passed on.

	Mother	
	a	a
a	aa	aa
A	Aa	Aa

Father (a, A)

In the example, the father has an autosomal dominant condition, and therefore has one normal chromosome (a) and one abnormal chromosome (A). The mother has two normal chromosomes. There are four possible ways that the genes can be passed on to the offspring (aa, aa, Aa and Aa).

Thus for autosomal dominant conditions:

- both males and females can be affected
- if one parent is affected, there will be a 50% chance that a child will also be affected.

Autosomal recessive inheritance

For an autosomal recessive disorder to be manifest, both chromosomes in a pair must carry the abnormal gene. One abnormal gene must therefore be passed on from each parent.

If a person has one normal and one abnormal chromosome, he or she is a termed 'a carrier' and does not exhibit any features of the disorder, and therefore will appear normal (ie normal phenotype).

The inheritance pattern for one carrier parent and one normal parent will be as follows (remember 'a' is the normal chromosome, and 'A' the abnormal).

	Mother	
	a	a
a	aa	aa
A	Aa	Aa

Father (a, A)

For autosomal recessive conditions with one carrier parent:

- both male and female offspring can be carriers
- 50% of the offspring will be carriers.

The inheritance pattern for two carrier parents will be as follows.

		Mother	
		a	A
	a	aa	aA
Father			
	A	Aa	AA

For autosomal recessive conditions with two carrier parents:

- both male and female offspring can be carriers or be affected
- 50% of the offspring will be carriers
- 25% of the offspring will be normal (ie not carriers)
- 25% of the offspring will have the condition.

The inheritance pattern for one affected parent will be as follows.

		Mother	
		a	a
	A	Aa	Aa
Father			
	A	Aa	Aa

For autosomal recessive conditions with an affected parent:

- both male and female offspring can be carriers
- all offspring will be carriers.

Sex chromosomal conditions

X-linked recessive inheritance

X-linked disorders involve faulty genes found on the X chromosome. Since females have two X chromosomes, having one faulty chromosome is of minor consequence with a recessive disorder, because the other X chromosome is normal. Males, however, have only one X (but also one Y) chromosome. A faulty X chromosome in a male will therefore result in phenotypical effects.

If a female has one abnormal X chromosome, they are termed 'a carrier' and generally do not exhibit any features of the disorder. Occasionally mild signs of disease may be present.

The inheritance pattern for a carrier mother and a normal father will be as follows (X = normal chromosome, X = abnormal chromosome):

		Mother	
		X	X
Father	X	XX	XX
	Y	YX	YX

For X-linked recessive disorders with a carrier mother:

- only males can be affected
- 50% of male offspring will have the disorder
- 50% of female offspring will be carriers
- 50% of all offspring will be normal.

The inheritance pattern for an affected father and a normal mother will be as follows:

		Mother	
		X	X
Father	X	XX	XX
	Y	YX	YX

For X-linked recessive disorders with an affected father:

- no offspring will be affected
- all daughters will be carriers
- all sons will be normal.

X-linked dominant inheritance

In these disorders, only one faulty X chromosome is necessary for the disease to be manifest. Thus, diseases can occur in both male and females.

The inheritance pattern for an affected mother and a normal father will be as follows:

		Mother	
		X	X
Father	X	XX	XX
	Y	YX	YX

For X-linked dominant disorders with an affected mother:

- both males and females can be affected
- 50% of male offspring will have the disorder
- 50% of female offspring will have the disorder.

The inheritance pattern for an affected father and a normal mother will be as follows:

		Mother	
		X	X
Father	X	XX	XX
	Y	YX	YX

For X-linked dominant disorders with an affected father:

- only female offspring can be affected
- all daughters will have the disorder
- all sons will be normal.

Other modes of inheritance

Mitochondrial inheritance

Mitochondria are cellular organelles that have a major role in energy production. They have their own DNA, which may undergo mutations. Diseases caused by mitochondrial genetic problems have an interesting inheritance pattern resulting from the fact that female ova all contain mitochondria; however, male sperm do not. Therefore, mitochondrial disorders can be passed on only by females. To summarise:

- both males and females can be affected
- affected females can pass on the disorder to all offspring
- affected males cannot pass on the disorder.

Genetic imprinting

This phenomenon relates to the fact that certain genes are expressed only if inherited from a particular parent. This can best be explained by looking at two conditions – Prader–Willi and Angelman syndromes. For Prader–Willi syndrome, only the paternal gene is important. Failure to inherit the paternal copy will therefore result in the syndrome. Angelman syndrome results from failure to inherit the maternal gene. The disorders may result from gene deletion mutations, where the gene from a particular parent is deleted. Alternatively, they may arise when two chromosomes are inherited from one parent rather than one from each. This is known as uniparental disomy.

> **MEMORY AID**
>
> In **P**rader–Willi syndrome – the **P**aternal gene is inactive
> In Angel**m**an syndrome – the **M**aternal gene is inactive

Other points

Variable expression relates to the fact that a person may carry the necessary genetic make-up for a condition, but not exhibit all the phenotypical features. At the extreme of this is 'non-penetrance' where the person has no features of the condition.

Genetic disorders may appear to arise out of the blue, with no family members being affected. This is most commonly due to a new genetic mutation, but can also result from gonadal mosaicism where a parent carries the mutated genes only in the germ cells.

Family tree interpretation

When faced with a family tree, and asked to comment on inheritance patterns, the flow diagram below should be helpful.

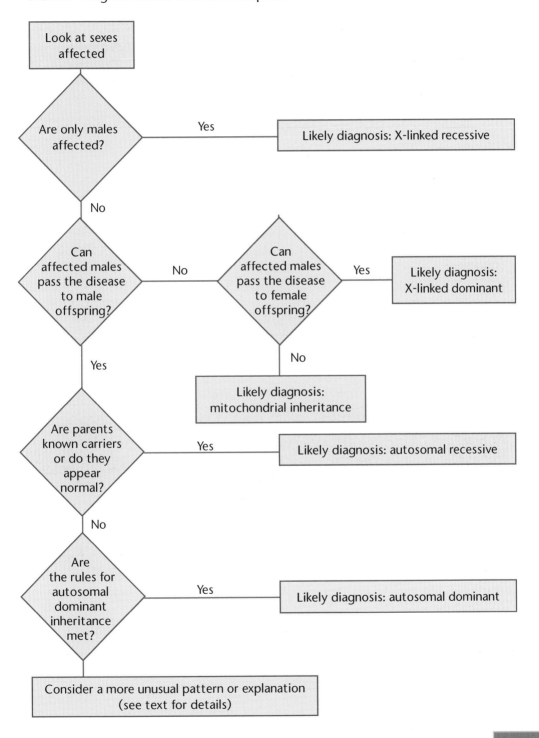

Examples of genetic conditions with different inheritance patterns

Those most commonly tested in undergraduate examinations are highlighted in bold in the following table.

MODE OF INHERITANCE	EXAMPLES
Autosomal dominant	Achondroplasia **Adult polycystic kidney disease** **Dystrophia myotonica** Ehlers–Danlos syndrome Familial adenomatous polyposis **Familial hypercholesterolaemia** Hereditary haemorrhagic telangiectasia **Huntington disease** **Marfan syndrome** **Neurofibromatosis** Noonan syndrome Osteogenesis imperfecta Otosclerosis **Tuberous sclerosis**
Autosomal recessive	Albinism Congenital adrenal hyperplasia **Cystic fibrosis** Friedreich ataxia Galactosaemia Glycogen storage diseases **Hereditary haemochromatosis** Hurler syndrome Oculocutaneous albinism Phenylketonuria **Sickle cell disease** Tay–Sachs disease Thalassaemia Wilson's disease
X-linked dominant	Vitamin D-resistant rickets

X-linked recessive	Alport syndrome
	Becker muscular dystrophy
	Duchenne muscular dystrophy
	Fragile X syndrome
	Glucose-6-phosphate dehydrogenase deficiency
	Haemophilia A
	Haemophilia B
	Hunter syndrome
Mitochondrial	Leber hereditary optic neuropathy

Karyotype analysis

The following table lists the common chromosomal abnormalities that you would be expected to recognise.

CHROMOSOMAL ABNORMALITY	CONDITION
Trisomy 21	Down syndrome
Trisomy 18	Edward syndrome
Trisomy 12	Patau syndrome
45, XO	Turner syndrome
47, XXY	Klinefelter syndrome
47, XXX	Triple X syndrome
47, XXY	Associated with behavioural problems
5p−	Cri-du-chat syndrome
Microdeletion at 22q11	DiGeorge syndrome
Microdeletion at 7q11	Williams syndrome

Common mutations

DISEASE	COMMON MUTATION
Cystic fibrosis	ΔF508 mutation on long arm of chromosome 7. This codes for the cystic fibrosis transmembrane conductance regulator
Haemochromatosis	C282Y mutation on the *HFE* gene on the short arm of chromosome 6. The H63D mutation can also be found

Case 12.1

What is the inheritance pattern in the following family tree?

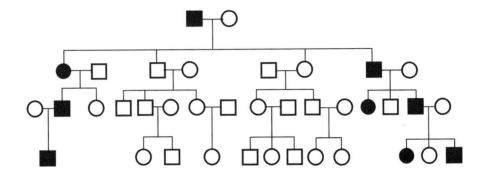

Key

☐ unaffected male   ■ affected male

◯ unaffected female   ● affected female

Answer 12.1

- Both males and females are affected
- Male-to-male inheritance is possible
- One of the parents of all affected cases is also affected.
- If one parent is affected, there appears to be approximately a 50% chance that a child will also be affected.

The inheritance pattern is therefore autosomal dominant.

Case 12.2

Some members of the following family suffer from a rare bone disease. What is the inheritance pattern?

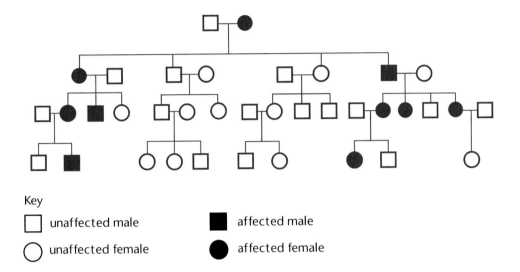

Key

☐ unaffected male   ■ affected male

○ unaffected female   ● affected female

Answer 12.2

- Both males and females are affected
- There are no instances of male-to-male transmission
- Male-to-female transmission is possible, with all daughters of an affected male having the condition.

The likely diagnosis is vitamin D-resistant rickets, with the inheritance pattern being X-linked dominant.

Case 12.3

Some family members have a rare genetic disorder. This is their family tree. What is the likely inheritance pattern?

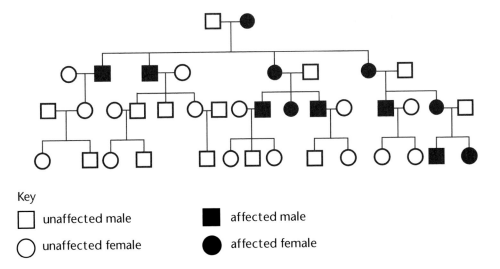

Key

☐ unaffected male   ■ affected male

○ unaffected female   ● affected female

Answer 12.3

- Both males and females are affected
- Male-to-male and male-to-female transmission do not occur
- Affected females pass the condition on to all offspring.

The inheritance pattern is mitochondrial.

RESPIRATORY MEDICINE

13

RESPIRATORY MEDICINE

Arterial blood gas analysis

Arterial blood gas (ABG) analysis provides a wealth of information about a patient's state of health. The test is most commonly used in acute illness but may also be used in the assessment of patients with chronic respiratory disease. In acute situations, multiple analyses are often made to assess response to treatment. Trends are usually more helpful than one-off readings. Never forget to consult old medical records if possible, since the patient's baseline may be well outside 'normal' limits.

Interpretation of four key indices – pH, partial pressure of oxygen (PaO_2), partial pressure of carbon dioxide ($PaCO_2$) and bicarbonate (HCO_3^-) – will provide most of the information needed in clinical practice. A fifth index, base excess (BE), can also be used, but will not be discussed here in detail.

Sophisticated blood gas analysers will provide other useful information such as blood levels of lactate and methaemoglobin.

NORMAL RANGES (BREATHING ROOM AIR AT SEA LEVEL)	
pH	7.35–7.45
PaO_2	11–13 kPa
$PaCO_2$	4.7–6.0 kPa
HCO_3^-	24–30 mmol/l
Base excess	−2 to +2 mmol/l
Anion gap	12–16 mmol/l

Of all the normal ranges for values listed in this book, it is recommended that all students learn the normal values in an ABG sample. This is for two reasons:

1. ABGs are commonly tested, so knowing the normal values will help you as an undergraduate.

2. More importantly, in real medical practice, ABGs are often encountered in stressful situations involving critically unwell patients. Knowing normal values can speed up analysis and reduce stress.

Oxygen levels in the air fall with increasing altitude. Bear this in mind if you are interpreting ABGs taken at any significant height above sea level. For the purposes of simplicity, for the remainder of this chapter, it will be assumed that samples have been taken at sea level.

Systematic interpretation of an ABG

The two main steps involved are to assess oxygenation, then acid–base status.

Assess oxygenation

You will note that the normal range for PaO_2 given in the box above was 11–13 kPa. This value holds true for a patient breathing room air that contains 21% oxygen. It is crucial to appreciate that a patient with normal lungs will have a much higher PaO_2 if their inspired oxygen concentration (FiO_2) is increased. The physiology behind this is summarised in the alveolar gas equation, which will be dealt with shortly.

Unless you are someone who particularly enjoys equations, a useful rule of thumb is that, for a healthy person at sea level, the expected PaO_2 (kPa) is roughly 10 less than the FiO_2 (%). This will not compute exactly, but will highlight patients with serious problems. Exact expected values are shown in the table below. Thus, if a patient is receiving 85% oxygen and the PaO_2 is 11 kPa, there is a serious problem.

INSPIRED OXYGEN CONCENTRATION (%)	RULE OF THUMB METHOD FOR ESTIMATING PaO_2	EXPECTED PaO_2 WITH HEALTHY LUNGS (kPa)
28	18	21
35	25	27
40	30	32
60	50	51
85	75	75
100	90	89

MEMORY AID

As a rule of thumb, the expected PaO_2 (kPa) is roughly 10 less than the FiO_2 (%).

It is therefore impossible to interpret the PaO_2 without knowing the FiO_2. If the PaO_2 is lower than expected, this implies that a disease process in the lungs is interfering with gas exchange. This can occur with a variety of conditions, from pulmonary fibrosis to pulmonary embolism, and pneumonia to pulmonary oedema, to name but a few.

.

The first step in interpreting an ABG sample is to assess oxygenation. So, with the above in mind, decide whether oxygenation is normal or abnormal.

The label of 'respiratory failure' is used when the PaO_2 is less than 8 kPa. It is divided into two types depending on the $PaCO_2$, as follows:

RESPIRATORY FAILURE TYPE	PaO_2 (kPa)	$PaCO_2$ (kPa)
Type 1	<8	<6.5
Type 2	<8	>6.5

MEMORY AID

In type **ONE** respiratory failure, **ONE** gas is abnormal (ie low O_2, without high CO_2). In type **TWO** respiratory failure, **TWO** gases are abnormal (low O_2 and high CO_2).

COMMON CAUSES OF RESPIRATORY FAILURE

TYPE 1	TYPE 2
Pulmonary oedema	Chronic obstructive pulmonary disease (COPD)
Pneumonia	Respiratory centre depression
Pulmonary embolism	Respiratory muscle weakness
Pulmonary fibrosis	Abnormal chest wall architecture

THE ALVEOLAR GAS EQUATION AND THE ALVEOLAR–ARTERIAL GRADIENT

The assessment of oxygenation described above will suffice in most situations. It is possible to be more precise, however, so, if you are particularly interested in this subject, there are two further equations that are of interest.

The alveolar gas equation

This equation allows the calculation of the expected oxygen level in the alveoli of an individual (P_AO_2). It is rarely used in clinical practice:

$$P_AO_2 = FiO_2(P_{atm} - PH_2O) - \frac{PaCO_2(1 - FiO_2) \times (1 - RQ)}{RQ}$$

where P_{atm} = atmospheric pressure, PH_2O = saturated vapour pressure of water at that particular temperature and pressure, and RQ = respiratory quotient (a ratio of CO_2 eliminated to O_2 consumed).

So, for example, for someone breathing 21% oxygen at sea level with $PaCO_2$ of 5 kPa:

$$P_AO_2 = 0.21 \times (101\,kPa - 6.25\,kPa) - \frac{5\,kPa(1 - 0.21) \times (1 - 0.8)}{0.8}$$

$$P_AO_2 = 0.21 \times 94.75\,kPa - 5.99$$

$$P_AO_2 = 13.91\,kPa$$

The alveolar–arterial gradient

This equation allows the calculation of the difference in oxygen concentration between alveoli and the arterial system:

$$\text{A–a gradient} = \left[FiO_2 \times (P_{atm} - PH_2O) - \left(\frac{PaCO_2}{0.8} \right) \right] - PaO_2$$

So for example, for someone breathing 40% oxygen at sea level with PaO_2 12 kPa and $PaCO_2$ 5 kPa:

$$\text{A--a gradient} = \left[0.4 \times (101\ kPa - 6.25\ kPa) - \left(\frac{5\ kPa}{0.8} \right) \right] - 12$$

A--a gradient = $(0.4 \times 94.75\ kPa - 6.25\ kPa) - 12$

A--a gradient = 19.65 kPa

There is no established normal range for A--a gradient. It has been defined in the following ways:

- No more than 2.66 kPa. This is a simplistic approach, however, as the A--a gradient normally increases with age.

- No more than ($\frac{\text{Age in years}}{4}$ + 4) x 0.13 kPa.

- Or compare the value with 'normal' age-based values in the literature.

Stein PD et al. (1995) Alveolar–arterial oxygen gradient in the assessment of acute pulmonary embolism. *Chest* **107**:139–43.

Assess acid–base status
This has five main components.

Look at the pH
Is it:

- normal (7.35–7.45)?
- low (<7.35) indicating acidosis?
- high (>7.45) indicating alkalosis?

Small deviations from normal are extremely relevant. Abnormalities of pH can be due to a problem with either respiration (respiratory acidosis or alkalosis) or metabolism (metabolic acidosis or alkalosis). The body's homeostatic mechanisms will attempt to correct pH problems, so evidence of compensation might be seen. In general, for respiratory problems, metabolic compensation occurs but this can take some time. For metabolic problems, respiratory compensation occurs, which can happen quickly.

Once you have identified a problem, next try to decide on the cause by proceeding with the next stages.

Look at the $PaCO_2$
Is it normal, low or high?

Carbon dioxide is an acidic gas (remember that carbon dioxide plus water → carbonic **acid**), so:

- If the pH is acid and the CO_2 is high, the problem is a respiratory acidosis (excess acidic CO_2).

- If the pH is alkaline and the CO_2 is low, the problem is a respiratory alkalosis (lack of acidic CO_2).

Look at the HCO_3^-
Is it normal, low or high?

Bicarbonate is an alkaline substance (remember that some people take sodium bicarbonate to combat stomach acid), so:

- If the pH is acid and the bicarbonate is low, the problem is a metabolic acidosis (lack of alkaline bicarbonate).

- If the pH is alkaline and the bicarbonate is high, the problem is a metabolic alkalosis (excess alkaline bicarbonate).

DON'T FORGET

In some circumstances, patients can have more than one abnormality, eg a combined respiratory and metabolic acidosis.

Look for compensation
As mentioned above, the body will attempt to compensate for a pH abnormality. Respiratory compensation happens faster than metabolic compensation. **The body will never overcompensate.** The following patterns are commonly seen:

- In an acute metabolic acidosis, the body responds by getting rid of extra CO_2, thus losing acid and shifting the pH towards normality.

- In a chronic respiratory acidosis, the body responds by holding onto extra bicarbonate, thus retaining alkalinity and shifting the pH towards normality.

Fig 13.1: Interpretation of common arterial blood gas abnormalities

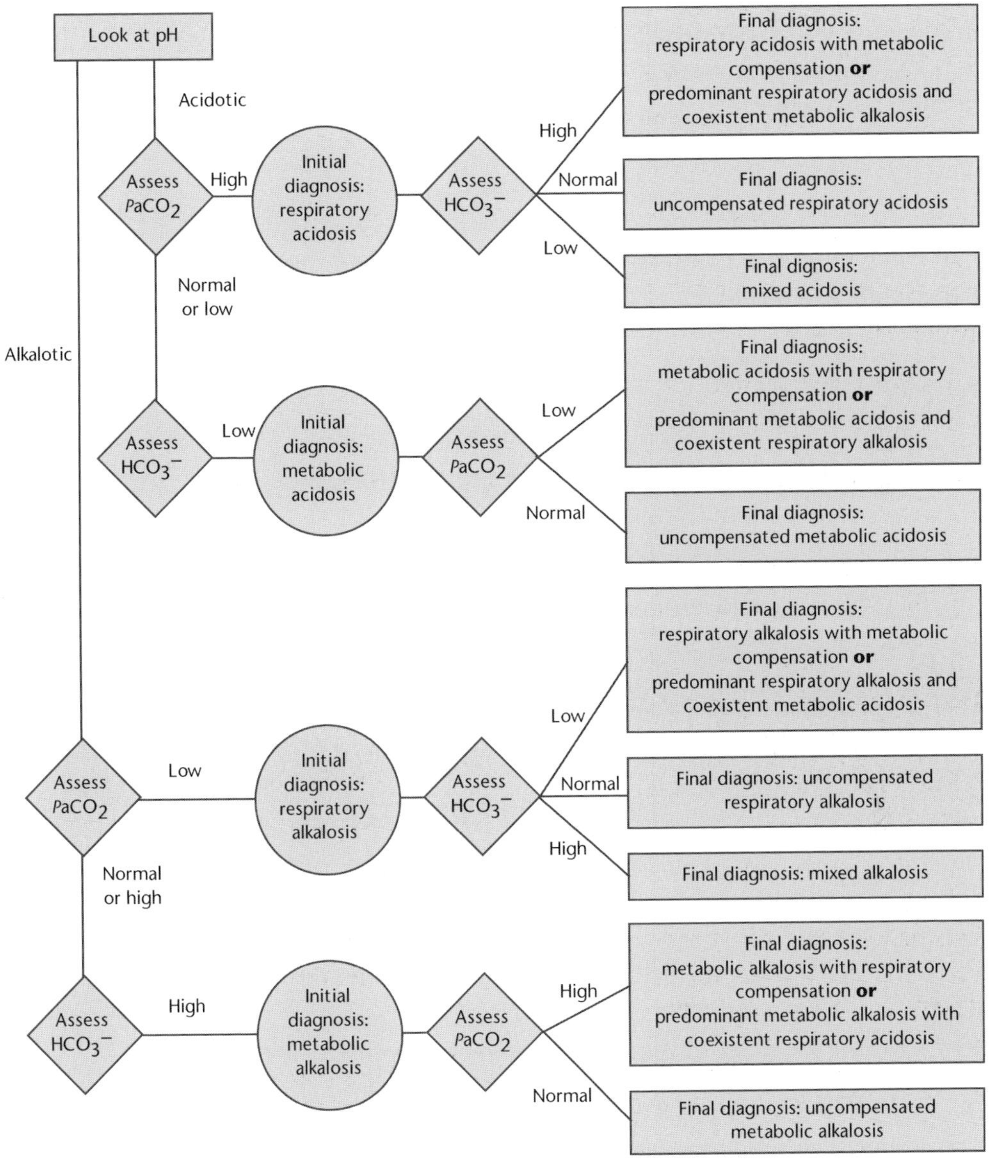

Try to determine the cause

Respiratory acidosis

Respiratory acidosis can be due to any of the causes of respiratory failure.

Respiratory alkalosis

Respiratory alkalosis is always due to hyperventilation. Be wary of attributing hyperventilation exclusively to anxiety, however, since it may occur secondary to an underlying severe disease process, such as sepsis or stroke.

Metabolic acidosis

There are a wide range of causes for a metabolic acidosis. To narrow down this list, and help you come to a diagnosis, it is helpful to calculate the anion gap. If this is high (>16 mmol/l), the acidosis is due to the presence of excess acids in the body that are not routinely analysed in the laboratory. The anion gap is calculated as follows:

Anion gap = $(Na^+ + K^+) - (Cl^- + HCO_3^-)$

A patient with the following biochemical findings — Na^+ 136 mmol/l, K^+ 3.5 mmol/l, Cl^- 100 mmol/l, HCO_3^- 24 mmol/l — would therefore have an anion gap of 15.5 mmol/l.

DON'T FORGET

Always calculate the anion gap in a patient with a metabolic acidosis.

COMMON CAUSES OF A METABOLIC ACIDOSIS

NORMAL ANION GAP	RAISED ANION GAP
HCO_3^- loss from gut, eg diarrhoea Renal tubular acidosis	Ketoacidosis Renal failure Lactic acidosis Salicylate toxicity Methanol ingestion Ethylene glycol (antifreeze) ingestion

Metabolic alkalosis

There are several causes of metabolic alkalosis (see box below). Most commonly, it is seen in patients with excessive vomiting.

COMMON CAUSES OF A METABOLIC ALKALOSIS

Losses from the gut, particularly vomiting (classically pyloric stenosis)
Primary or secondary hyperaldosteronism
Hypercalcaemia
Use of diuretics
Bicarbonate ingestion

Pulmonary function tests

Peak expiratory flow rate

Peak expiratory flow rate (PEFR) is a simple bedside test that gives a useful insight into the respiratory function of a patient. The PEFR is measured in litres per minute using a basic plastic device. An average recording of three attempts is documented on a peak flow chart. The trend in PEFR and its relationship to symptoms are a guide to the severity of illness and the effectiveness of treatment.

Some patients with asthma will keep records of their PEFR. For comparative purposes recordings should be taken at the same time each day. This will eliminate changes due to normal diurnal variation. There is a normal variation in PEFR in people with asthma, with a typical dip first thing in the morning.

It is important to appreciate when interpreting values that the normal PEFR varies with age, height and sex.

PATIENT	HEIGHT (cm)	NORMAL PEFR (l/min)
25-year-old man	175	630
25-year-old woman	175	505
60-year-old man	160	545
60-year-old woman	160	445

DON'T FORGET

PEFR varies with age, sex and height.

Spirometry

Spirometry provides a wealth of information about lung volumes and function. Spirometry reports can appear confusing. However, by looking at four indices, most of the important patterns of lung disease can be distinguished.

KEY RESULTS IN SPIROMETRY		
INDEX	**ABBREVIATION**	**INTERPRETATION**
Forced expiratory volume in 1 second	FEV_1	The volume of air that can be expired in 1 second
Forced vital capacity	FVC	The volume of air expired in a complete expiration
Ratio of FEV_1 to FVC	FEV_1/FVC	—
Carbon monoxide transfer coefficient	K_{CO}	A measure of the rate of diffusion of carbon monoxide from the alveoli into the capillary blood

Values obtained by spirometry should always be compared with age- and sex-matched control values. Often results are converted into percentages of the predicted value in order to simplify interpretation.

Arguably the most useful index is the FEV_1/FVC. This test can be used to distinguish between obstructive airway disease (eg asthma, COPD) and restrictive lung disease (eg pulmonary fibrosis). In an obstructive defect, the FEV_1/FVC will be less than 70%. The percentage is greater than 80% with a restrictive defect.

COMMON PATTERNS OF FEV_1/FVC
<70% in obstructive airway disease >80% in restrictive lung disease

The theory underlying these patterns is easily understood. In a patient with obstructive airway disease, airway obstruction makes expiration slow (and usually wheezy). The FEV_1 is therefore typically low, since only a small volume of air can be expired in 1 second. These patients also 'trap air' so the FVC will usually be high. A low FEV_1 and a high FVC combine to give a low FEV_1/FVC. In other words, the volume of air in the lungs is normal or high, but it is not easily forced out.

In restrictive lung disease, on the other hand, there is no airway obstruction. The FEV_1 is therefore typically higher than with an obstructive defect (although it is still usually reduced compared with normal). Small lung volumes contribute to a low FVC. A relatively high FEV_1 and a low FVC combine to give a high FEV_1/FVC. Put simply, the patient can force air out of their lungs, but as the lung volume is reduced there is less of it to force out.

The three main patterns of lung function (normal, obstructive and restrictive) are shown pictorially on Fig 13.2.

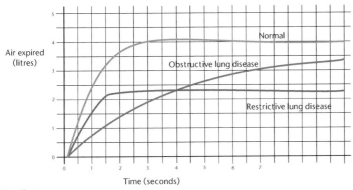

Fig 13.2

The Kco measures the ease of diffusion of carbon monoxide from alveolar air to capillary blood. Anything that hinders gas transfer from alveolus into blood will therefore result in a low Kco. Common causes of low Kco are shown in the box below.

CAUSES OF A LOW Kco

Interstitial lung disease
Emphysema
Pulmonary oedema
Pulmonary embolism
Anaemia

In rare cases, the Kco can be raised. In such circumstances, gas transfers more easily than normal from alveolus into blood. Examples include polycythaemia (see Chapter 1) or in cases of pulmonary haemorrhage (eg Goodpasture syndrome).

Note that anaemia is the classic case where a patient will have a low Kco with normal spirometry. The Kco is low because there is less haemoglobin present to carry gas away from the alveoli.

Case 13.1

The blood gas below was taken following admission of an elderly patient to the acute medical unit. He was breathing room air.

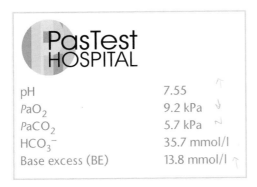

PasTest HOSPITAL	
pH	7.55 ↗
PaO_2	9.2 kPa ↓
$PaCO_2$	5.7 kPa N
HCO_3^-	35.7 mmol/l
Base excess (BE)	13.8 mmol/l ↗

1. **Outline the abnormalities on this ABG.**

2. **What are the likely causes for these abnormalities?**

Answer 13.1

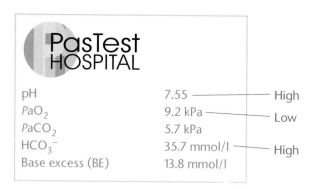

1. Oxygenation is abnormal, ie the PaO_2 is lower than normal for a patient breathing room air.

   The pH is high, indicating an alkalosis. The $PaCO_2$ is normal, and the HCO_3^- is high. Using the flow diagram on page 427, you can work out that this represents an uncompensated metabolic alkalosis.

2. Poor oxygenation could reflect any disease process affecting the lungs. Common causes would be pulmonary oedema or pneumonia.
   The causes of a metabolic alkalosis are listed in the box on page 428.
   The patient in this case had a lower respiratory tract infection and vomiting.

Case 13.2

A 68-year-old man with a 40-pack-year smoking history was admitted short of breath and with a cough productive of green sputum. On examination he was tachypnoeic and using his accessory muscles of respiration. Auscultation of his chest revealed widespread expiratory wheeze with bibasal coarse crepitations. He was placed on 28% oxygen and his initial ABG is shown below.

PasTest
HOSPITAL

pH	7.28 ↓
PaO_2	7.8 kPa ↓
$PaCO_2$	6.7 kPa ↑
HCO_3^-	35.4 mmol/l ↑
BE	−5 mmol/l

1. **Outline the abnormalities on this ABG.** *resp acidosis partial met comp*

2. **What is the likely diagnosis?** *COPD*

3. **What type of assisted ventilation could be considered in the management of this condition?** *NIV*

Answer 13.2

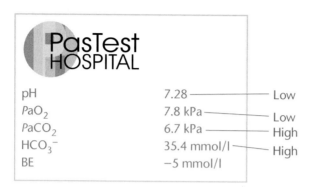

PasTest HOSPITAL		
pH	7.28	Low
PaO_2	7.8 kPa	Low
$PaCO_2$	6.7 kPa	High
HCO_3^-	35.4 mmol/l	High
BE	−5 mmol/l	

1. Oxygenation is abnormal. The patient has type 2 respiratory failure, with low PaO_2 and high $PaCO_2$.

   The pH is low, indicating an acidosis. The $PaCO_2$ is high, as is the HCO_3^-. Using the flow chart you can see that this pattern could represent either respiratory acidosis with metabolic compensation, or a predominant respiratory acidosis with a coexistent metabolic alkalosis.

2. The most likely diagnosis is an acute exacerbation of chronic obstructive pulmonary disease (COPD). This would be in keeping with the clinical findings. The acid–base disturbance would therefore represent respiratory acidosis with metabolic compensation. Note that the compensation is only partial, since the patient remains acidotic. An acute exacerbation of COPD is the most common cause of a respiratory acidosis with a raised HCO_3^-.

   Many patients with COPD have high resting CO_2 levels, causing a respiratory acidosis. However, with time, the kidneys compensate for this acidosis by retaining HCO_3^-. Thus, in the 'normal' state, many patients with COPD have a normal pH, with a raised $PaCO_2$ and a raised HCO_3^-, such as that shown in the ABG below:

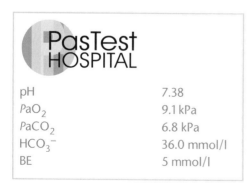

PasTest HOSPITAL	
pH	7.38
PaO_2	9.1 kPa
$PaCO_2$	6.8 kPa
HCO_3^-	36.0 mmol/l
BE	5 mmol/l

During an acute exacerbation, however, the $PaCO_2$ levels increase, giving rise to a respiratory acidosis.

3. Patients may often benefit from non-invasive ventilation (NIV) using bilevel positive airway pressure (BiPAP). If deterioration occurs, intubation and ventilation may be required.

Case 13.3

An anxious 27-year-old student was admitted with shortness of breath and tingling in her hands. On examination, she had a respiratory rate of 28 breaths per minute. Chest examination was unremarkable. Chest X-ray and routine blood tests were normal. An ECG showed sinus tachycardia. An ABG was taken on 35% oxygen.

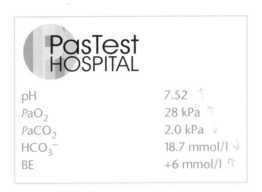

PasTest HOSPITAL	
pH	7.52 ↑
PaO_2	28 kPa ↑
$PaCO_2$	2.0 kPa ↓
HCO_3^-	18.7 mmol/l ↓
BE	+6 mmol/l ↑

1. **Outline the abnormalities on this ABG.**   resp alcalosis partial met comp

2. **What is the likely cause?**   ↑RR

3. **How might one treat this woman?**

Answer 13.3

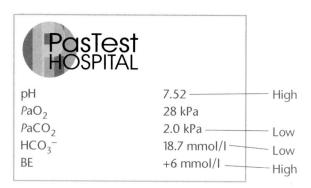

pH	7.52	High
PaO_2	28 kPa	
$PaCO_2$	2.0 kPa	Low
HCO_3^-	18.7 mmol/l	Low
BE	+6 mmol/l	High

1. Oxygenation is normal given that the FiO_2 is 35%.

    The pH is high indicating an alkalosis. The $PaCO_2$ and HCO_3^- are both low. Using the flow chart, you can see that this pattern could be due to either a respiratory alkalosis with metabolic compensation or a predominant respiratory alkalosis with coexistent metabolic acidosis.

2. The likely cause for this ABG given the clinical history is hyperventilation. Thus the acid–base disturbance is a respiratory alkalosis with metabolic compensation. One of the most common causes is anxiety, but it may occur as a result of organic pathology such as a stroke or subarachnoid haemorrhage affecting the respiratory centre.

    A full history and examination would be essential to help rule out a serious cause of this acid–base disturbance.

3. Reassurance would be a key aspect of treatment in the case of anxiety. Re-breathing one's own exhaled air, using a paper bag, may also be beneficial.

Case 13.4

A 32-year-old French tourist is brought to A&E feeling generally unwell. No history is available. He appears dehydrated and has a respiratory rate of 22 breaths per minute. The following ABG and biochemical profile are taken on admission, breathing room air.

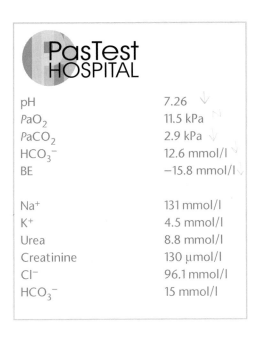

PasTest
HOSPITAL

pH	7.26
PaO_2	11.5 kPa
$PaCO_2$	2.9 kPa
HCO_3^-	12.6 mmol/l
BE	−15.8 mmol/l
Na^+	131 mmol/l
K^+	4.5 mmol/l
Urea	8.8 mmol/l
Creatinine	130 μmol/l
Cl^-	96.1 mmol/l
HCO_3^-	15 mmol/l

1. **Outline the abnormalities seen.**
2. **What tests should you request?**
3. **Which drugs or substances taken in overdose could give a similar pattern?**

Answer 13.4

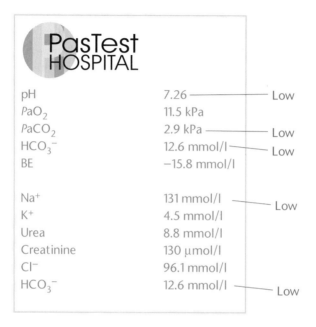

PasTest HOSPITAL

pH	7.26	Low
PaO_2	11.5 kPa	
$PaCO_2$	2.9 kPa	Low
HCO_3^-	12.6 mmol/l	Low
BE	−15.8 mmol/l	
Na^+	131 mmol/l	Low
K^+	4.5 mmol/l	
Urea	8.8 mmol/l	
Creatinine	130 µmol/l	
Cl^-	96.1 mmol/l	
HCO_3^-	12.6 mmol/l	Low

1. Oxygenation is normal.

   The pH is low indicating an acidosis. The $PaCO_2$ and HCO_3^- are both low. Using the flow chart you can see that this indicates either a metabolic acidosis with respiratory compensation or a predominant metabolic acidosis with coexistent respiratory alkalosis.

   Remember to calculate the anion gap with any case of metabolic acidosis. In this case the anion gap is calculated as follows: $(131 + 4.5) − (96.1 + 12.6) = 26.8$. Thus this is a raised anion gap metabolic acidosis.

2. Bearing in mind the causes of a raised anion gap metabolic acidosis shown in the box on page 428, the following tests would be helpful: urinalysis for ketones, plasma lactate levels and salicylate levels.

3. This pattern can be seen when salicylates (eg aspirin), methanol or ethylene glycol is taken in excess.

Case 13.5

A 57-year-old man is medically retired from his former job in the local shipyard. For the past 6 years his health has deteriorated with an exercise tolerance now reduced to 10 metres on the flat. He is a life-long non-smoker. A recent high-resolution CT (HRCT) scan of the chest demonstrated diffuse bibasal interstitial changes. His ABG was taken on room air without any intercurrent illness.

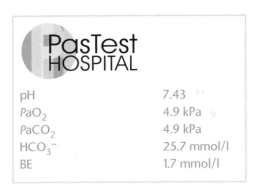

pH	7.43
PaO_2	4.9 kPa
$PaCO_2$	4.9 kPa
HCO_3^-	25.7 mmol/l
BE	1.7 mmol/l

1. **Outline the abnormalities seen.**
2. **What are the likely causes for an ABG such as this?**
3. **What long-term therapy might be considered?**

Answer 13.5

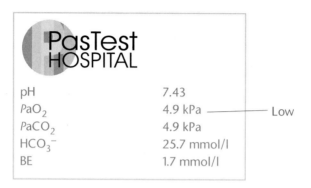

PasTest
HOSPITAL

pH	7.43	
PaO_2	4.9 kPa	———— Low
$PaCO_2$	4.9 kPa	
HCO_3^-	25.7 mmol/l	
BE	1.7 mmol/l	

1. Oxygenation is abnormal. The patient has type 1 respiratory failure, with a low PaO_2 and normal $PaCO_2$.

   The pH is normal, as is the HCO_3^-.

2. This man's clinical history when taken in conjunction with his clinical signs and ABG is highly suggestive of pulmonary fibrosis. The fact that he worked in a shipyard may suggest exposure to asbestos, which is a potential cause of pulmonary fibrosis – especially at the lung bases as the CT scan suggests. Other causes for type 1 respiratory failure are listed in the box on page 423.

3. Long-term oxygen therapy (LTOT) could be considered. However, there are strict guidelines that must be met before LTOT is commenced.

Case 13.6

The following chart plots changes in PEFR of a patient with asthma during her hospital stay.

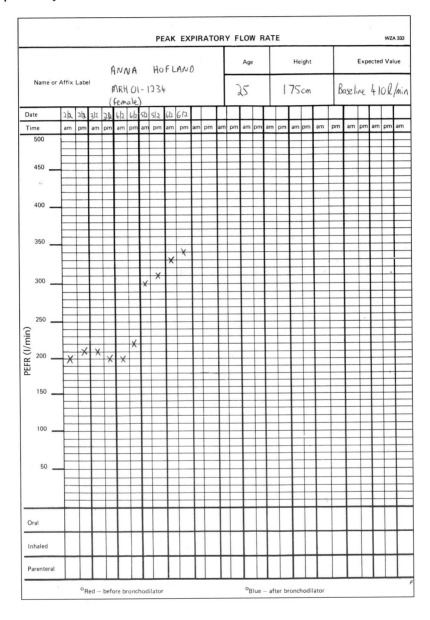

How would you interpret this chart?

Answer 13.6

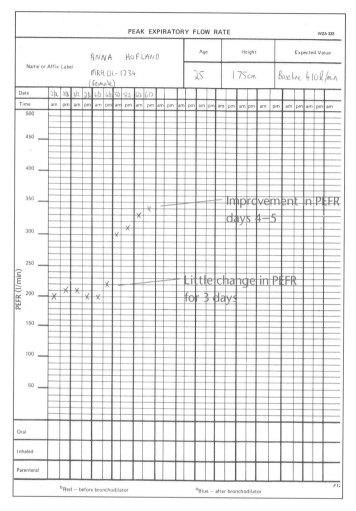

In this bedside chart, the patient's known baseline PEFR of 410 l/min has been documented. Using the patient details at the top of the chart, one can look up the predicted PEFR, which is 505 l/min. Thus, even when at 'her best' she has a reduction in expiratory flow compared with a 'normal' adult of the same build. At the time of admission her PEFR is only 200 l/min – less than half of her baseline. Over the course of the next 2 days there is little change in her PEFR. Her condition has stabilised. Days 4 and 5 of her stay show a significant and sustained increase in her readings. A steady rise to 340 l/min is seen. Either there has been a natural resolution of her asthma attack or the instigation of effective treatment has caused this change.

Case 13.7

A 70-year-old man with a long history of rheumatoid disease is reviewed at clinic. He complains that he is unable to make it to the newsagents any longer without having to stop to catch his breath. He has no history of chest or cardiovascular disease. He has no other symptoms. On examination, fine end-inspiratory crepitations are heard at both lung bases. Spirometry is requested.

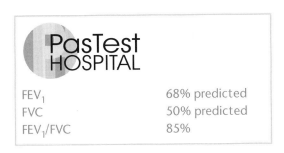

PasTest HOSPITAL	
FEV$_1$	68% predicted
FVC	50% predicted
FEV$_1$/FVC	85%

1. Outline the abnormal findings in the results above.

2. What is the most likely cause for these abnormalities in this patient?

3. What imaging test would be most useful here?

Answer 13.7

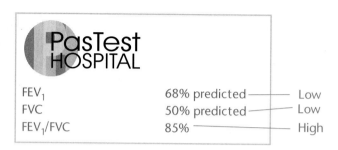

FEV$_1$	68% predicted	Low
FVC	50% predicted	Low
FEV$_1$/FVC	85%	High

1. This man has a restrictive defect on spirometry as shown by the raised FEV$_1$/FVC.

2. The most likely cause would be pulmonary fibrosis, either secondary to his rheumatoid disease or as a side effect of its treatment with methotrexate.

3. An HRCT scan of the chest would best aid diagnosis and management. This would identify any pulmonary changes associated with fibrosis.

Case 13.8

A 68-year-old man who has been a life-long smoker is admitted with a lower respiratory tract infection. He was noted to be wheezy at the time of admission to hospital, and was treated with antibiotics and nebulised bronchodilators. His inflammatory markers settled, but he remained wheezy. Pulmonary function tests were performed 3 weeks later after resolution of his acute illness.

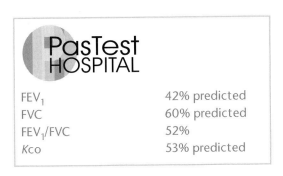

PasTest
HOSPITAL

FEV_1	42% predicted
FVC	60% predicted
FEV_1/FVC	52%
Kco	53% predicted

1. **Outline the abnormal findings in the results above.**

2. **What is the most likely cause for these abnormalities in this patient?**

Answer 13.8

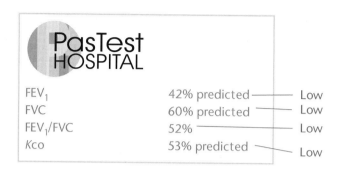

1. This patient's spirometry shows an obstructive pattern. His *K*co is low, indicating that something is interfering with gas transfer in the lungs. In this case, it is a reflection of his airway disease.

2. Given that this patient is a life-long smoker, it is likely that he has COPD. Consideration should be given to optimising inhaled bronchodilator therapy before discharge.

Case 13.9

A 64-year-old woman is admitted from A&E complaining of increasing shortness of breath. This has been increasing over a period of 2 months. There is little of note on examination. The admitting doctor arranges for pulmonary function tests to assess her symptom.

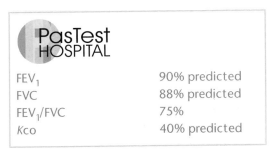

PasTest
HOSPITAL

FEV$_1$	90% predicted
FVC	88% predicted
FEV$_1$/FVC	75%
Kco	40% predicted

1. **Outline the abnormal findings in the results above.**

2. **What blood test would you order?**

Case 13.10

A 36-year-old woman has been attending the respiratory outpatient department for 5 years because of sarcoidosis. Her disease has been well controlled recently, and her dose of oral steroids has been gradually reduced over a period of several months. On her most recent visit, she complains of increasing shortness of breath over the preceding 3 weeks. Her pulmonary function tests are shown alongside a set taken when she was feeling well.

PasTest
HOSPITAL

	2 months before	Present day
FEV$_1$	69% predicted	63% predicted
FVC	52% predicted	49% predicted
FEV$_1$/FVC	68%	65% predicted
Kco	90% predicted	61% predicted

What parameter has changed significantly between the two sets of readings, and how would you account for this?

Answer 13.9

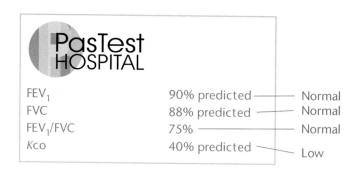

PasTest
HOSPITAL

FEV₁	90% predicted	Normal
FVC	88% predicted	Normal
FEV₁/FVC	75%	Normal
Kco	40% predicted	Low

1. FEV_1 and FVC are considered normal unless they are less than 80% of the predicted value. Spirometry is essentially normal in this example. The only abnormality shown is a low Kco.

2. A classic cause of reduced Kco with normal spirometry is anaemia. This patient should have a full blood picture analysed as a first-line measure.

Answer 13.10

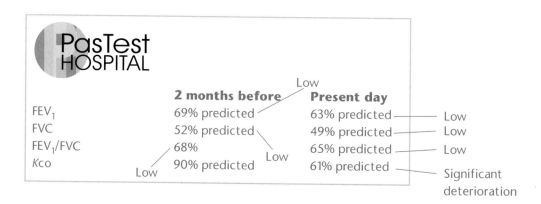

PasTest
HOSPITAL

	2 months before	Present day	
FEV₁	69% predicted	63% predicted	Low
FVC	52% predicted	49% predicted	Low
FEV₁/FVC	68%	65% predicted	Low
Kco	90% predicted	61% predicted	Significant deterioration

The FEV_1 and FVC remain fairly similar between both sets of readings, indicating a restrictive lung defect. The major deterioration lies with the Kco, which has taken a marked turn for the worse. This is most likely due to a deterioration in the underlying disease process because of the reducing dose of steroids. Consideration should be given to increasing the steroid dose.

INTERPRETING BEDSIDE CHART DATA

14

INTERPRETING BEDSIDE CHART DATA

The most easily measured and readily available data on a patient lie at the bedside on a series of observation charts. Nursing staff dutifully complete a number of observations on a regular basis. The nature of these and the frequency at which they are taken vary, depending on the clinical status of the patient. Analysis and interpretation of bedside chart data are an extension of the clinical assessment of a patient, and may provide the first evidence of a downward trend in clinical condition. The best way to learn from bedside charts is to pick them up and try to interpret them during your clinical attachments.

> **DON'T FORGET**
> Data interpretation begins at the end of the bed.

Vital signs

The so-called 'vital signs' represent the basic set of observations that are recorded regularly for all patients and include the parameters listed in the box below.

BASIC OBSERVATIONS MEASURED (WITH NORMAL RANGES)	
Pulse rate	60–100 beats/min
Blood pressure	Abnormally high – >140 mmHg systolic or 90 mmHg diastolic
	Abnormally low – <90 mmHg systolic or a drop of 20 mmHg or more systolic from the patient's baseline
Respiratory rate	14–18 breaths per minute
Oxygen saturation	96–100% on room air
Temperature	36.5–37.5°C

Looking at how a particular physiological parameter varies with time can be highly informative. For example, taking a one-off temperature recording may or may not be useful in a patient with a particular symptom, but much more useful is the way in which the patient's temperature varies with time. In the example in Fig 14.1, the temperature can be seen to be 'swinging' and this pattern is highly suggestive of a serious infection or inflammatory process.

Fig 14.1: Swinging fever

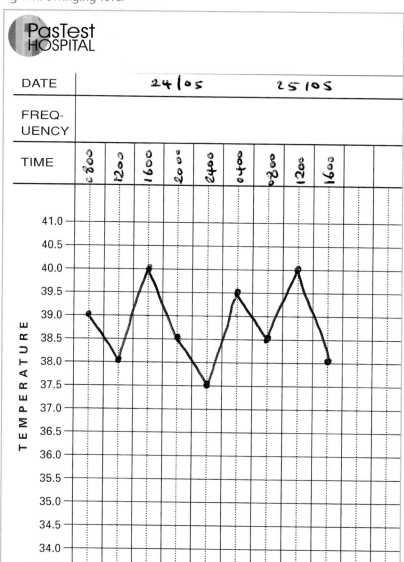

Similarly, a steadily rising respiratory rate or pulse rate, or a falling blood pressure can highlight evolving physiological changes much more readily than can a snapshot recording at one moment in time.

Early warning scores

'Early warning scores' are becoming increasingly used. Examples are the Physicians' Early Warning Score (PEWS) and the Medical Early Warning Score (MEWS). To calculate such a score, weightings are given for deviations in set physiological parameters away from normality. The higher the deviation, the greater the score. An example is shown in the table below. There are several advantages to such a system. A patient with seemingly minor abnormalities in several parameters will be identified as acutely unwell because their score will be quite high. Also, nursing staff who might not be confident in knowing when to call for medical assistance can be assured that a high score equates to a seriously unwell patient who requires urgent help from a senior doctor. As with any vital sign measurement, a change in early warning score is more informative than a one-off reading.

	3	2	1	0	1	2	3
Pulse (beats/min)		<40	41–50	51–90	91–110	111–130	≥131
Breathing rate (beats/min)	≤8		9–11	12–20		21–24	≥25
Temperature (°C)	≤35		35.1–36	36.1–38.0	38.1–39	≥39.1	
Systolic BP (mmHg)	≤90	91–100	101–110	111–249	≥250		
SaO$_2$ (%)	≤91	92–93	94–95	≥96			
Inspired O$_2$				Air			Any O$_2$
CNS (use AVPU scale)				Alert (A)			Voice (V) Pain (P) Unresponsive (U)

Prytherch DR, Smith GB, Schmidt PE, Featherstone PI. ViEWS – Towards a national early warning score for detecting adult inpatient deterioration. *Resuscitation* 2010;**81**:932–7.

Neurological observations

Neurological observations are recorded at intervals in patients who are at risk of deterioration in their level of consciousness. Two commonly used systems are described.

1. AVPU

This is a quickly recorded summary measure of neurological status. The patient is graded as:

A – if they are **A**lert
V – if they respond to **V**oice
P – if they respond only to **P**ain
U – if they are **U**nresponsive.

2. Glasgow Coma Scale (GCS)

This is more time-consuming to measure than the AVPU score, but also provides more information. It is scored out of 15, with a minimum score of 3 and a maximum of 15. The patient's best response at the time of assessment should be recorded.

TASK	PERFORMANCE	SCORE
Eyes open	Spontaneously	4
	To speech	3
	To pain	2
	None	1
Best verbal response	Oriented	5
	Confused	4
	Inappropriate words	3
	Incomprehensible sounds	2
	None	1
Best motor response	Obey commands	6
	Localises pain	5
	Flexion withdrawal	4
	Abnormal flexion	3
	Extension to pain	2
	None	1

Figure 14.2 shows a GCS chart from a patient who exhibits a sudden drop in GCS at 11am.

Fig 14.2: Sudden drop in GCS.

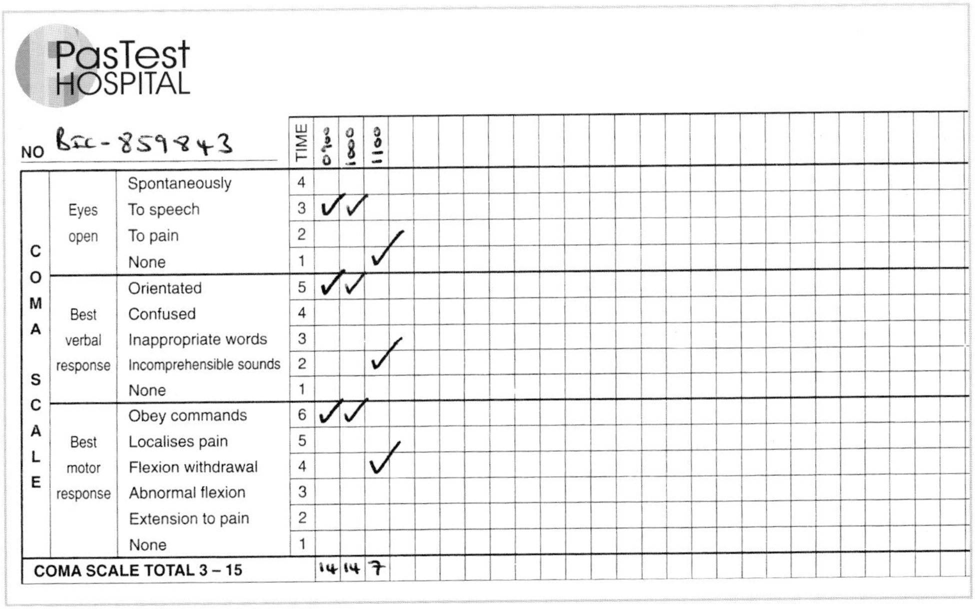

Fluid balance chart

A carefully completed fluid balance chart can be extremely helpful in making management decisions for patients. In essence, these charts record the quantity and type of all fluid entering and leaving the body.

Examples of fluid entering the body:

- Food and drink taken orally

- Intravenous fluid

- Nutrition given enterally (eg via a nasogastric or percutaneous gastrostomy tube) or parenterally (ie intravenous feeding)

- Blood products (eg packed red cells, platelets, cryoprecipitate, fresh frozen plasma)

- Intravenous drugs.

Examples of fluid leaving the body:

- Urine
- Bowel motions
- Blood (from any orifice, including blood loss during surgery)
- Fluid from drains (eg chest drain).

One should also bear in mind insensible fluid loss. This refers to fluid that is lost but not normally recorded and includes moisture lost in expired air and sweat. A general rule of thumb is that, in normal circumstances, a patient loses approximately 500 ml/day of fluid through insensible losses. These losses can increase massively, eg if a patient has extensive burns or if they have a fever.

Interpreting a fluid balance chart should incorporate several steps:

1. Compare total input to total output, remembering to account for insensible losses. Are they equal, or is there a positive or negative fluid balance? A positive fluid balance means that more fluid has entered the patient than has left, and would be entirely appropriate, for example, in a patient being treated for dehydration. A negative fluid balance means that more fluid has left the patient than has entered, and would be entirely appropriate, for example, in a patient with heart failure who is fluid overloaded and being treated with diuretics. Is the total volume of fluid entering the patient too little, adequate or too much for requirements? This will depend on the age, sex and weight of the patient, and also on the state of health (particularly current illnesses, cardiac and renal function).

2. Look at the type of fluid that the patient has received and correlate this with the clinical circumstances.

3. Think about electrolytes. Is the patient receiving enough electrolyte replacement to account for his or her body's daily requirements as well as compensating him or her for any abnormal electrolyte losses. For example, an elderly person might require 40 mmol potassium per day to maintain potassium equilibrium when healthy. If he develops severe diarrhoea, however, he will lose a lot of potassium from the gut and may well need much more than 40 mmol potassium per day to prevent him becoming hypokalaemic. Output from drains can often be important sources of electrolyte losses and can easily be overlooked.

Drug charts

A great deal of information about a patient can be gleaned by examining their drug chart. Errors are common and doctors at all levels should be vigilant and watch for potentially dangerous mistakes or oversights in drug prescriptions.

Other bedside data

Stool chart

Patients with altered bowel activity often have bowel movements recorded using a stool chart based on the 'Bristol Stool Chart' (Fig 14.3). Although not very appealing, a chart such as this allows staff to record the frequency and nature of bowel activity.

Bristol Stool Chart

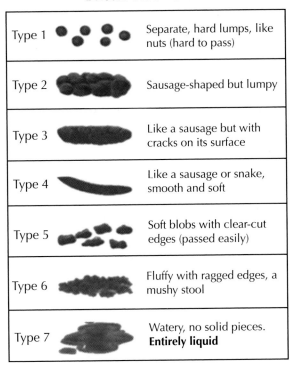

Type 1		Separate, hard lumps, like nuts (hard to pass)
Type 2		Sausage-shaped but lumpy
Type 3		Like a sausage but with cracks on its surface
Type 4		Like a sausage or snake, smooth and soft
Type 5		Soft blobs with clear-cut edges (passed easily)
Type 6		Fluffy with ragged edges, a mushy stool
Type 7		Watery, no solid pieces. **Entirely liquid**

Fig 14.3: Bristol Stool Chart. (From Lewis SJ, Heaton KW. Stool form scale as a useful guide to intestinal transit time. *Scand J Gastroenterol* 1997;**32**:920–4.)

Weight chart

It is often helpful to monitor a patient's weight with time. Malnourished patients might be monitored for weight gain after the establishment of a feeding programme, whereas patients with fluid overload are often monitored for weight loss as they are treated with diuretics and their oedema improves. Sudden dramatic changes in weight are, however, uncommon. Unless the patient has had a procedure (eg a large quantity of fluid drained or limb amputation), be wary that a sudden change in weight might simply be an error.

Blood glucose (and ketones)

Patients with diabetes mellitus will have their blood glucose level checked frequently during their stay using finger-prick blood draws and glucometers. Adjustments to their treatment may be required if they have either hyper- or hypoglycaemia. Patients with diabetic ketoacidosis will also have measurements taken of ketone levels in the blood or urine. Blood ketone levels are increasingly being measured with bedside ketometers, which work like glucometers. Urinary ketones are measured using urinalysis. As treatment for diabetic ketoacidosis is administered, ketone levels should fall into the normal range.

Blood glucose recording is not limited to patients with diabetes, however. Other examples of patients who should have blood glucose measured include:

- Patients who have been treated with insulin for hyperkalaemia
- Patients who are malnourished and are at risk of hypoglycaemia
- Patients with liver failure who are at risk of hypoglycaemia
- Patients on high doses of corticosteroids who are at risk of hyperglycaemia.

Respiratory function

Patients with respiratory difficulty often have simple respiratory tests performed at regular intervals. The most common example would be the peak expiratory flow rate (PEFR) in patients with obstructive airway disease such as asthma. In addition, patients at risk of neuromuscular weakness affecting respiration should have their vital capacity checked regularly. A falling vital capacity can indicate the need for assistance with ventilation.

Cardiac telemetry

Patients with cardiac disease and critical illness are at risk of cardiac arrhythmia and cardiac arrest, and their heart's electrical activity is often monitored using a bedside ECG machine. Interpretation of such data is included in Chapter 10. A useful function of many telemetry machines is that the heart rhythm strips are stored for several days. Patients who exhibit intermittent cardiac arrhythmias can have their heart rhythms analysed retrospectively, thus allowing the identification of serious problems.

Other information at the bedside

The area around a patient's bed often has a wealth of additional information for the astute observer to note. Therapists who have assessed a patient may record information such as the following on signs around the bed:

- Details about mobility, including devices to be used when mobilising or how many staff members will be required to help a patient mobilise.

- Communication difficulties: patients with deafness, dysphasia or who do not speak the native language may therefore be identified.

- Swallowing difficulties: signs such as 'nil orally' or 'yoghurt consistency foods only' might be seen.

- Dietary and fluid requirements such as fluid restrictions, salt restrictions, etc.

Case 14.1

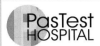 **FAECES CHART**

NAME	A PATIENT	HOSPITAL NUMBER	123456
DATE OF BIRTH	1 / 1 / 1970	WARD	BUTTERCUP

DATE	TIME	STOOL TYPE	CONSISTENCY	BLOOD	MUCUS	PUS	SIGN
10/06	0800	MODERATE	6 or 7	✓	✓		
	1000	"	7	✓			
	1230	"	6	✓			
	1425	"	6		✓		
	1615	"	7	✓			
	1845	"	7	✓			
	2105	LARGE	7	✓	✓		
	2330	"	6	✓			
11/06	0200	"	7	✓	✓		
	0530	MODERATE	6	✓			
	0720	"	6	✓			
	0930	"	7	✓	✓		
	1145	"	7	✓	✓		
	1355	LARGE	7	✓	✓		
	1605	MODERATE	7	✓			
	1830	"	6	✓			
	2010	"	6	✓			
	2235	"	7	✓			
	2355	"	7	✓			

Summarise the findings on the stool chart and list the potential causes

Answer 14.1

This patient is having bowel motion activity recorded formally using a faeces chart. At least eight motions each day have been passed. The consistency has been Bristol type 6 and 7 indicating very soft, watery motions. Furthermore it is mucoid and bloody. It would be important clinically for the fluid balance sheet to be assessed in conjunction with the stool chart to assess for adequate hydration. Possible causes for this pattern of bowel activity are listed in the box below.

> Inflammatory bowel disease
> Infective diarrhoea (eg *Shigella*, *Salmonella*)
> Colorectal malignancy
> Ischaemic colitis

Case 14.2

DAILY WEIGHTS

PasTest
HOSPITAL

DATE	TIME	WEIGHT
10/06/05	0800 HRS	125 kg
11/06/05	0800	124 kg
12/06/05	0800	123.1 kg
13/06/05	0800	122.2 kg
14/06/05	0800	115.4 kg
15/06/05	0800	115.9 kg
16/06/05	0800	116.6 kg
17/06/05	0800	118.1 kg

1. **Explain the findings on this daily weight chart for this patient with liver cirrhosis and ascites.**

2. **What could be the reason for the sudden loss of nearly 7 kg on 14/06/05?**

Answer 14.2

DAILY WEIGHTS   PasTest HOSPITAL

DATE	TIME	WEIGHT	
10/06/05	0800 HRS	125 kg	
11/06/05	0800	124 kg	
12/06/05	0800	123.1 kg	
13/06/05	0800	122.2 kg	Steady weight loss until here
14/06/05	0800	115.4 kg	Dramatic weight loss
15/06/05	0800	115.9 kg	
16/06/05	0800	116.6 kg	
17/06/05	0800	118.1 kg	Gradual weight gain

1. Daily weight charts are an extension of the standard fluid balance ('input/output') chart. In the short term (hours and days) changes usually reflect a change in body fluid content. It is paramount (as seen from the chart) that the recordings are taken at the same time each day. Dietitians keep weight records for those who are undernourished, receiving enteral or parenteral nutritional supplementation, or enrolled in dietary programmes. In such cases, changes in the longer term become more important. The common reasons for recording daily weight are conditions in which excess fluid is retained by the body – severe congestive cardiac failure, ascites or renal failure being prime examples.

   A response to treatment, in particular diuretics, and dietary sodium restriction may be monitored using a weight chart in conjunction with a fluid balance chart.

   This example documents a patient with significant ascites (excess fluid in the peritoneal cavity) over a period of several days after treatment. Over the initial 4 days a steady, albeit relatively small, daily reduction in weight is observed. This is in response to the introduction or increased dosing of diuretic therapy.

2. On 14/06/05 a more substantial reduction of 6.8 kg is observed. This is due to paracentesis with the removal of a substantial volume of fluid.

Case 14.3

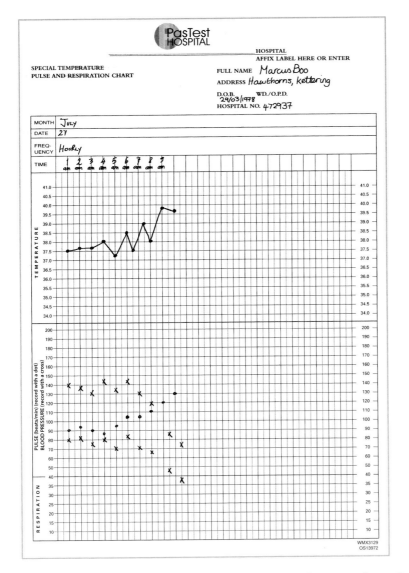

1. **Describe each abnormality on the observation chart and the overall impression.**

2. **Where should this patient be cared for?**

Answer 14.3

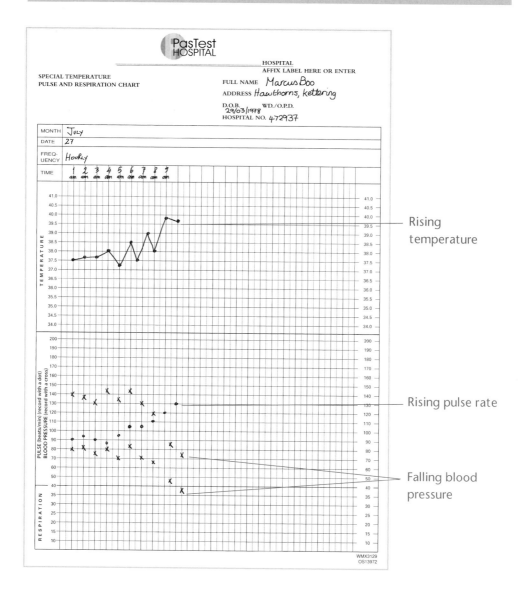

1. The diagnosis of sepsis requires a full patient assessment. However, the bedside chart may provide the first evidence of impending sepsis. Taking an assessment of the chart over several hours, rather than a snapshot, aids in the diagnosis as one views the alteration of three key parameters – blood pressure, pulse rate and temperature. A persistent pyrexia or swinging fever is seen in the context of haemodynamic instability (hypotension and tachycardia).

   This example clearly shows a rising and sustained pyrexia with a maximum temperature of 39.9°C. A falling blood pressure, to a low of 78/38 mmHg, with an accompanying tachycardia of 130 beats/min, demonstrates a haemodynamically unstable state.

2. If this patient fails to respond to initial treatment with fluids and antibiotics they should be transferred to an HDU/ICU environment where inotropic support (eg noradrenaline) may be administered to support the cardiovascular system until the underlying infection has been identified and treated.

Case 14.4

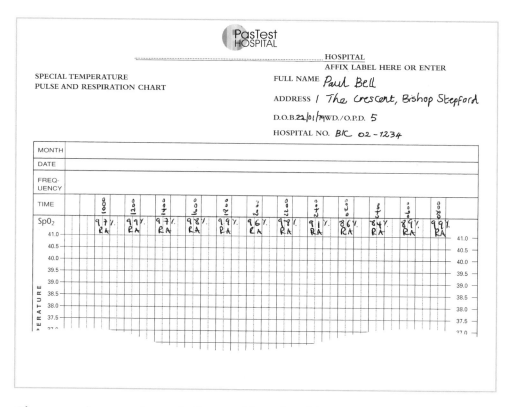

Give your impression of the problem in this patient.

Answer 14.4

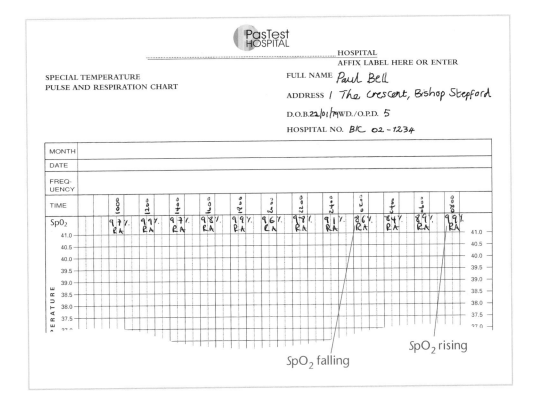

This chart outlines the blood oxygen saturations taken at 2-h intervals by pulse oximetry throughout a 24-h period. The vast majority are normal while breathing room air. If one was not to record the saturations during sleeping hours the patient may be deemed to be entirely normal. However, during the period 02:00–06:00 hours there is evidence of significant deoxygenation with a low of 84% at 04:00 hours.

The likely diagnosis here is obstructive sleep apnoea (OSA). If one was to waken the patient purposefully and then record the oxygen saturations they would probably return to normal. This diagnosis may be confirmed through formal sleep studies.

Case 14.5

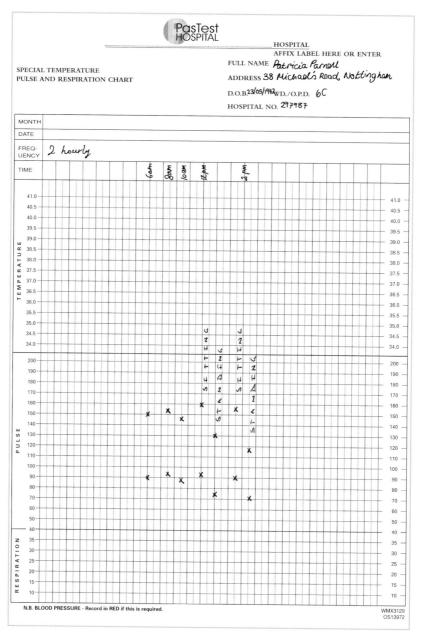

1. **What abnormality is seen?**

2. **Suggest a list of potential underlying diagnoses.**

Answer 14.5

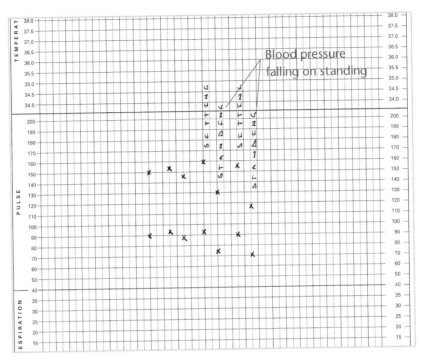

Blood pressure falling on standing

1. This basic chart demonstrates a series of blood pressure measurements. Unlike a conventional recording it indicates that some have been taken in different positions of posture. The likely indication for this is a patient with a history of falls, especially an elderly patient. For changes to be deemed significant, there must be a change in systolic blood pressure of greater than 20 mmHg when the patient changes from lying to standing. This patient has postural (orthostatic) hypotension.

2. Potential diagnoses are listed below:

CAUSES OF POSTURAL HYPOTENSION

Idiopathic
Dehydration (hypovolaemia)
Drug induced (eg diuretics, vasodilators, anti-parkinsonian medication)
Addison's disease
Autonomic neuropathy
Multisystem atrophy

Case 14.6

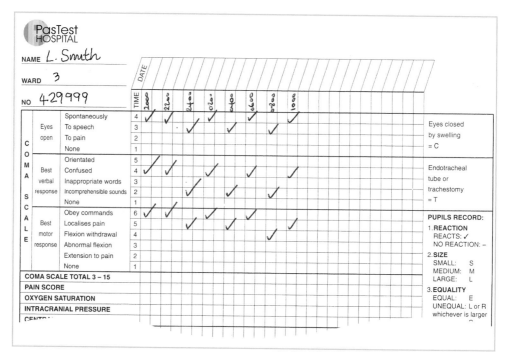

1. **Explain the findings on the neuro-observation chart.**

2. **What are the potential causes?**

Answer 14.6

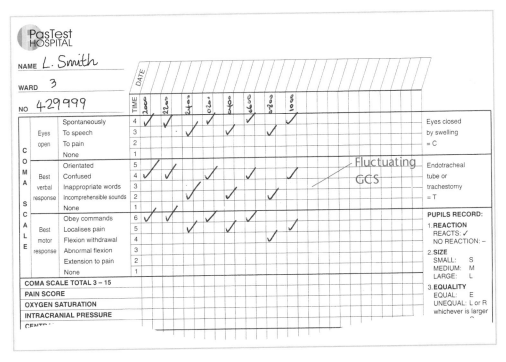

PasTest
HOSPITAL

NAME L. Smith

WARD 3

NO 429999

1. The GCS is a routinely used method of accurately and objectively recording a patient's level of consciousness. It is an easy-to-use scoring system which may be recorded in a reproducible fashion by nursing or medical staff. It comprises three independent categories – EYE OPENING, VERBAL RESPONSE and MOTOR RESPONSE. It is scored out of 15. The GCS must be measured in patients with head injury and after any neurosurgical intervention. This bedside chart illustrates its use in a patient after a fall.

On admission the GCS is 14/15 on the basis of the patient being confused. At midnight the conscious level takes a drop from 14/15 to 10/15. Two hours later one can observe that the GCS has returned to its admission level of 14/15. Further frequent monitoring throughout the morning shows a repeat of this pattern – the GCS IS FLUCTUANT. An intracranial cause should be sought with urgent imaging.

2. This pattern is typically seen in subdural haematoma. Following a fall, the patient is lucid at times but the conscious level is variable. Extracranial causes, eg sepsis or hypoglycaemia, may also account for such patterns.

Case 14.7

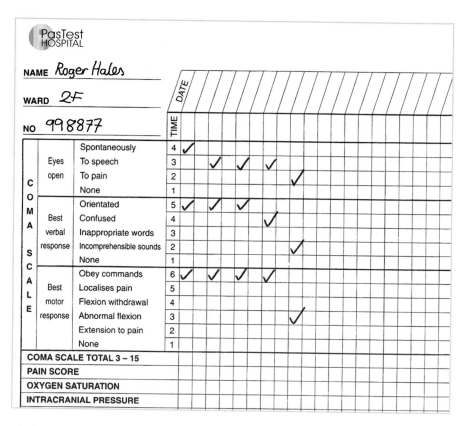

Explain what action one would take on becoming aware of these observations.

Answer 14.7

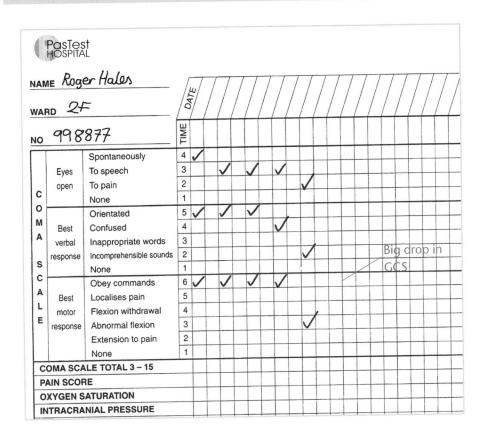

Changes in conscious level may be sudden and permanent as well as fluctuant. A significant drop in the GCS should be acted upon without delay. This bedside chart records a large drop from 13 to 7. This sudden change requires both a fast answer to establish the cause, and action to be taken to ensure the welfare of the patient. A GCS of less than 8/15 is an indication for consideration of intubation as the patient's airway is likely to become compromised .

CAUSES OF LARGE SUDDEN DROP IN GCS	
Intracerebral bleed (including subarachnoid haemorrhage) Cerebral oedema Drugs and alcohol	Trauma – diffuse axonal injury Metabolic causes (such as hypoglycaemia)

Case 14.8

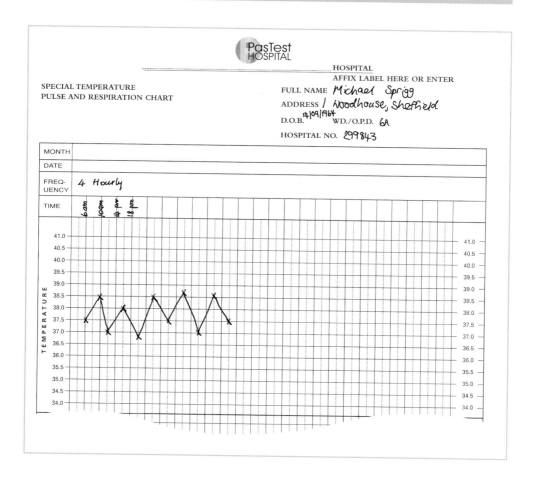

Describe the findings on this chart.

Answer 14.8

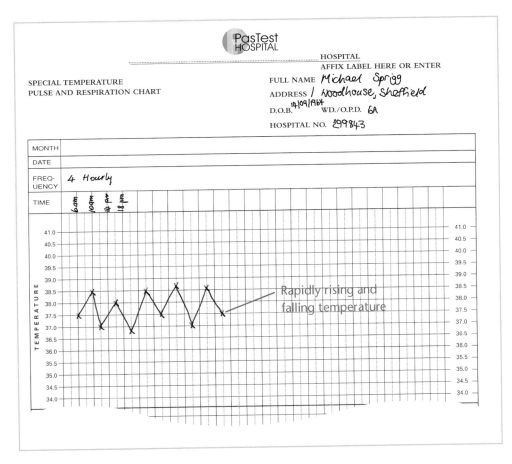

There is a simple but striking finding on the general observation chart over a period of several hours. The trend in temperature recordings is highly abnormal. It can be seen that the patient is apyrexic at times but has a significantly elevated temperature on other occasions. This is a swinging or spiking fever. Each temperature peak probably represents the shedding of bacterial toxins into the bloodstream. This finding may be due to any underlying infective source – although the pattern is characteristically seen in the setting of an abscess. A similar pattern can be seen in several rheumatological diseases e.g. Still's disease.

Case 14.9

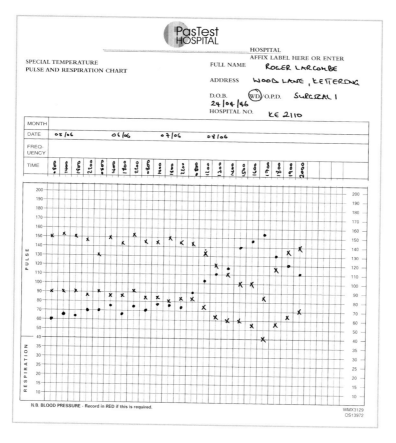

PasTest HOSPITAL

HOSPITAL

SPECIAL TEMPERATURE
PULSE AND RESPIRATION CHART

AFFIX LABEL HERE OR ENTER

FULL NAME   ROGER LARCOMBE

ADDRESS   WOOD LANE, KETTERING

D.O.B.   WD/O.P.D.   SURGICAL 1
24/04/46
HOSPITAL NO.   KE 2110

NAME	ROGER LARCOMBE	HOSPITAL NUMBER	KE 2110
DATE OF BIRTH	24/04/1946	WARD	SURGICAL 1

DATE	TIME	AMOUNT	CONSISTENCY	BLOOD	MUCUS	PUS	SIGN
5/6	08 00	SMALL	4				Mudgate
	16 00	MODERATE	5				Mudgate
6/6	10 00	SMALL	5	DARK			Mudgate
	20 00	SMALL	4	DARK			Mudgate
7/6	0900	MODERATE	5	DARK			Mudgate
	1300	SMALL	4				Mudgate
	2100	MODERATE	4	DARK			Mudgate
8/6	06 00	LARGE	5	BLACK+FOUL			Mudgate
	07 00	MODERATE	5	"			Mudgate
	09 00	LARGE	5	"			Mudgate
	13 00	MODERATE	5	"			Mudgate
	1700	MODERATE	5	"			Mudgate

Describe the findings on these charts and what investigation(s) are needed to confirm the cause.

Answer 14.9

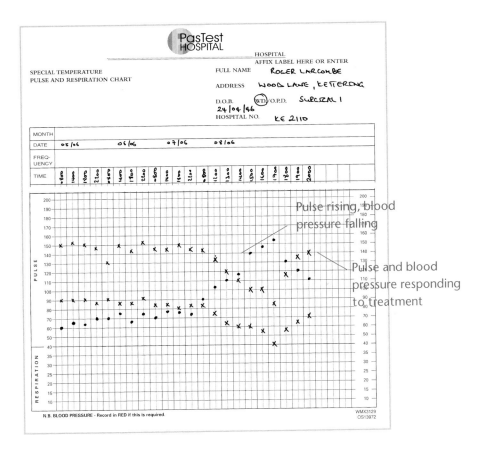

Most patients will have several observation charts at the end of the bed. These should all be viewed in a systematic fashion to maximise the information obtained. In this scenario, both the vital signs chart and the bowel habit chart reveal the likely diagnosis.

An inpatient for several days following admission with dark stools and rectal bleeding, this patient has remained stable, albeit with persistently abnormal bowel motions. It can be seen that on occasion the motion is both loose and dark in nature, but is always relatively small in volume and the patient's general observations initially remain normal.

Fluid resuscitation, possibly with blood products, has occurred. Note on day 4 (08/06) that the patient becomes progressively more tachycardic and with this the blood pressure falls. This corresponds to an increase in the frequency of the motions, which are noted to be black and foul smelling in nature – this patient has melaena.

The melaena has been present to an extent since admission; however, on this occasion the patient has become haemodynamically unstable. There has been a significant upper gastrointestinal tract bleed. The patient should now undergo emergency endoscopy to locate and if possible treat the cause. In the meantime, intravenous fluids and packed cells should be administered. Any coagulopathy should be corrected. One can see the blood pressure and tachycardia respond to fluid replacement (08/06 from 18:00 hours onwards).

Case 14.10

Start date
22/09/2005

PasTest HOSPITAL

Drug Prescription and Administration Record (DPAR1)

Andrew Brown

Patient details
Affix label
RFC 293949
DoB 22/06/1959

Drug allergies:

NKDA

| Weight | Date | Signature |
| Weight | Date | Signature |

REGULAR PRESCRIPTIONS

Date, month and year →	Times ↓	22/09	23/09	24/09	25/09									
Drug ATENOLOL **Frequency** OD	08	TIB	RA	SM	EM									
Dose 50 MG **Route** Po **Start date** 22/09/05 **Stop date**														
Signature Mickle **Stop signature**														
Additional information														
Drug SPIRONOLACTONE **Frequency** OD	08	CM	CM	SM	EM									
Dose 100 MG **Route** Po **Start date** 22/09/05 **Stop date**														
Signature Mickle **Stop signature**														
Additional information														
Drug LISINOPRIL **Frequency** OD	08	/	CM	SM	EM									
Dose 5 MG **Route** Po **Start date** 23/09/05 **Stop date**														
Signature Mickle **Stop signature**														
Additional information														
Drug SLOW – K **Frequency** BD	08			SM	EM									
Dose TT **Route** Po **Start date** 24/09 **Stop date**														
Signature Mickle **Stop signature**														
Additional information	22			TRJ	RHT									
Drug LACTULOSE **Frequency** BD	08			SM	EM									
Dose 10 MLS **Route** Po **Start date** 24/09 **Stop date**														
Signature Mickle **Stop signature**														
Additional information	22			TRJ	RHT									

What electrolyte is likely to be deranged in this patient?

Answer 14.10

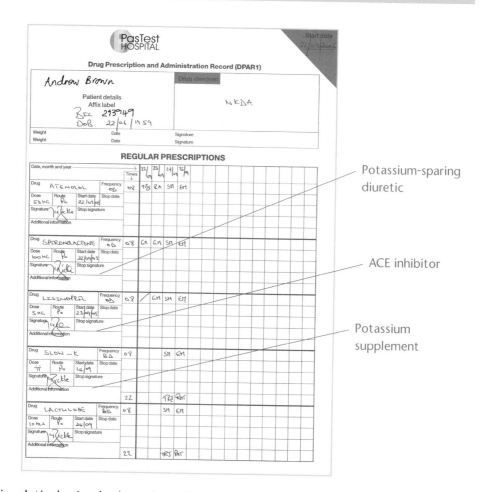

This relatively simple drug chart illustrates the importance of appreciating the actions of common medications and the problems that can arise. On admission, the patient is on a K$^+$-sparing diuretic (spironolactone) at a dose that suggests an indication for liver disease rather than heart failure. On day 1 of his admission, an angiotensin-converting enzyme (ACE) inhibitor is introduced. The combination of an ACE inhibitor (lisinopril) and spironolactone, although acceptable, should be appreciated and initially the serum potassium should be checked to ensure that it does not rise to a dangerous level. Therefore, when supplemental potassium is started the following day – perhaps by a busy doctor who does not usually cover this patient and who has limited understanding of the patient's overall case – we have a potential disaster. If left unchecked the K$^+$ may increase to a level causing cardiac dysrhythmias or, worse, cardiac arrest.

Case 14.11

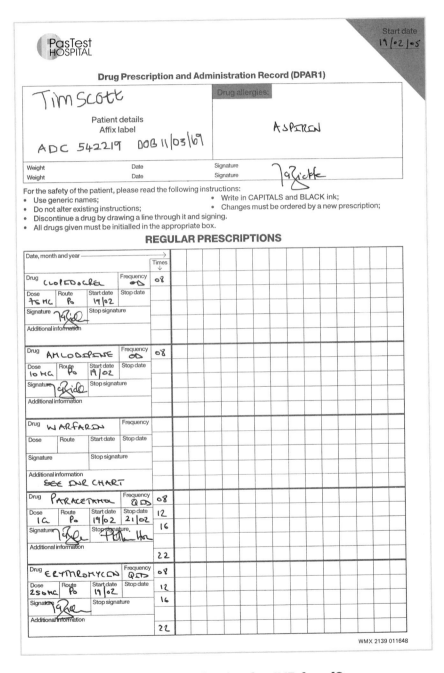

What has caused the difficulties in the INR level?

PasTest
HOSPITAL

Tim Scott

ADC 542219   DOB 11/05/69

Date	INR result	Warfarin dose	Prescribed by	Given by	Time	Date	INR result	Warfarin dose	Prescribed by	Given by	Time
19/02	2.35	4 mg	Jaz	CM	2200						
20/02	—	4 mg	Jaz	CM	2200						
21/02	2.98	3 mg	PKH	EFF	2200						
22/02	—	3 mg	Jaz	KRT	2200						
23/02	3.99	2 mg	PKH	NHY	2200						

Answer 14.11

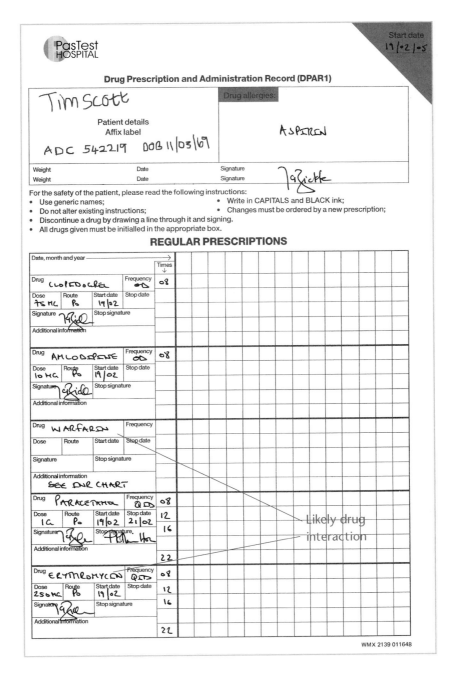

Start date
19/02/05

PasTest HOSPITAL

Drug Prescription and Administration Record (DPAR1)

Tim Scott

Patient details
Affix label

ADC 542219 DOB 11/03/69

Drug allergies:

ASPIRIN

| Weight | Date | Signature |
| Weight | Date | Signature |

For the safety of the patient, please read the following instructions:
- Use generic names;
- Do not alter existing instructions;
- Discontinue a drug by drawing a line through it and signing.
- All drugs given must be initialled in the appropriate box.
- Write in CAPITALS and BLACK ink;
- Changes must be ordered by a new prescription;

REGULAR PRESCRIPTIONS

Date, month and year →   Times ↓

Drug CLOPIDOGREL **Frequency** OD 08
Dose 75 MG **Route** Po **Start date** 19/02 **Stop date**
Signature **Stop signature**
Additional information

Drug AMLODIPINE **Frequency** OD 08
Dose 10 MG **Route** Po **Start date** 19/02 **Stop date**
Signature **Stop signature**
Additional information

Drug WARFARIN **Frequency**
Dose **Route** **Start date** **Stop date**
Signature **Stop signature**
Additional information SEE OUR CHART

Drug PARACETAMOL **Frequency** QDS 08
Dose 1 G **Route** Po **Start date** 19/02 **Stop date** 21/02 12
Signature **Stop signature** 16
Additional information 22

Likely drug interaction

Drug ERYTHROMYCIN **Frequency** QDS 08
Dose 250 MG **Route** Po **Start date** 19/02 **Stop date** 12
Signature **Stop signature** 16
Additional information 22

WMX 2139 011648

PasTest
HOSPITAL

Tim Scott

ADC 542219   DOB 11/03/69

Date	INR result	Warfarin dose	Prescribed by	Given by	Time	Date	INR result	Warfarin dose	Prescribed by	Given by	Time
19/02	2·35	4 mg	7.9/8	CM	2200						
20/02	—	4 mg	7.9/8	CM	2200						
21/02	2·98	3 mg	PKH	EFF	2200						
22/02	—	3 mg	7.9/8	KRT	2200						
23/02	3·99	2 mg	PKH	NHY	2200						
			Rising INR								

This scenario is based upon both a patient's drug chart and warfarin chart. Those patients on warfarin while in hospital should be placed on a dedicated warfarin chart. This generally outlines the indication for its prescription, the desired target INR (international normalised ratio) range and the daily warfarin dose and INR if taken. It is easy, but also dangerous, to view this chart in isolation. Following admission this patient is started on erythromycin and the warfarin dose remains at the usual level from admission. The INR was recorded before the first inpatient dose and was 2.35, perfectly placed in the desired range for the indication, atrial fibrillation. On day 3 it is checked again and found to be 2.98. The dose is decreased by 1 mg, but again 2 days later the INR has continued to rise to 3.99. This is not in the highly dangerous range, but is enough to warrant consideration. The drug erythromycin is the cause. A macrolide antibiotic, it is known to enhance the anticoagulant effect of warfarin through its effect as an enzyme inhibitor in the liver.

Case 14.12

A patient's heart rate is monitored frequently after an admission with a suspected myocardial infarction.

What is your interpretation, and what would you do for the patient?

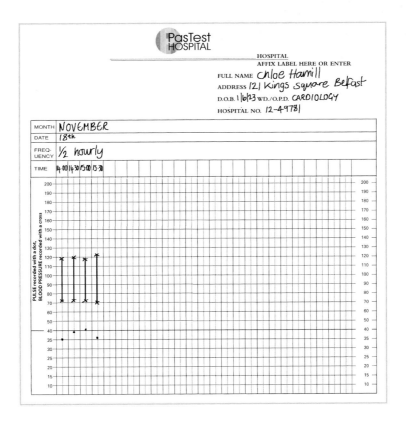

Answer 14.12

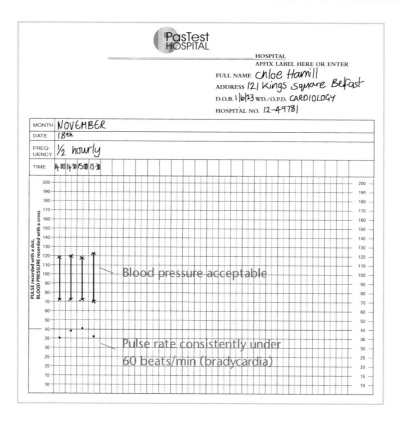

The patient has a marked bradycardia. The blood pressure seems acceptable, so gathering more information seems most appropriate at this stage. You should record a 12-lead ECG and attach the patient to a cardiac monitor.

After a short time, you are called to interpret the cardiac monitor. You see the following on the screen:

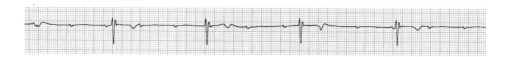

What is your interpretation of the heart rhythm?

The rhythm is complete heart block (or third-degree heart block) (see page 350 for further details). The patient requires drug treatment to speed the heart up, and will probably require the insertion of a pacemaker.

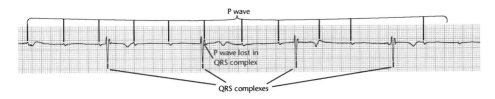

MISCELLANEOUS 15

MISCELLANEOUS

Ankle brachial pressure index

The ankle brachial pressure index (ABPI) is an easily measured clinical parameter that is often used to assess the adequacy of blood flow to the lower limbs.

The patient should lie flat on a bed when having an ABPI measured. The systolic blood pressure in the brachial artery is measured using a stethoscope and sphygmomanometer. The systolic blood pressure at the ankle is then measured using a sphygmomanometer wrapped around the calf and a Doppler probe positioned over the posterior tibial or dorsalis pedis artery. Cuff pressure is inflated until blood flow to the foot is cut off. Flow is slowly re-established by deflating the cuff, and the pressure at which the first Doppler signal is obtained is noted.

After performing these tests, the observer will have two figures – the systolic blood pressures in the brachial artery and at the ankle. The ABPI is calculated simply by finding their ratio. In health, the ratio should be greater than or equal to 1. As the value decreases, symptoms and signs of arterial insufficiency to the lower limbs would be expected. Values lower than 0.5 may result in critical ischaemia. ABPIs of lower than 0.2 can be associated with ulceration and gangrene.

ABPI	INTERPRETATION
>1	Normal
<0.5	At risk of critical ischaemia
<0.2	At risk of ulceration and gangrene

One potentially complicating factor relates to the fact that some patients (particularly those with long-standing diabetes mellitus) have calcified arteries which cannot be compressed with a blood pressure cuff. In such cases, Doppler signals will be obtained even when the cuff is inflated to very high pressures. ABPIs cannot be reliably measured in these patients.

DON'T FORGET
The ABPI must be interpreted with caution in patients with diabetes mellitus.

Synovial fluid analysis

Patients with acute monoarthritis often have synovial fluid aspirated for diagnostic purposes. It is important to be able to differentiate between the common causes of the acutely red, hot and swollen joint on the basis of fluid analysis.

DIAGNOSIS	APPEARANCE	LEUKOCYTE COUNT (/mm^3)	APPEARANCE ON PLANE POLARISED LIGHT MICROSCOPY
Septic arthritis	Purulent	>750 000	
Haemarthrosis	Heavily blood stained		
Gout	Cloudy	3000–40 000	Negatively birefringent needle-shaped crystals
Pseudogout	Cloudy	3000–40 000	Weakly positively birefringent rhomboidal crystals

MEMORY AID

Gout – remember the letter 'N' – **N**egatively birefringent, **N**eedle-shaped crystals of sodium urate

Pseudogout – remember the letter 'P' – weakly **P**ositively birefringent rhomboidal crystals of sodium **P**yrophosphate

Schirmer test

Keratoconjunctivitis sicca is the term used to describe dry eyes. This phenomenon can occur in isolation (primary Sjögren syndrome) or in association with many other rheumatological conditions.

The test is performed by attaching a specially shaped piece of filter paper to the lower eyelid. This is left for 5 min, and the distance that has become wet is then measured. Normally 10 mm or more of the paper will become wet.

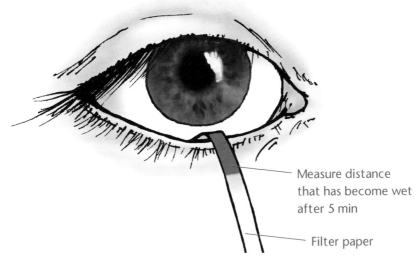

Measure distance
that has become wet
after 5 min

Filter paper

Fig 15.1

It is important to bear in mind, however, that normal tear production is reduced in old age. Also, drugs with anticholinergic properties, such as tricyclic antidepressants, reduce tear production and may result in a false-positive Schirmer test.

PABA test

The PABA test is used to detect pancreatic exocrine insufficiency, ie failure of the pancreas to produce sufficient enzymes for complete digestion.

The principle behind the test is simple. After fasting overnight, the patient is given a fixed dose of a peptide comprising *N*-benzoyl-L-tyrosyl-*pa*-aminobenzoic acid (NBT-PABA). In a patient with normal pancreatic exocrine function, pancreatic enzymes break down NBT-PABA into the smaller compound PABA, which is then absorbed and excreted in the urine. Normally more than 70% of the dose administered appears in the urine. Less than 70% excretion implies that the exocrine activity of the pancreas is impaired.

DON'T FORGET
Normally >70% of the oral PABA dose is detected in the urine.

Tests for the presence of *Helicobacter pylori*

The Gram-negative bacillus *H. pylori* can infect the stomach and predispose to the development of peptic ulcer disease. Testing for the presence of the organism should be carried out in all patients with a peptic ulcer, and eradication should be attempted in affected individuals.

There are several methods that can be used to test for the presence of *H. pylori*.

Breath testing

This test relies on the fact that *H. pylori* organisms produce urease, an enzyme that breaks down urea to form ammonia and carbon dioxide. The ammonia produced raises the pH and helps the organism survive the acidic environment in the stomach.

In a *H. pylori* breath test, the patient is given a tablet containing radiolabelled urea ($[^{13}C]$urea). If infection is present, the organisms act on the urea to liberate radiolabelled carbon dioxide ($^{13}CO_2$). A sample of breath is collected (eg in a tube or balloon), and analysed for the presence of $^{13}CO_2$. If this is detected, the test is positive and the patient can be assumed to be infected.

This test rapidly becomes negative if *H. pylori* is eradicated.

Detection of *H. pylori* antibodies

A sample of blood can be tested for the presence of IgG antibodies to *H. pylori*. The test can remain positive for up to a year after eradication therapy, and so it is not a particularly useful way of testing for clearance.

Campylobacter-like organism (CLO) test

This test also requires a biopsy sample obtained at oesophagogastro-duodenoscopy (OGD). The sample of tissue is placed into a medium that contains urea and phenol red. Phenol red is a dye that turns red in alkaline conditions. If *H. pylori* is present in the biopsy sample, its urease enzyme will liberate ammonia from the urea in the medium, causing the pH to rise. The colour of the medium will therefore turn red (Fig 15.2).

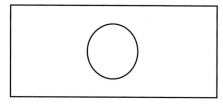

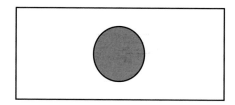

CLO test negative   *CLO test positive (red circle)*

Fig 15.2

Tissue histology

A stomach biopsy sample can be stained and examined under a microscope. This may reveal curved organisms at the mucosal surface.

Tissue culture

A biopsy sample obtained at OGD can be cultured to look for the presence of offending organisms.

Audiograms

Audiograms illustrate, in graphic form, how well a person can hear noises at different frequencies. A healthy ear can hear sounds transmitted in the air better than those conducted by bone. This is because the ossicles in the middle ear amplify sound waves in the air.

Several patterns of abnormalities should be recognised.

1. **Conductive deafness**
   Anything that impedes the progression of sound waves down the ear canal can result in conductive deafness. The classic example of this is the patient with severe ear wax. In these conditions, sounds conducted by bone will be heard louder than those conducted by air. The audiogram will show a gap between the hearing level for air and bone conduction. This is termed a wide air–bone gap.

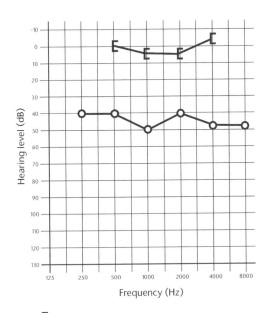

Fig 15.3

2. Sensorineural deafness

A patient with unilateral auditory nerve damage (eg due to an acoustic neuroma) will have reduced hearing for both air conduction and bone conduction.

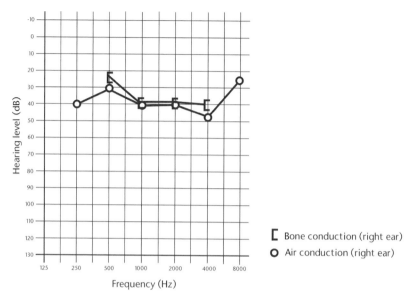

[Bone conduction (right ear)

O Air conduction (right ear)

Fig 15.4

3. Presbyacusis

This describes the loss of hearing of sounds at high frequencies that is a common finding in elderly patients. It represents a form of sensorineural deafness.

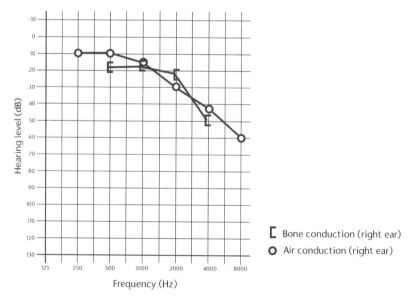

[Bone conduction (right ear)

O Air conduction (right ear)

Fig 15.5

4. **Noise-induced hearing loss**

Patients with noise-induced hearing loss typically have difficulty hearing sounds with a frequency around 4000 Hz. Their audiograms usually have a trough at this frequency level.

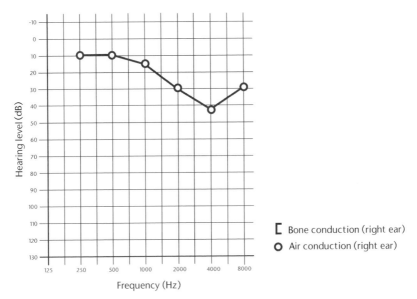

Fig 15.6

Cardiovascular risk

Until relatively recently, clinical judgement has been the main method of deciding which patients require drug therapy for primary prevention against cardiovascular disease. Guidelines are now available that aim to help doctors decide which patients require treatment. One part of a cardiovascular risk assessment chart is shown here.

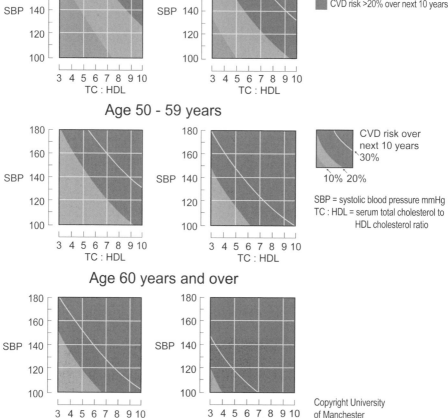

Fig 15.7 Reproduced with kind permission of Manchester University Press.

These charts are easily interpreted as follows.

1. Choose the correct chart using the patient's sex, smoking status and age group. Whether or not a patient is classified as a smoker depends on their lifetime exposure to smoke, not just their current smoking status. Thus, patients who are ex-smokers, but gave up smoking within the last 5 years, should be classified as smokers for the purposes of interpreting these charts.

2. Knowledge of the patient's systolic blood pressure and details of their lipid profile are plotted to obtain the patient's cardiovascular risk over the next 10 years. Note that the x-axis on the charts plots the ratio of total cholesterol to high-density-lipoprotein (HDL) cholesterol, and this value should be used when available. When only the serum cholesterol concentration is known, assume that the HDL level is 1 mmol/l.

Ambulatory blood pressure monitoring

Ambulatory blood pressure monitoring (ABPM) is being increasingly used as an investigative tool in the management of people with high blood pressure. It gives a lot more information than a one-off office blood pressure measure, and can help identify people with various blood pressure patterns, such as:

- White-coat hypertension: blood pressure 'artificially' high when measured by a doctor or nurse, ie ABPM lower than clinic pressure.

- Masked hypertension: blood pressure 'artificially' low when measured by a doctor or nurse, ie ABPM higher than clinic pressure.

- Nocturnal dipping: it is normal for the blood pressure to drop overnight when sleeping. The mean arterial pressure should drop by at least 10 mmHg.

- Non-dipping: blood pressure that does not fall in sleep.

- Reverse dipping: blood pressure that increases during sleep.

To interpret an ABPM results summary take the following steps:

- Look at how many of the attempted readings were successful. If the vast majority of readings were successful, the study is useful. If only a few readings were successful, the results of the study are of questionable value.

- Look at the average daytime pressure. Apply a 'correction factor' of 10/5 mmHg to this to calculate an equivalent clinic blood pressure, eg if the average daytime pressure is 140/80 mmHg on the ABPM, the equivalent clinic pressure would be 150/85 mmHg. This is the value that should be used for making treatment decisions.

- Compare the average daytime pressure with the most recent clinic readings and decide if the patient is 'normal', or has 'white-coat' or 'masked' hypertension.

- Look at the overnight blood pressure. Compare the mean arterial pressure overnight with that obtained during the day. If the blood pressure does not dip normally, the patient should be questioned. A poor night's sleep or obstructive sleep apnoea are common causes for blood pressure failing to dip at night. If the patient slept well on the night of the study, one can use the ABPM result to classify them into having normal-, non- or reverse-nocturnal dipping.

An ABPM record can also provide much more information, such as detail about the pulse pressure and heart rate at various times of the day. These data may also be helpful in stratifying a patient's cardiac risk.

Case 15.1

A 74-year-old woman attends the diabetes clinic for a routine appointment. Her medical history includes type 2 diabetes (diagnosed 15 years previously), two previous myocardial infarctions and previous varicose vein surgery. She has noticed an ulcer on her left leg. Examination reveals the presence of varicose eczema, and a shallow ulcer of diameter 4 cm affecting the medial aspect of the left leg.

1. **How would you manage this woman?**

The ABPI was 0.9.

2. **What treatment should the patient receive?**

Answer 15.1

1. Leg ulcers can be the result of several underlying disease processes. Most commonly, ulcers can be due to venous insufficiency, arterial insufficiency or a combination of both. The patient's medical history puts her at risk of both venous (previous varicose vein surgery) and arterial (diabetes and ischaemic heart disease) ulcers. Findings on examination are, however, more in keeping with a venous ulcer.

    Management of venous ulceration is complex, but the mainstay relies on graduated pressure bandages. However, these bandages can exacerbate arterial insufficiency, and should not be routinely applied to all patients without first performing an ABPI measurement. The first step in the management of this patient's ulcer should therefore involve measurement of the ABPI.

2. The patient should be treated with graduated pressure bandages. Patients with an ABPI of less than 0.8 should not, in general, have compression bandages applied.

COMPLETE CLINICAL CASES

16

Use your understanding and interpretative skills from the rest of the book to approach these complete cases. The cases represent full patient pathways in which data from a multitude of investigations are available for interpretation. These holistic cases will test your skills in real-life scenarios.

COMPLETE CLINICAL CASES

Case 16.1

DATA COVERED IN THIS CLINICAL CASE SCENARIO

- Haematology: full blood picture
- Biochemistry: urea and electrolytes, amylase, glucose, ketones
- Respiratory: arterial blood gas
- Urinalysis
- Bedside chart: vital signs

An 18-year-old shop assistant is admitted with generalised abdominal pain that has been worsening for 36 hours. On examination, you find the abdomen to be generally tender, although there is no clinical evidence of peritonism. The nurse hands you her observations recording sheet.

PasTest
HOSPITAL

.... HOSPITAL

AFFIX LABEL HERE OR ENTER

SPECIAL TEMPERATURE
PULSE AND RESPIRATION CHART

FULL NAME Julie Smyth
ADDRESS 101 Clifton Road, Bangor
D.O.B. 31/12/92 WD./O.P.D. Admissions ward
HOSPITAL NO. PH11-12345

MONTH	November
DATE	21st
FREQ-UENCY	Hourly
TIME	1500

SpO₂ 97% RA

TEMPERATURE

41.0	41.0
40.5	40.5
40.0	40.0
39.5	39.5
39.0	39.0
38.5	38.5
38.0	38.0
37.5	37.5
37.0	37.0
36.5	36.5
36.0	36.0
35.5	35.5
35.0	35.0
34.5	34.5
34.0	34.0

PULSE recorded with a dot,
BLOOD PRESSURE recorded with a cross

200	200
190	190
180	180
170	170
160	160
150	150
140	140
130	130
120	120
110	110
100	100
90	90
80	80
70	70
60	60
50	50
40	40

RESPIRATION

35	35
30	30
25	25
20	20
15	15
10	10

1. **What parameters are notably abnormal? Does this narrow your differential diagnosis?**

Shortly, you receive her initial blood results.

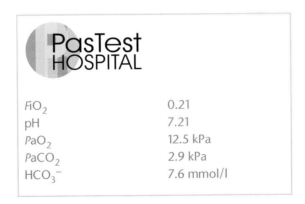

PasTest HOSPITAL	
Hb	13.2 g/dl
MCV	84 fl
WCC	$7.6 \times 10^9/l$
Plt	$368 \times 10^9/l$
Na$^+$	142 mmol/l
K$^+$	3.9 mmol/l
Urea	6.2 mmol/l
Creatinine	46 µmol/l
Cl$^-$	94 mmol/l
HCO$_3^-$	8 mmol/l
Amylase	52 U/l

2. **What is the major abnormality? Are any possible diagnoses less likely bearing these results in mind?**

On account of the abnormalities seen, you perform a blood gas analysis. The results are shown. The patient is breathing room air.

PasTest HOSPITAL	
FiO$_2$	0.21
pH	7.21
PaO$_2$	12.5 kPa
PaCO$_2$	2.9 kPa
HCO$_3^-$	7.6 mmol/l

3. **What are the causes of the acid–base abnormality demonstrated and what tests might you arrange to differentiate between them?**

You request urinalysis. The results are shown.

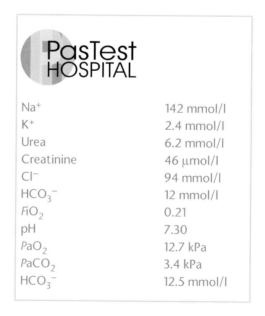

Glucose	++++
Bilirubin	Neg
Ketones	++++
Specific gravity	1.005
Blood	Neg
Protein	Neg
Nitrite	Neg
Leukocytes	Neg

4. Based on all the results so far, what is the apparent cause of the abdominal pain?

Treatment is commenced, and the patient appears to improve. You are asked to review her in 4 hours. Her bedside charts on the opposite page show the trend of vital signs.

5. Are you satisfied that the patient is improving?

Repeat blood tests show the following:

Na^+	142 mmol/l
K^+	2.4 mmol/l
Urea	6.2 mmol/l
Creatinine	46 μmol/l
Cl^-	94 mmol/l
HCO_3^-	12 mmol/l
FiO_2	0.21
pH	7.30
PaO_2	12.7 kPa
$PaCO_2$	3.4 kPa
HCO_3^-	12.5 mmol/l

6. What action would you take now?

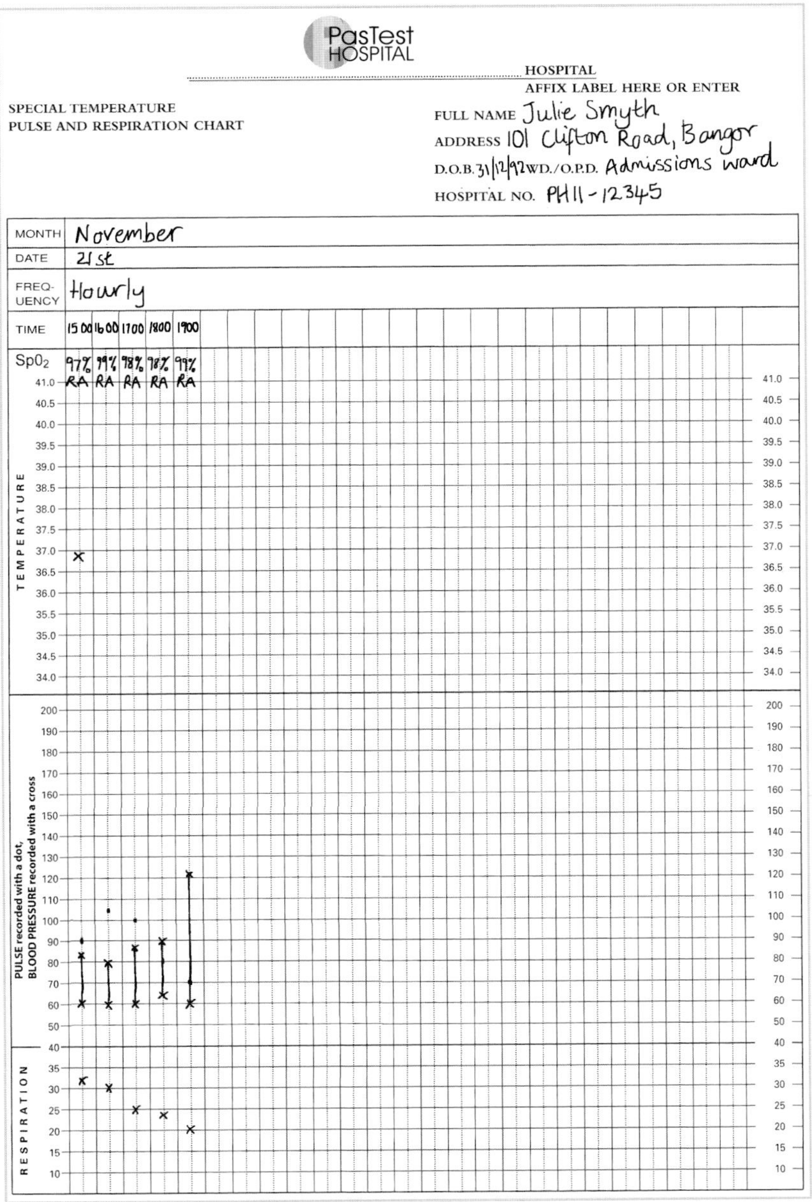

PasTest
HOSPITAL

.... HOSPITAL

AFFIX LABEL HERE OR ENTER

SPECIAL TEMPERATURE
PULSE AND RESPIRATION CHART

FULL NAME Julie Smyth
ADDRESS 101 Clifton Road, Bangor
D.O.B. 31/12/42 WD./O.P.D. Admissions ward
HOSPITAL NO. PH11 - 12345

MONTH	November
DATE	21st
FREQUENCY	Hourly
TIME	1500 1600 1700 1800 1900

SpO2: 97% 99% 98% 98% 99%
RA RA RA RA RA

TEMPERATURE (41.0 – 34.0)

X at 37.0 (1500)

PULSE recorded with a dot, BLOOD PRESSURE recorded with a cross

RESPIRATION

Time	Glucose (mmol/l)	Ketones (mmol/l)
1500	28.2	7.2
1600	26.3	6.1
1700	19.5	4.9
1800	12.7	4.1
1900	8.6	2.8

Answer 16.1

1. The patient's respiratory rate is increased. Your first thought might be that the patient has a problem with breathing, and indeed this could be the case. A basal pneumonia, for example, can present with abdominal discomfort. However, there are many reasons for tachypnoea outside the chest, eg patients breathe faster when they are in pain or if they have a metabolic acidosis (to facilitate respiratory compensation). As a result of the wide range of problems that can manifest with increased respiratory rate, this sign is often regarded as the most sensitive parameter that something serious is wrong with a patient.

    The patient's blood pressure is low. Again this could be due to a wide variety of reasons. Commonly, blood pressure falls with blood loss, sepsis and dehydration. Bearing in mind the abdominal pain, sensible suggestions would include a bleeding peptic ulcer, appendicitis or colitis.

    Taking abdominal pain in context with tachypnoea and hypotension, the range of possible diagnoses remains wide and further tests are required.

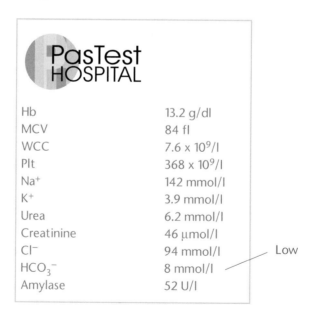

Hb	13.2 g/dl
MCV	84 fl
WCC	7.6×10^9/l
Plt	368×10^9/l
Na+	142 mmol/l
K+	3.9 mmol/l
Urea	6.2 mmol/l
Creatinine	46 µmol/l
Cl−	94 mmol/l
HCO3−	8 mmol/l — Low
Amylase	52 U/l

2. The major abnormality is the very low bicarbonate level. This is highly suggestive of a metabolic acidosis, although a measure of pH and $PaCO_2$ would be required to be sure of this.

    The normal haemoglobin is reassuring in terms of the fact that major blood loss would seem less likely. It should be borne in mind, however, that, after an acute bleed, it takes some time before the haemoglobin concentration falls – bleeding cannot therefore be ruled out using this test alone. The normal white cell count makes an infective cause less likely. The normal amylase level makes acute pancreatitis less likely, although sometimes the level can rise after a few hours, so if there is suspicion of pancreatitis, the level should be repeated.

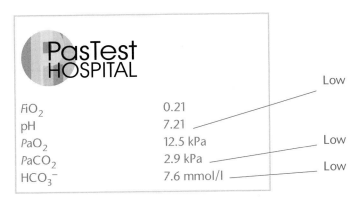

PasTest HOSPITAL		
FiO_2	0.21	
pH	7.21	Low
PaO_2	12.5 kPa	Low
$PaCO_2$	2.9 kPa	Low
HCO_3^-	7.6 mmol/l	Low

3. The blood gas analysis shows first that oxygenation is adequate. There is a metabolic acidosis present with respiratory compensation. You should then proceed to calculate the anion gap based on information presented earlier in the case. This is calculated as $(142 + 3.9) - (94 + 7.6) = 44.3$ mmol/l, and is therefore markedly raised. Note that it would also be reasonable to use the bicarbonate level from the initial set of blood tests for your calculation, although it is good practice always to use the most up-to-date results when making impressions about a patient's current state. Please refer to page 428 for a list of causes of this pH abnormality. Tests that would be useful at this stage could include; blood glucose, urinary glucose, blood ketones, urinary ketones, blood lactate and blood salicylate level if there is any suggestion of poisoning.

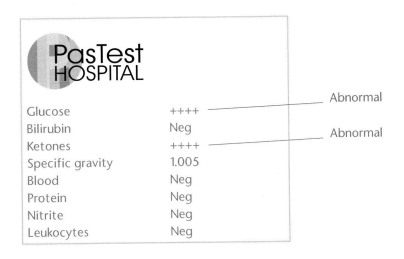

PasTest HOSPITAL		
Glucose	++++	Abnormal
Bilirubin	Neg	Abnormal
Ketones	++++	
Specific gravity	1.005	
Blood	Neg	
Protein	Neg	
Nitrite	Neg	
Leukocytes	Neg	

4. The presence of significant quantities of glucose and ketones on urinalysis, taken in context with an increased anion gap metabolic acidosis, is highly suggestive of diabetic ketoacidosis (DKA). This is recognised as an uncommon cause of abdominal pain and should always be borne in mind because it can be easily missed. The diagnosis should be confirmed by measuring blood glucose and ketone levels.

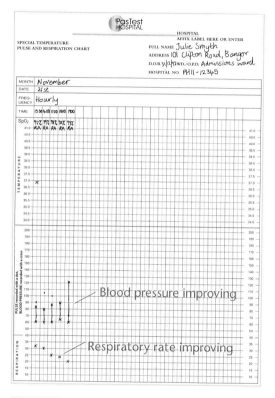

Time	Glucose (mmol/l)	Ketones (mmol/l)
1500	28.2	7.2
1600	26.3	6.1
1700	19.5	4.9
1800	12.7	4.1
1900	8.6	2.8

Glucose and ketone levels falling

5. The chart shows an improving respiratory rate and blood pressure. This is good evidence that the patient is improving. The administration of fluid and insulin to a patient with DKA is life saving and can result in a dramatic improvement in condition. The falling blood ketone level is more important than the normalisation of glucose levels. It would be important to see that the patient's acid–base status is normalising as a result of the treatment that you are giving.

An important point to note is that there is often a precipitating factor for DKA. Sometimes, as in this case, DKA can represent the first presentation of type 1 diabetes. More commonly, in patients with known diabetes, DKA results from missing insulin doses or an infection. In a case such as this one, you should be very vigilant not to miss an underlying intra-abdominal precipitant for the DKA (eg appendicitis).

Repeat blood tests show the following:

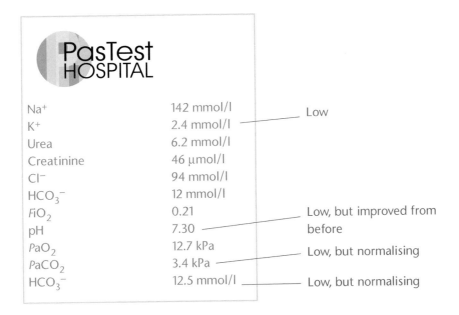

PasTest HOSPITAL		
Na+	142 mmol/l	Low
K+	2.4 mmol/l	
Urea	6.2 mmol/l	
Creatinine	46 μmol/l	
Cl−	94 mmol/l	
HCO₃−	12 mmol/l	
FiO₂	0.21	Low, but improved from
pH	7.30	before
PaO₂	12.7 kPa	Low, but normalising
PaCO₂	3.4 kPa	
HCO₃−	12.5 mmol/l	Low, but normalising

6. The patient's potassium level has fallen to an extremely low level due to the insulin given to treat the DKA. This could result in a cardiac arrhythmia. The patient should have a 12-lead ECG recorded to look for evidence of hypokalaemia, and should be connected to a bedside cardiac monitor. The patient should then receive an intravenous infusion of potassium.

The patient still has a high anion gap metabolic acidosis, but this is improving as the DKA is treated. This would be expected to normalise entirely when the ketone level is back to normal and the patient has received sufficient fluid replacement. If it does not, another concomitant cause for the acidosis should be sought.

CASE SUMMARY

Wide anion gap metabolic acidosis due to diabetic ketoacidosis
Hypokalaemia due to insulin treatment

Case 16.2

A 72-year-old man with a history of hypertension and ischaemic heart disease was admitted 90 minutes after the witnessed onset of acute right-sided arm and leg weakness, and right-sided facial droop.

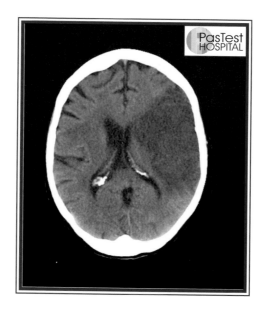

1. What is the diagnosis, and what treatment should be considered?

Treatment is administered and the patient makes a reasonable recovery in the first few hours. You are then called to assess him due to a deterioration in his condition. This is his neurological observations chart:

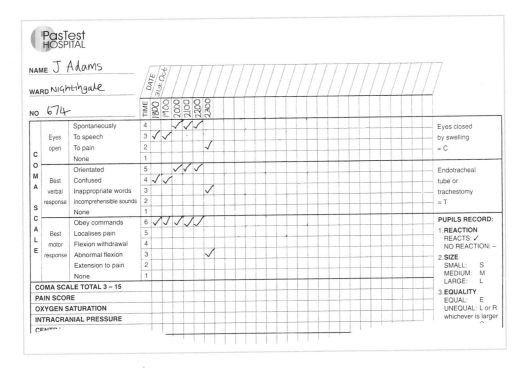

2. What do you think has happened, and what are your priorities?

You arrange another CT scan which shows haemorrhagic transformation in the same region as the abnormality seen on the first scan.

3. What are your priorities now?

A blood test result comes back showing the following:

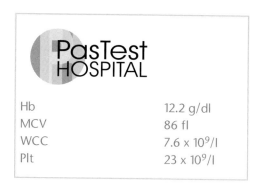

PasTest HOSPITAL

Hb	12.2 g/dl
MCV	86 fl
WCC	$7.6 \times 10^9/l$
Plt	$23 \times 10^9/l$

4. How will this affect your management?

The patient stabilises, and over the course of 2 weeks makes a reasonable improvement in conscious level. The limb weakness remains profound. You review him because he has developed anterior chest pain that reminds him of a previous myocardial infarction.

5. How would you interpret his ECG?

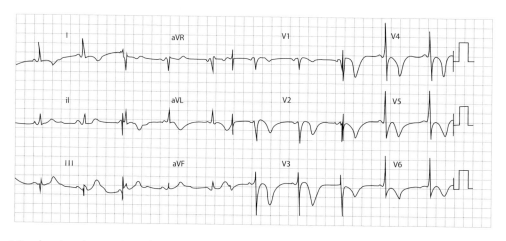

His chest pain settles after 1 hour; 12 hours later you request a blood test that shows the following:

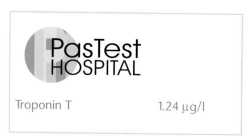

PasTest HOSPITAL

Troponin T	1.24 μg/l

6. What has happened and what are the challenges in management?

Answer 16.2

1. The patient has had a stroke caused by infarction in the territory of the left middle cerebral artery. All patients presenting with infarction strokes should be considered for thrombolytic therapy. It is important to ensure that there are no contraindications for thrombolysis. These include, but are not limited to, recent trauma or surgery, bleeding disposition and uncontrolled hypertension. Thrombolysis must be administered relatively soon after symptom onset (current evidence suggests within 4.5 h).

2. The patient's level of consciousness has dramatically worsened. The integrity of the patient's airway should be assessed and the airway protected if necessary. Breathing and circulation should be assessed next. A sudden drop in blood pressure might be indicative of a large amount of bleeding somewhere in the body, precipitated by the thrombolytic agent. A bedside blood glucose reading should be taken because hypoglycaemia could present like this. Assuming that all these parameters are satisfactory, you should then rapidly consider the intracranial status. Options include extension of the infarction or intracerebral haemorrhage. A repeat CT scan of the brain should be performed without delay.

3. The CT scan confirms that the patient's infarct has undergone haemorrhagic transformation. The priorities always start with ensuring that the 'ABCs' are stable. The patient may require airway protection if the level of consciousness means that it is not secure. The next priority would be to correct any problem that might increase bleeding propensity and increase blood loss into the brain. Blood tests of coagulation and a platelet count should be arranged urgently. A haematologist should be contacted about blood product replacement. A neurosurgeon should also be contacted for an opinion as to whether surgical intervention with evacuation of haemorrhage might be helpful.

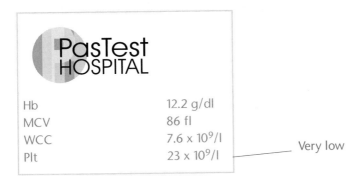

PasTest
HOSPITAL

Hb	12.2 g/dl
MCV	86 fl
WCC	$7.6 \times 10^9/l$
Plt	$23 \times 10^9/l$ ——— Very low

4. A patient with intracranial bleeding in the setting of thrombocytopenia should receive an infusion of platelets with the intention of increasing the platelet count to a safe level. In the longer term, the patient should be investigated to find out why the platelet count was so low.

5. This ECG shows horizontal ST depression in the anterior and lateral leads. This might simply represent myocardial ischaemia (angina) but the possibility of a non-ST elevation myocardial infarction (NSTEMI) should be borne in mind. Biochemical testing for cardiac troponin will be necessary to distinguish between these two possibilities.

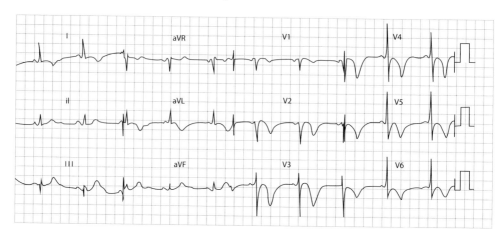

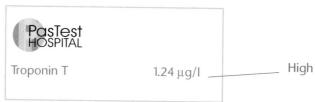

PasTest HOSPITAL		
Troponin T	1.24 µg/l	High

6. The elevated blood troponin level would suggest that the patient has had a myocardial infarction. Given the ECG noted earlier, the most likely diagnosis is NSTEMI. In 'normal circumstances' the patient would receive anti-platelet therapy and heparin. The complicating factor in this case is that the patient is recovering from a recent intracerebral haemorrhage and any treatment given for the heart might result in further bleeding in the brain. Difficult decisions will have to be made by senior clinicians.

CASE SUMMARY

Stroke (infarction)
Haemorrhagic transformation of ischaemic stroke post-thrombolysis
Thrombocytopenia

Case 16.3

DATA COVERED IN THIS CLINICAL CASE SCENARIO

- Bedside chart: fluid balance chart
- Haematology: full blood picture, ESR
- Biochemistry: urea and electrolytes, glucose, protein, immunoglobulins
- Imaging: skull X-ray

A 64-year-old man is admitted for investigation of generalised aches and pains, and lethargy. He is previously healthy and is on no prescribed medication. His fluid balance is monitored and, for the first day of hospitalisation, is as follows:

Time	Intake					Output				
	By mouth		IV or other			Urine	Faeces	Vomit (ml)	Gast. Asp. (ml)	Drain (ml)
	Amount (ml)	Type	Amount (ml)	Type	Add.					
08:00										
09:00	150					450				
10:00										
11:00	400									
12:00	100					400				
13:00										
14:00	300					350				
15:00										
16:00	250									
17:00	150					400				
18:00	300									
19:00										
20:00	150					400				
21:00	300									
22:00										
23:00						350				
24:00										
01:00										
02:00						500				
03:00										
04:00						350				
05:00										
06:00										
07:00						300				

Total	By Mouth	IV or other	Urine	Faeces	Vomit	Gast. Asp.	Drain
Day	1800 ml		2350 ml				
Night	300 ml		1150 ml				
Total	2100 ml		3500 ml				
Total Intake		2100 ml	Total Output		3500 ml		

1. How would you interpret the fluid balance chart? What is your differential diagnosis?

You request a panel of blood tests that come back showing the following. His kidney function had been found to be normal 4 months before.

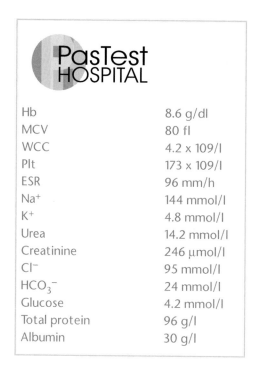

Hb	8.6 g/dl
MCV	80 fl
WCC	4.2×10^9/l
Plt	173×10^9/l
ESR	96 mm/h
Na^+	144 mmol/l
K^+	4.8 mmol/l
Urea	14.2 mmol/l
Creatinine	246 μmol/l
Cl^-	95 mmol/l
HCO_3^-	24 mmol/l
Glucose	4.2 mmol/l
Total protein	96 g/l
Albumin	30 g/l

2. What are the abnormalities, and what is the likely diagnosis?

A skeletal survey is performed. Here is the skull x-ray.

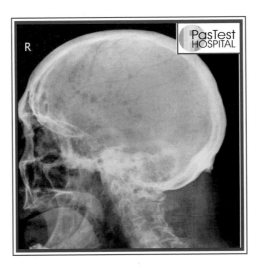

3. How does the X-ray appearance relate to the likely diagnosis?

After several days, the laboratory phones through the following results:

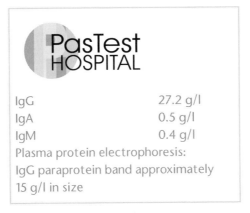

PasTest
HOSPITAL

IgG	27.2 g/l
IgA	0.5 g/l
IgM	0.4 g/l

Plasma protein electrophoresis:
IgG paraprotein band approximately
15 g/l in size

You request a blood calcium level. It is returned as 2.59 mmol/l.

4. What is the cause of the abnormality seen on the fluid balance chart at the start of the case?

Answer 16.3

1. The patient's urinary output seems excessive when compared with the amount of fluid consumed. The most common cause for this pattern is treatment with diuretics (eg for oedema in heart failure). We are told, however, that the patient is on no treatment, so this is not the cause. Other causes of polyuria include diabetes mellitus, diabetes insipidus, hypercalaemia and following the relief of urinary tract obstruction.

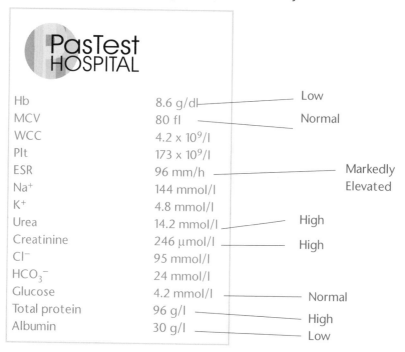

PasTest HOSPITAL		
Hb	8.6 g/dl	Low
MCV	80 fl	Normal
WCC	4.2 x 10⁹/l	
Plt	173 x 10⁹/l	
ESR	96 mm/h	Markedly Elevated
Na⁺	144 mmol/l	
K⁺	4.8 mmol/l	
Urea	14.2 mmol/l	High
Creatinine	246 µmol/l	High
Cl⁻	95 mmol/l	
HCO₃⁻	24 mmol/l	
Glucose	4.2 mmol/l	Normal
Total protein	96 g/l	High
Albumin	30 g/l	Low

2. Several abnormalities are demonstrated, and the key to making the diagnosis is thinking of a condition that could explain all the results. It is possible that several disease processes coexist in the patient, but a single unifying diagnosis would be much more likely. The abnormalities are: normocytic anaemia, elevated ESR, acute kidney injury, high total protein and low albumin. The glucose level is normal making diabetes mellitus less likely. The normal sodium concentration makes diabetes insipidus less likely, but does not exclude it.

The key to suspecting the correct diagnosis here lies with correct interpretation of the protein and albumin results. Total protein is a measure of albumin plus globulins. As this patient's albumin level is low and the total protein level is high, one can extrapolate that the globulin (IgG, IgA and

IgM) level must be high. The disease most likely to give an elevated globulin level along with all the other abnormalities documented is multiple myeloma.

3. Lytic bone lesions are a recognised feature of multiple myeloma. Patients would routinely undergo a 'skeletal survey' to identify bony pathology in this condition.

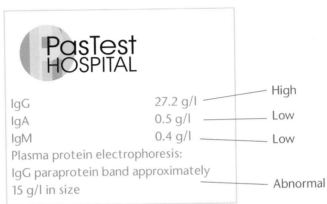

You request a blood calcium level. It is returned as 2.59 mmol/l.

4. The IgG level is highly elevated, and the levels of other immunoglobulins are suppressed. The particular type of myeloma in this patient is one in which abnormal plasma cells are producing massive quantities of IgG. This test confirms myeloma as the diagnosis.

Although the blood calcium level is apparently normal, the cause of the polyuria documented is hypercalcaemia. Don't forget to correct calcium levels for abnormalities with serum albumin. As this patient's albumin level is 30 g/l, the 'corrected calcium' level is 2.84 mmol/l which is high (see page 67 for details).

CASE SUMMARY

Multiple myeloma
Hypercalcaemia

Case 16.4

A 51-year-old male teacher is referred for investigation of high blood pressure. He has been started on an ACE inhibitor by his GP after two readings showing moderate hypertension. He does not smoke. You arrange ambulatory blood pressure monitoring.

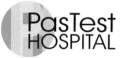

PasTest HOSPITAL

Ambulatory Blood Pressure Monitor – Summary of Results

Name of patient: Mr Richard Eakin
Age: 51 years
Hospital Number: PH99-29283
Number of Attempted Readings: 50
Number of Successful Readings: 48 (96%)

	Minimum (mmHg)	Maximum (mmHg)	Mean (mmHg)
Wake period	136/72	212/108	162/88
Sleep period	122/80	216/108	174/92
Overall	122/80	216/108	164/89

1. What is your interpretation of this recording?

As a result of this investigation, you arrange a series of tests, the results of which are shown below.

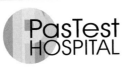

Na$^+$	144 mmol/l
K$^+$	3.3 mmol/l
Urea	4.3 mmol/l
Creatinine	46 µmol/l
Cl$^-$	93 mmol/l
HCO$_3^-$	25 mmol/l
Glucose	7.2 mmol/l
Total cholesterol	5.2 mmol/l
HDL-cholesterol	0.9 mmol/l
LDL-cholesterol	4.1 mmol/l
Cholesterol:HDL ratio	5.78
Urinary albumin:creatinine ratio	67

Chest X-ray report
Cardiac contour normal. Lungs clear.

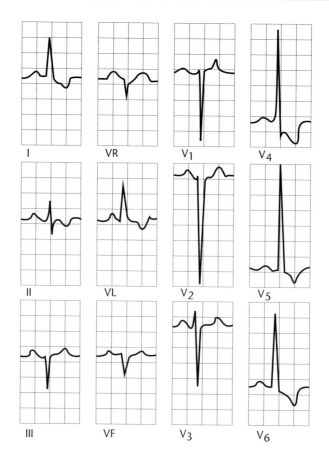

I   VR   V₁   V₄

II   VL   V₂   V₅

III   VF   V₃   V₆

Transthoracic echocardiogram report

Moderate concentric left ventricular hypertrophy. Left ventricular function appears normal. No significant valvular disease. Other chambers appear normal.

Renal ultrasonography and Doppler ultrasonography: report of study of renal vessels

Both kidneys appear normal in size, shape and echogenicity. Normal Doppler waveform tracings were obtained from vessels on both sides.

2. **What are your conclusions based on these results? What further tests would be helpful?**

3. **Calculate the 10-year cardiovascular risk using the prediction chart on page 504.**

You arrange an oral glucose tolerance test, which shows the following:

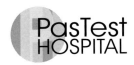

Fasting glucose	5.6 mmol/l
2-hour glucose post-75 g glucose load	9.7 mmol/l

4. **How would you interpret the test, and how does this affect cardiovascular risk?**

You decide to stop treatment to allow a hormone test to be carried out.

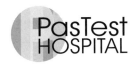

Plasma renin activity	0.3 ng/ml per h
Aldosterone	24 ng/dl
Aldosterone:renin ratio	80

5. **What are the implications of this test, and how might you investigate further?**

Answer 16.4

1. Ninety-six per cent of blood pressure readings were successful, meaning that the study is valid and its results meaningful. The average daytime pressure was 162/88 mmHg. Applying a correction factor of 10/5 mmHg, we might assume that the equivalent clinic blood pressure is 172/93 mmHg and is in keeping with significant hypertension. The other major finding on the report is that the patient's blood pressure rises at night. This is abnormal. Assuming that the patient had a good night's sleep on the night of the study and that he does not have obstructive sleep apnoea, this is a worrying finding. 'Reverse dipping' of blood pressure at night increases the chances of finding a secondary cause for the hypertension.

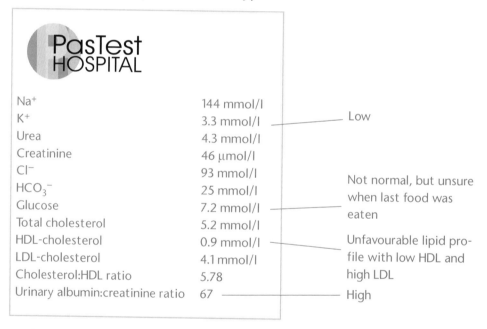

PasTest		
HOSPITAL		
Na⁺	144 mmol/l	
K⁺	3.3 mmol/l	Low
Urea	4.3 mmol/l	
Creatinine	46 µmol/l	
Cl⁻	93 mmol/l	
HCO₃⁻	25 mmol/l	Not normal, but unsure
Glucose	7.2 mmol/l	when last food was eaten
Total cholesterol	5.2 mmol/l	
HDL-cholesterol	0.9 mmol/l	Unfavourable lipid pro-
LDL-cholesterol	4.1 mmol/l	file with low HDL and
Cholesterol:HDL ratio	5.78	high LDL
Urinary albumin:creatinine ratio	67	High

2. A chest X-ray in a patient with hypertension can potentially show evidence of coarctation of the aorta, in the form of rib notching. More commonly, cardiomegaly or signs of cardiac failure might be seen. The absence of cardiomegaly on a chest X-ray does not rule out the possibility of left ventricular hypertrophy (LVH). The ECG has findings in keeping with LVH. The ECG is, however, only really a screening test for LVH, and echocardiography is necessary to establish its presence with certainty. LVH is confirmed on the echocardiogram. This signifies evidence of target organ damage from hypertension and suggests that measures should be taken to

lower the pressure as soon as possible. The ultrasound study was normal, but might have shown findings such as a renal tumour, echobright kidneys (common in 'medical' kidney disease) or abnormal Doppler tracings (associated with renal artery stenosis).

The biochemistry results show mild hypokalaemia and a sodium concentration towards the upper end of the normal range. The hypokalaemia is particularly surprising as the patient is taking an ACE inhibitor, which would be expected to cause hyperkalaemia if anything. The finding of hypokalaemia in a patient with hypertension should raise suspicions of an underlying diagnosis of primary hyperaldosteronism.

The glucose level is raised, but we are not given any information explaining whether this is a fasting level or whether in fact the patient had just eaten a sugary substance. It is not in the 'normal' range, however, and further steps should be taken to clarify the patient's glycaemic status. The lipid profile is suboptimal for a patient at risk of cardiovascular disease.

The urinary albumin:creatinine ratio is a measure of protein excretion from the kidneys. The level seen in this patient is in the 'microalbuminuric' range. The level requires repeating to ensure that it is truly abnormal. Assuming that it is a true value, however, this would be further evidence of target organ damage – this time to the kidney.

3. Using the chart for a non-diabetic, non-smoking, 51-year-old man, and plotting the 'corrected' ambulatory daytime systolic blood pressure and cholesterol:HDL ratio, it should be apparent that this patient's 10-year cardiovascular risk is in the 'greater than 20%' zone (>30% if the line is used).

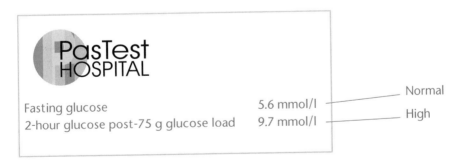

PasTest HOSPITAL		
Fasting glucose	5.6 mmol/l	Normal
2-hour glucose post-75 g glucose load	9.7 mmol/l	High

4. The patient has impaired glucose tolerance because, although the fasting glucose level is normal, the level after glucose loading is between 7.8 and 11.0 mmol/l.

We have already estimated the cardiovascular risk as more than 20% in the next 10 years. The particular risk tool that was used did not, however, have any way for impaired glucose tolerance to be taken into consideration. As this is a further cardiovascular risk factor, we can assume simply that the patient's risk is even higher than that calculated. If the fact that the patient has LVH and microalbuminuria is also taken into consideration, the actual risk will be considerably higher than 20%.

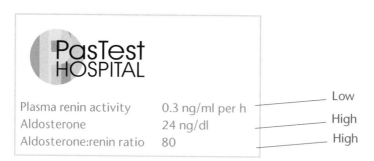

Plasma renin activity	0.3 ng/ml per h	Low
Aldosterone	24 ng/dl	High
Aldosterone:renin ratio	80	High

5. The test was performed in a patient suspected of having primary hyperaldosteronism. In this condition, aldosterone levels will be high and, because of negative feedback, renin levels will be low. The suggested cut-off value for an abnormal ratio, as detailed on page 146, is 30. In this case, the hormone patterns are in keeping with primary hyperaldosteronism and the ratio is greatly increased.

The patient should be investigated further by arranging a further test such as a saline suppression test. Imaging of his adrenal glands to search for a tumour (could be a carcinoma or more likely an adenoma) should then be undertaken. Adrenal hyperplasia can also cause this hormone abnormality. A CT scan would be the first imaging modality used in most instances. Nuclear imaging can also be used, and adrenal vein hormone sampling may also be required.

CASE SUMMARY

Hypertension
Left ventricular hypertrophy
Impaired glucose tolerance
Primary hyperaldosteronism

Case 16.5

DATA COVERED IN THIS CLINICAL CASE SCENARIO

- Respiratory: blood gas analysis
- Biochemistry: U&Es, liver function tests, glucose
- Cardiology: ECG, cardiac arrest rhythm recognition
- Toxicology blood levels

A 45-year-old woman with a history of depression is admitted at 1.30am after the ingestion of an unknown quantity of antidepressants (specific type unknown) 5 hours before. She is fully conscious on arrival at the hospital and insists that she does not want to live, but is refusing to answer your questions.

You perform a blood gas analysis:

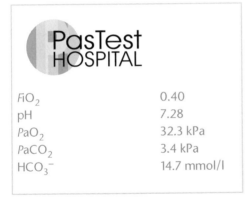

PasTest HOSPITAL	
FiO_2	0.40
pH	7.28
PaO_2	32.3 kPa
$PaCO_2$	3.4 kPa
HCO_3^-	14.7 mmol/l

1. **How would you interpret this test? What else would you like to measure?**

The biochemistry laboratory phones through her initial results to a member of the team:

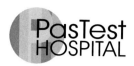

PasTest
HOSPITAL

Na$^+$	142 mmol/l
K$^+$	3.8 mmol/l
Urea	4.6 mmol/l
Creatinine	55 µmol/l
Cl$^-$	95 mmol/l
HCO$_3^-$	15 mmol/l
Glucose	5.2 mmol/l
Total bilirubin	10 µmol/l
ALP	62 U/l
AST	22 IU/l
ALT	31 IU/l
GGT	132 IU/l
Paracetamol	45 mg/l
Salicylate	<20 mmol/l
Alcohol	126 mmol/l

2. **How would you interpret these tests, and how would your management change?**

An ECG is performed and a rhythm strip printed.

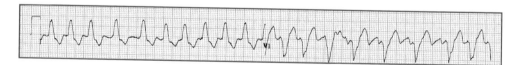

3. **What substance has she taken in overdose, and what is the priority in management?**

While you are preparing to give her a drug, her monitor starts to alarm. There is no response from the patient and there is no pulse. Her bedside cardiac monitor shows the following rhythm:

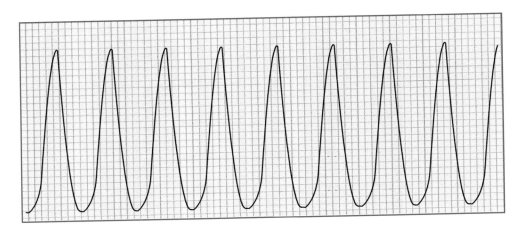

4. **What is the rhythm and how will you manage the patient?**

Answer 16.5

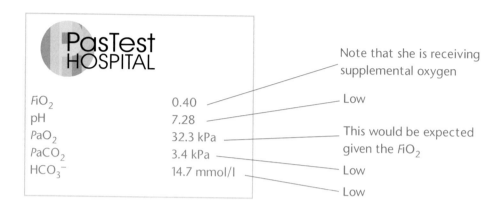

1. Oxygenation is adequate given that the patient is breathing 40% oxygen. The pH is low in keeping with an acidosis. The bicarbonate and carbon dioxide levels are also low, so the patient has a metabolic acidosis with respiratory compensation. It would be helpful to perform a U&E profile, so that the anion gap can be calculated. Given the clinical scenario, however, a raised anion gap acidosis would be expected. You should also measure paracetamol concentrations, because, although the patient denies taking paracetamol, its level should generally be measured in all patients presenting after an overdose (as the treatment of paracetamol toxicity is simple, and not treating could have catastrophic consequences).

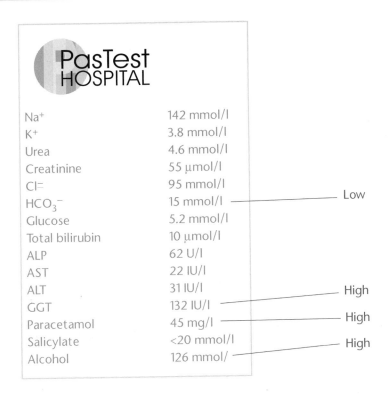

2. The bicarbonate is low in keeping with the known metabolic acidosis. The anion gap is 35.8 mmol/l which is raised. Please note that the list of causes for acid–base abnormalities listed in Chapter 13 is not exhaustive. The GGT is high, and this is often the case in patients who have consumed alcohol recently. The patient has taken some paracetamol as the blood level was 45. It would be important to consult the paracetamol overdose nomogram to check if treatment is required. As we have few details to go on (because the patient is uncooperative), we must assume that she is at high risk of paracetamol liver toxicity when plotting her blood value on the chart shown on page 170. Given that the blood sample was drawn at 5 hours post-ingestion, we can be confident that treatment for paracetamol poisoning is not required in this case. Her blood alcohol level is reasonably high, indicating that she has recently consumed alcohol.

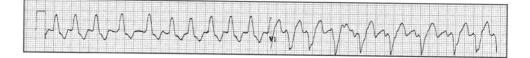

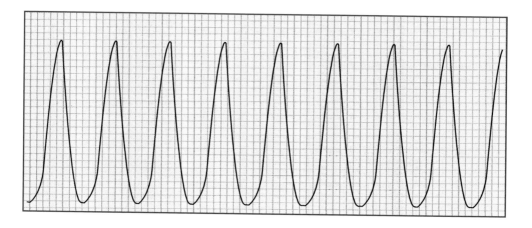

3. The major abnormality with the ECG is the broadening of the QRS complexes. Taken in the context of a patient who has ingested an antidepressant and has a metabolic acidosis, we can be fairly certain that she has taken a tricyclic antidepressant. Given the ECG abnormalities, she is at high risk of cardiac arrhythmia and/or seizures. She should be placed on a cardiac monitor and intravenous sodium bicarbonate administered to correct the cardiac arrhythmia and the acidosis.

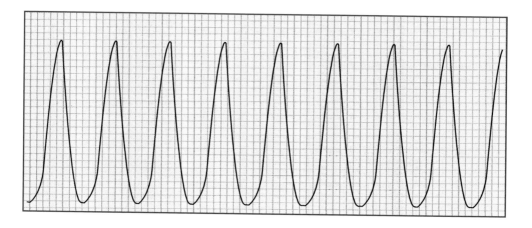

4. You should instantly recognise this rhythm tracing as ventricular tachycardia. On occasion, this rhythm can generate sufficient cardiac output such that a pulse is felt. In this case, no pulse can be felt and the patient is in cardiac arrest. The cardiac arrest treatment algorithm should be started without delay (treatment details outside the scope of this text). As this rhythm often responds to defibrillation, this should be a treatment priority. Sodium bicarbonate should also be administered to the patient.

CASE SUMMARY

Tricyclic antidepressant overdose
Ventricular tachycardia

Case 16.6

DATA COVERED IN THIS CLINICAL CASE SCENARIO

- Toxicology: blood levels
- Biochemistry: liver function tests, U&Es
- Haematology: coagulation
- Imaging: chest X-ray
- Respiratory: arterial blood gas
- Microbiology: sputum
- Bedside chart: vital signs

An 18-year-old student is found by her housemates. She is in a confused state on the floor and is surrounded by several packets of paracetamol. It is 22:00 hours and they are able to ascertain that she took the tablets around 15:30 hours that day. She smells of alcohol. She had been on medications for low mood but is otherwise healthy. On arrival at hospital half an hour later blood tests were taken which are shown.

PasTest HOSPITAL

Na^+	139 mmol/l
K^+	3.7 mmol/l
Urea	5.1 mmol/l
Creatinine	52 µmol/l
Cl^-	105 mmol/l
HCO_3^-	25 mmol/l
Paracetamol	160 mg/l
Alcohol	25 mmol/l
Salicylates	Nil
Bilirubin	12 µmol/l
AST	78 IU/l
ALT	65 IU/l
GGT	99 IU/l
ALP	67 U/l
Albumin	39 g/l
Prothrombin time	18.7 s
APTT	35.4 s
Fibrinogen	6.7 g/l

1. With the above results in mind outline the treatment approach for this patient.

Following the commencement of her treatment blood tests are taken on a regular basis and are shown below.

PasTest HOSPITAL

Time (hours)	Bilirubin (μmol/l)	AST (IU/l)	ALT (IU/l)	ALP (U/l)	GGT (IU/l)	Albumin (g/l)	PT (s)
4	13	44	56	65	64	42	16.05
12	15	44	56	65	64	41	17.05
20	16	8001	7056	55	64	39	17.15
28	16	9977	10 230	75	54	38	18.55
36	19	12 333	11 156	65	61	34	19.05
44	23	12 993	12 333	64	62	32	21.05
52	27	13 144	12 456	75	73	28	21.44
56	29	13 111	12 346	77	74	24	24.05
60	36	13 244	12 153	85	77	22	30.05

2. Outline the trend and significance of these results. What treatment should be considered now?

She is transferred to a regional centre where she undergoes surgery. In the initial days postoperatively she progresses well, but on day 5 becomes short of breath and a chest X-ray is taken which is shown below.

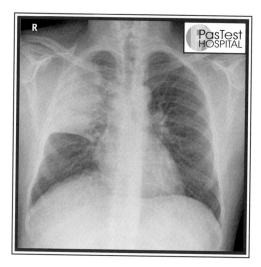

3. Report the findings on this chest X-ray.

At the same time a sample is sent for arterial blood gas analysis. The patient was breathing room air.

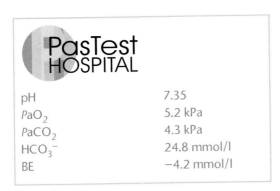

pH	7.35
PaO_2	5.2 kPa
$PaCO_2$	4.3 kPa
HCO_3^-	24.8 mmol/l
BE	−4.2 mmol/l

4. What abnormality is observed on the arterial sample?

She is commenced on antimicrobial therapy and sputum is sent for analysis. The following day the results of her sputum analysis are conveyed from microbiology.

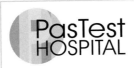

Gram-positive cocci in keeping with
Streptococcus pneumoniae

During the middle of the night you are called by the nurse to see her as some of her vital signs are concerning. Her bedside chart is shown.

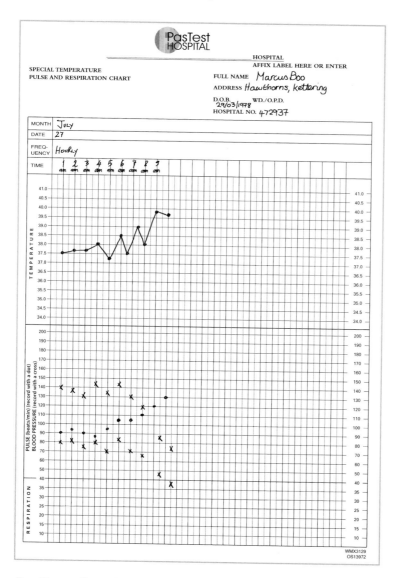

5. **Describe the findings on the chart and the underlying cause.**

Answer 16.6

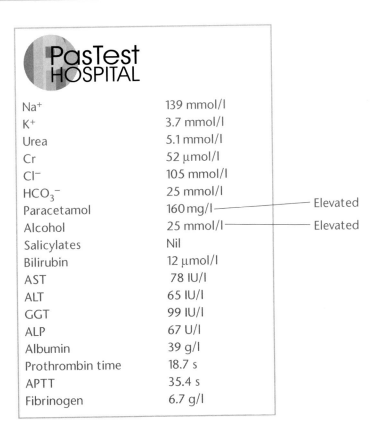

PasTest
HOSPITAL

Na$^+$	139 mmol/l
K$^+$	3.7 mmol/l
Urea	5.1 mmol/l
Cr	52 µmol/l
Cl$^-$	105 mmol/l
HCO$_3^-$	25 mmol/l
Paracetamol	160 mg/l ——— Elevated
Alcohol	25 mmol/l ——— Elevated
Salicylates	Nil
Bilirubin	12 µmol/l
AST	78 IU/l
ALT	65 IU/l
GGT	99 IU/l
ALP	67 U/l
Albumin	39 g/l
Prothrombin time	18.7 s
APTT	35.4 s
Fibrinogen	6.7 g/l

1. The following should have been interpreted from the data provided in this
    scenario.

This woman has probably taken a substantial overdose of paracetamol in combination with alcohol.

The level of 160 mg/l is 6½ hours after ingestion. The significance of this is seen below on the paracetamol nomogram. At 6½ hours, the line intersects the normal treatment line of the graph at 125 mg/l making treatment necessary at levels higher than this: 160 mg/l is well above this line.

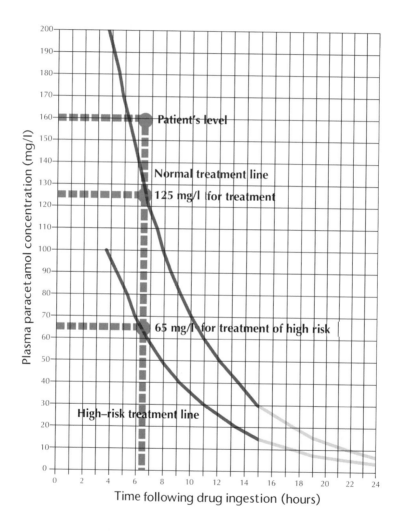

2. The patient should be treated with an intravenous infusion of N-acetylcysteine. The exact dose depends on the weight of the patient.

Time (hours)	Bilirubin (μmol/l)	AST (U/l)	ALT (U/l)	ALP (U/l)	GGT (IU/l)	Albumin (g/l)	PT (s)
4	13	44	56	65	64	42	16.05
12	15	44	56	65	64	41	17.05
20	16	8001	7056	55	64	39	17.15
28	16	9977	10 230	75	54	38	18.55
36	19	12 333	11 156	65	61	34	19.05
44	23	12 993	12 333	64	62	32	21.05
52	27	13 144	12 456	75	73	28	21.44
56	29	13 111	12 346	77	74	24	24.05
60	36	13 244	12 153	85	77	22	30.05

PasTest HOSPITAL

Falling trend

Rising trend

This chart shows the changes in liver function over the 2–3 days following overdose. A huge surge in transaminases is seen from 20 hours indicating substantial hepatocellular damage from the toxic effects of paracetamol. Hepatic necrosis is taking place and the liver is failing. This can be seen because the prothrombin time is rising and the albumin is falling, as the ability of the liver to synthesise protein is diminishing. A liver transplantation should be considered.

3. Her transfer to a regional centre was to facilitate liver transplantation. Five days after her operation her chest X-ray, sputum analysis and ABG indicate that she had developed a postoperative pneumonia.

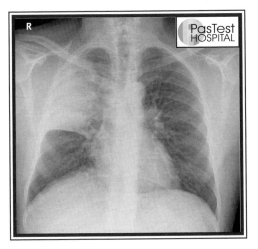
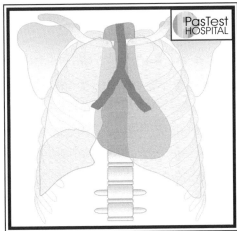

Chest X-ray report

This is a PA chest radiograph taken on 14 December 2005. It is the second in a series of postoperative films on this patient. The patient is 18 years of age and is an inpatient on the liver unit. The technical quality of the film is sound. The most obvious abnormality on this film is an area of increased radio-opacity in the right mid-zone. These findings are in keeping with consolidation. On review of the remainder of the film no other abnormalities are noted. These findings are in keeping with a right upper lobe pneumonia. I would like to view previous films for comparison.

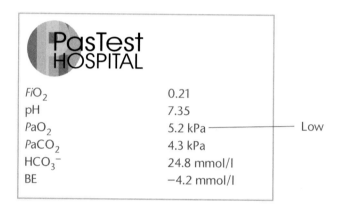

FiO_2	0.21	
pH	7.35	
PaO_2	5.2 kPa	Low
$PaCO_2$	4.3 kPa	
HCO_3^-	24.8 mmol/l	
BE	−4.2 mmol/l	

4. The arterial blood gas shows a marked hypoxia with a normal pH. She has type 1 respiratory failure, caused by pneumonia.

From the sputum analysis a specific causative organism has been identified – *Streptococcus pneumoniae*. It must be emphasised that culturing takes time. Treatment should be instigated with empirical therapy, and altered later, if necessary, on the basis of the growth and sensitivities.

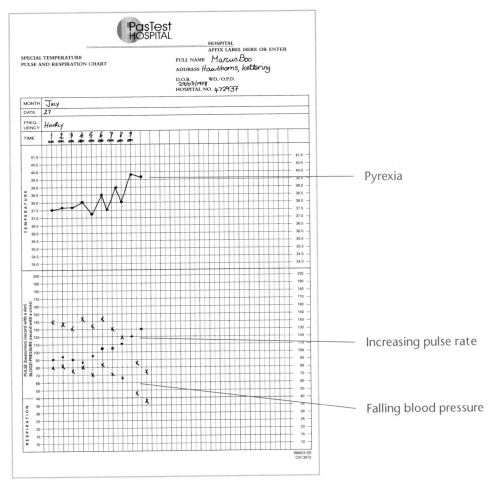

PasTest HOSPITAL

HOSPITAL
AFFIX LABEL HERE OR ENTER

SPECIAL TEMPERATURE
PULSE AND RESPIRATION CHART

FULL NAME Marcus Boo
ADDRESS Hawthorns, Kettering

D.O.B. WD./O.P.D.
29/03/1978
HOSPITAL NO. 472937

MONTH July
DATE 27
FREQ-UENCY Hourly

Pyrexia

Increasing pulse rate

Falling blood pressure

WMX3129
OS13972

5. The bedside chart shows three key findings:

1. Pyrexia

2. Hypotension

3. Tachycardia.

In the context of an established pneumonia this may be in keeping with septic shock.

CASE SUMMARY

Paracetamol overdose requiring treatment
Development of hepatic failure requiring liver transplantation
Postoperative type 1 respiratory failure due to pneumonia
Development of septic shock

Case 16.7

- Bedside chart: neurological observations
- Imaging: CT of the brain
- Neurology: CSF analysis
- Neurology: EEG

A 38-year-old teacher is brought to hospital by her concerned husband due to her unusual behaviour and sleepiness over the past 48 h. She has recently returned from supervising a school trip.

Her observation chart from the initial 6 h of her admission is shown.

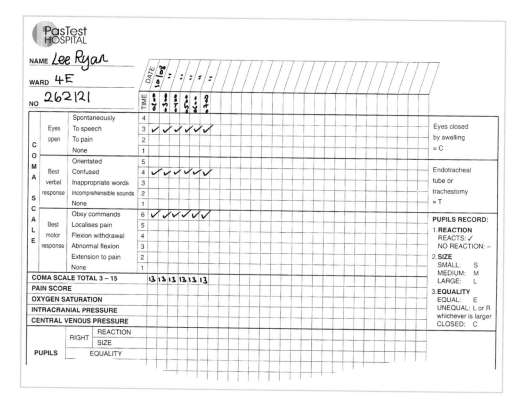

CT of the brain is arranged and the following report is telephoned to her doctor.

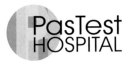

Neuroradiology Department

Routine unenhanced images of the brain performed. No mass lesion seen. There is the suggestion of mild oedema within the temporal lobes bilaterally. MRI recommended.

Clinical examination revealed no signs of raised intracranial pressure. After discussion with the patient's consultant, lumbar puncture is performed. The details are below.

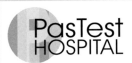

Opening pressure	16 cmCSF
Appearance	Clear
	No organisms seen on microscopy
WCC	121 /mm^3 (>95% lymphocytes)
RCC	3 /mm^3
Glucose	2.8 mmol/l (plasma glucose 5.6 mmol/l)
Total protein	0.89 g/l (plasma total protein 0.44 g/l)

1. **Summarise the findings from the CSF analysis and suggest one further specific test that might be performed on the CSF given the clinical history.**

In the meantime an electroencephalogram is also performed. The report is sent back with the patient.

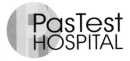

EEG Department

There is evidence of slow wave changes. Periodic complexes are seen

2. **Given the result of the EEG, CSF analysis and CT brain imaging what is the likely diagnosis?**

Answer 16.7

1. Given the finding of an altered conscious level, the patient is placed on a neuro-observation chart. The observation chart shows a stable Glasgow Coma Scale of 13/15. The patient is deemed to be confused and opens her eyes to speech.

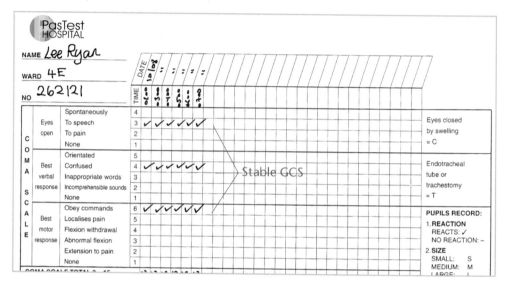

The CT brain imaging is abnormal. Lumbar puncture and an EEG are therefore performed to help come to a diagnosis.

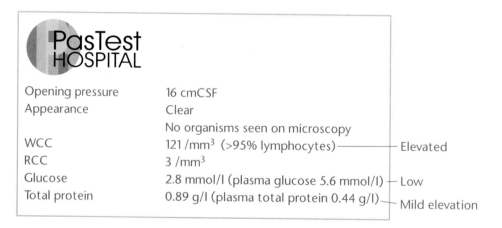

PasTest HOSPITAL	
Opening pressure	16 cmCSF
Appearance	Clear
	No organisms seen on microscopy
WCC	121 /mm³ (>95% lymphocytes) —— Elevated
RCC	3 /mm³
Glucose	2.8 mmol/l (plasma glucose 5.6 mmol/l) — Low
Total protein	0.89 g/l (plasma total protein 0.44 g/l) — Mild elevation

This collection of findings is termed a CSF pleocytosis.

CAUSES OF A CSF PLEOCYTOSIS

Viral meningitis
Encephalitis
Partially treated bacterial meningitis
TB or fungal meningitis
Intracranial abscess
Post-subarachnoid haemorrhage

One should have inferred from the clinical scenario so far that the cause of her symptoms and CSF findings is a viral meningitis/encephalitis. An additional test would be for PCR serology of the CSF to enable detection of viruses, especially herpes simplex virus (HSV).

2. The EEG findings demonstrate the characteristic neurophysiological findings of HSV encephalitis.
   Further tests in HSV encephalitis would include:

- **MRI of brain:**
  - Oedema within the temporal lobes bilaterally (better seen than on CT)

- **PCR serology of CSF:**
  - HSV-1: present.

CASES SUMMARY

A CSF pleocytosis
Herpes simplex encephalitis

Case 16.8

DATA COVERED IN THIS CLINICAL CASE SCENARIO

- Haematology: iron studies
- Biochemistry: liver function tests
- Genetics
- Peritoneal fluid analysis
- Haematology: coagulation

A 34 year-old oil-rig engineer is required to attend a medical before a secondment to his company's overseas operation in Brunei. He has been fortunate with his health with no previous attendance within the health service. He admits to smoking 20 cigarettes a day and drinking approximately 38 units of alcohol a week. His conscientious doctor sends several tests. The following results were of some concern.

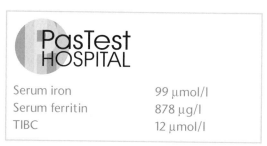

PasTest
HOSPITAL

Serum iron	99 μmol/l
Serum ferritin	878 μg/l
TIBC	12 μmol/l

1. **What can one infer from this iron profile?**

2. **Ferritin is an acute phase reactant. Name some other acute phase reactants.**

His liver function tests are recalled on the computer and are shown below.

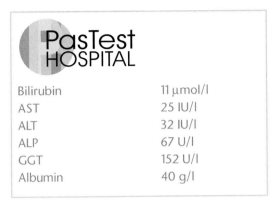

PasTest HOSPITAL	
Bilirubin	11 µmol/l
AST	25 IU/l
ALT	32 IU/l
ALP	67 U/l
GGT	152 U/l
Albumin	40 g/l

3. What do the liver function tests show?

The doctor is concerned about an underlying genetic disorder and a blood sample is sent to the genetics laboratory. The result below was obtained.

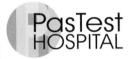

Genetics Laboratory
Homozygous abnormality on chromosome 6p – *HFE* gene – missense mutation *C282Y*

The doctor tries to arrange treatment, but unfortunately the patient leaves his job and no further medical action is taken. Nothing is heard of him for several years, until he is admitted to a local hospital with a distended abdomen and fever.

Physical examination demonstrates the presence of ascites. Peritoneal aspiration is performed and shown below.

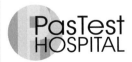

PasTest HOSPITAL	
Neutrophil count (WCC)	312 cells/mm³
Ascites albumin content	19 g/l
Serum albumin	32 g/l
Microscopy and Gram stain	Gram-negative rods
Culture	E. coli
Amylase	92 U/l

4. What is the diagnosis?

He is treated for the acute condition and further blood tests are performed to assess his liver function.

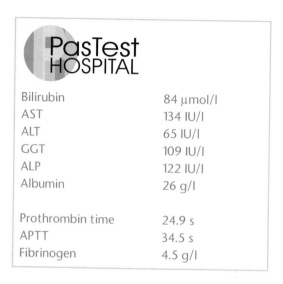

PasTest
HOSPITAL

Bilirubin	84 µmol/l
AST	134 IU/l
ALT	65 IU/l
GGT	109 IU/l
ALP	122 IU/l
Albumin	26 g/l
Prothrombin time	24.9 s
APTT	34.5 s
Fibrinogen	4.5 g/l

5. What do these liver function tests suggest?

Answer 16.8

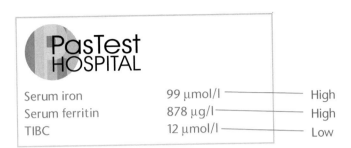

PasTest
HOSPITAL

Serum iron	99 μmol/l	High
Serum ferritin	878 μg/l	High
TIBC	12 μmol/l	Low

1. These results suggest a state of iron overload. The most likely reason for this in an otherwise healthy person found at screening is hereditary haemochromatosis. Haemochromatosis may present with:

    - Cardiomyopathy

    - Liver disease

    - Pituitary disease

    - Diabetes mellitus

    - Joint problems (pseudogout).

    All manifestations are related to the deposition of iron within organs.

2. Other acute phase reactants include:

    - CRP

    - ESR

    - Ceruloplasmin.

    Note that albumin acts as a 'negative acute phase reactant' – its levels decreasing with inflammation.

PasTest
HOSPITAL

Bilirubin	11 µmol/l
AST	25 IU/l
ALT	32 IU/l
ALP	67 U/l
GGT	152 U/l —————— High
Albumin	40 g/l

3. As is commonly the case, both at diagnosis and in established disease, the LFTs are essentially normal. The only abnormal LFT is the GGT which is mildly elevated. Given his clinical history this is likely to reflect heavy alcohol consumption rather than haemochromatosis.

   Idiopathic haemochromatosis is an inherited autosomal recessive condition. Only homozygotes develop clinically overt disease. There is now a gene test for haemochromatosis and screening of first-degree relatives of patients is offered. The most common genetic defect is homozygosity of the *C282Y* missense mutation of the *HFE* gene on chromosome 6p. In addition, a different mutation – *H63D* – can play a role in some cases.

   With appropriate management, patients with haemochromatosis should, in large part, not develop liver failure.

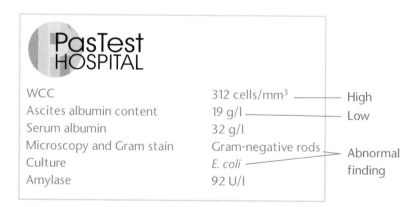

PasTest
HOSPITAL

WCC	312 cells/mm³ ————— High
Ascites albumin content	19 g/l ——————— Low
Serum albumin	32 g/l
Microscopy and Gram stain	Gram-negative rods
Culture	E. coli — Abnormal finding
Amylase	92 U/l

4. The presentation with ascites implies the development of liver cirrhosis with portal hypertension. The peritoneal aspiration performed tells us three things:

   - The serum–ascites albumin gradient (SAAG) is 32 − 19 = 13 g/l. This tells us that the patient probably has portal hypertension.

- The ascitic fluid is infected with the Gram-negative micro-organism *E. coli.*
- There is a high neutrophil count.

This all implies spontaneous bacterial peritonitis. In the acute setting, the most important result to note would be the WCC. An elevated WCC should be taken as evidence for peritonitis and appropriate therapy instituted before culture results are obtained. If the WCC had been normal, one should consider ascites secondary to the development of hepatocellular carcinoma. Haemochromatosis patients with cirrhosis are susceptible to this primary liver malignancy.

5. The accompanying LFTs show:

- Poor synthetic function (prothrombin time UP and albumin DOWN)
- Mildly deranged liver function
- The patient has developed liver failure as a result of the combined hepatotoxic insults of iron and alcohol.

PasTest HOSPITAL

Bilirubin	84 μmol/l	High
AST	134 IU/l	High
ALT	65 IU/l	High
GGT	109 IU/l	High
ALP	122 U/l	High
Albumin	26 g/l	High
		Low
Prothrombin time	24.9 s	
APTT	34.5 s	High
Fibrinogen	4.5 g/l	

CASE SUMMARY

Haemochromatosis
Spontaneous bacterial peritonitis
Liver failure

Case 16.9

DATA COVERED IN THIS CLINICAL CASE SCENARIO

- Haematology: full blood count
- Biochemistry: bone profile, urate and CRP
- Immunology: autoimmune screen
- Miscellaneous: knee aspirate analysis
- Respiratory: spirometry
- Imaging: chest X-ray and DEXA scan

A 39-year-old secretary attends hospital with a painful and swollen right knee, pains in the fingers and fatigue. The finger pains have been with her for several weeks and are especially bad first thing in the morning, making her work difficult. The knee is a more recent complaint.

On examination there is active synovitis in the small joints of the hands and a large effusion of the right knee.

Among the initial blood tests from the A&E officer are those shown.

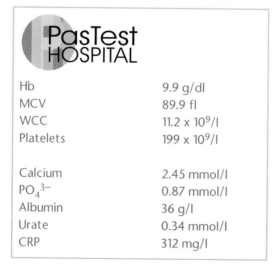

PasTest
HOSPITAL

Hb	9.9 g/dl
MCV	89.9 fl
WCC	11.2 x 10⁹/l
Platelets	199 x 10⁹/l
Calcium	2.45 mmol/l
PO$_4^{3-}$	0.87 mmol/l
Albumin	36 g/l
Urate	0.34 mmol/l
CRP	312 mg/l

1. **Describe the findings.**

An enthusiastic junior doctor carries out knee aspiration, to exclude septic arthritis. The results are shown.

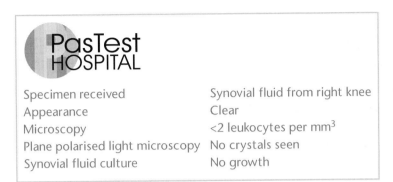

PasTest
HOSPITAL

Specimen received	Synovial fluid from right knee
Appearance	Clear
Microscopy	<2 leukocytes per mm^3
Plane polarised light microscopy	No crystals seen
Synovial fluid culture	No growth

A few days later the result of her autoimmune screen is sent to the ward.

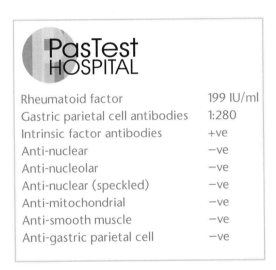

PasTest
HOSPITAL

Rheumatoid factor	199 IU/ml
Gastric parietal cell antibodies	1:280
Intrinsic factor antibodies	+ve
Anti-nuclear	−ve
Anti-nucleolar	−ve
Anti-nuclear (speckled)	−ve
Anti-mitochondrial	−ve
Anti-smooth muscle	−ve
Anti-gastric parietal cell	−ve

She is treated for her arthritis and attends regular review for many years with a variable course to her illness. On one occasion she complains of increasing shortness of breath and on auscultation of the chest there are inspiratory crepitations at the bases.

Spirometry is arranged. The results are shown.

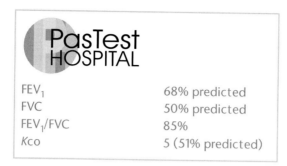

FEV$_1$	68% predicted
FVC	50% predicted
FEV$_1$/FVC	85%
Kco	5 (51% predicted)

The accompanying chest X-ray is shown.

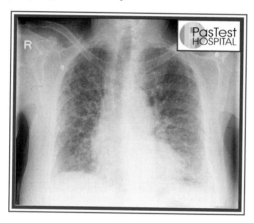

2. What problem does this patient now have and how may it be related to her treatment?

3. What further radiological investigation would be of benefit?

Six months later the patient sustains a forearm fracture. She is referred for a DEXA scan. The results can be seen below.

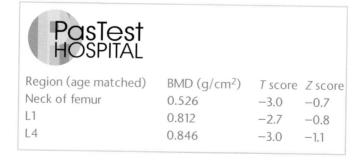

Region (age matched)	BMD (g/cm^2)	T score	Z score
Neck of femur	0.526	−3.0	−0.7
L1	0.812	−2.7	−0.8
L4	0.846	−3.0	−1.1

4. Outline the significance of these results.

Answer 16.9

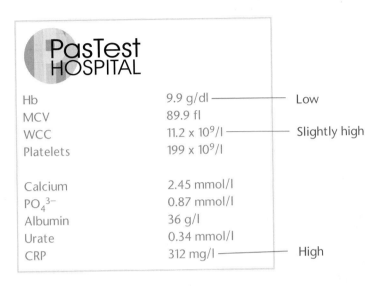

PasTest HOSPITAL

Hb	9.9 g/dl	Low
MCV	89.9 fl	
WCC	11.2 x 10^9/l	Slightly high
Platelets	199 x 10^9/l	
Calcium	2.45 mmol/l	
PO_4^{3-}	0.87 mmol/l	
Albumin	36 g/l	
Urate	0.34 mmol/l	
CRP	312 mg/l	High

1. The important findings from the FBC, bone profile and other biochemistry tests are:

   • A normocytic anaemia (low haemoglobin and normal MCV)

   • A substantially raised CRP

   • A normal urate

   • A normal bone profile.

   Sometimes normal blood results are as important as positive ones. In this case, gout is on the list of differential diagnoses for an acute-onset, painful, swollen joint so the urate level is important to measure. However, remember that the urate level can be normal in acute gout.

PasTest HOSPITAL

Specimen received	Synovial fluid from right knee
Appearance	Clear
Microscopy	<2 leukocytes per mm³
Plane polarised light microscopy	No crystals seen
Synovial fluid culture	No growth

The knee aspirate sample is normal. No white cells or organisms were identified, and culture was negative, excluding septic arthritis. Similarly, no crystals were seen to suggest a crystalline arthritis.

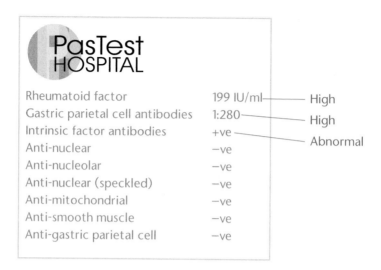

PasTest
HOSPITAL

Rheumatoid factor	199 IU/ml	High
Gastric parietal cell antibodies	1:280	High
Intrinsic factor antibodies	+ve	Abnormal
Anti-nuclear	−ve	
Anti-nucleolar	−ve	
Anti-nuclear (speckled)	−ve	
Anti-mitochondrial	−ve	
Anti-smooth muscle	−ve	
Anti-gastric parietal cell	−ve	

The result of the autoimmune screen is important. The rheumatoid factor is highly elevated, which in the context of the clinical symptoms and earlier finding of a raised CRP and normochromic anaemia implies a diagnosis of rheumatoid disease. There are three important points to remember about rheumatoid factor:

- Its level does not necessarily reflect disease activity.

- It can be raised in a number of states other than rheumatoid disease (ie poor specificity).

- It does not need to be positive for the diagnosis of rheumatoid disease to be made (20% of patients are rheumatoid factor negative).

Interestingly, the screen also has antibodies to gastric parietal cells and intrinsic factor in keeping with a diagnosis of pernicious anaemia. It is common for patients to suffer from several coexisting autoimmune diseases.

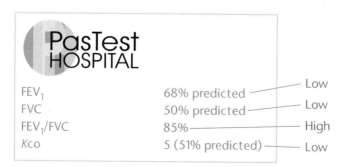

PasTest
HOSPITAL

FEV$_1$	68% predicted	Low
FVC	50% predicted	Low
FEV$_1$/FVC	85%	High
Kco	5 (51% predicted)	Low

2. The positive findings from spirometry with transfer factor are:

- A reduced FEV_1
- A reduced FVC
- A high FEV_1/FVC ratio
- A reduced transfer factor.

This demonstrates a restrictive pattern wholly in keeping with interstitial lung fibrosis.

Chest X-ray report

This is a PA chest X-ray of Mrs B taken on 2 January 2006. She is 39 years of age. The technical quality of the film is satisfactory. There is evidence of increased interstitial lung markings throughout both bases. The lung volumes appear reduced overall. These findings are typical of interstitial lung fibrosis. High-resolution computed tomography (HRCT) of the chest is advised.

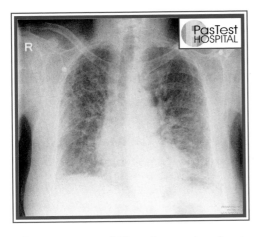
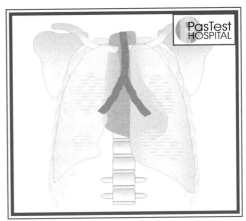

The presence of fibrosis may be due to:

- The disease itself – pulmonary fibrosis is one of the pulmonary manifestations of rheumatoid disease
- A side effect of treatment with methotrexate (first-line disease-modifying anti-rheumatic drug treatment for this condition).

3. As seen in the report above HRCT is advisable as this will help clarify in greater detail the nature and extent of the disease.

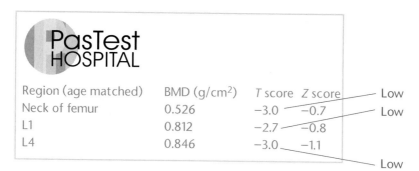

Region (age matched)	BMD (g/cm²)	T score	Z score	
				Low
Neck of femur	0.526	−3.0	−0.7	Low
L1	0.812	−2.7	−0.8	
L4	0.846	−3.0	−1.1	
				Low

4. Patients with rheumatoid disease often have exacerbations ('flares') of their disease requiring treatment with either intravenous or oral steroids. The disease itself and steroid treatment put such patients at risk of developing osteoporosis which is diagnosed by dual energy X-ray absorptiometry (DEXA) scanning. A T score of less than −2.5 indicates osteoporosis. A score of −1.5 to −2.5 implies the presence of osteopenia.

CASE SUMMARY

Knee effusion (due to rheumatoid disease)
Interstitial lung fibrosis (rheumatoid lung)
Steroid-induced osteoporosis

Case 16.10

- Respiratory: arterial blood gas
- Biochemistry: urea and electrolytes
- Bedside chart: fluid input/output
- Cardiology: ECG
- Imaging: abdominal X-ray

A 74-year-old man is admitted with a painful abdomen. He has a history of hypertension and atrial fibrillation. He had a laparotomy as a younger man for a gastric ulcer. He has not passed a motion in several days. On examination his abdomen is tender with rebound.

An abdominal X-ray is taken and shown below.

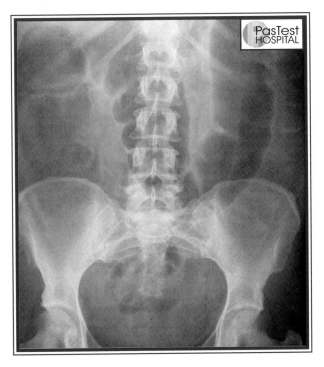

1. Interpret this X-ray.

The patient's condition rapidly deteriorates. An arterial blood gas is analysed.

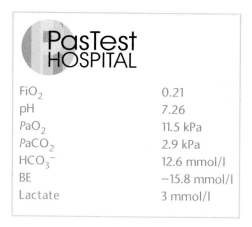

PasTest HOSPITAL	
FiO_2	0.21
pH	7.26
PaO_2	11.5 kPa
$PaCO_2$	2.9 kPa
HCO_3^-	12.6 mmol/l
BE	−15.8 mmol/l
Lactate	3 mmol/l

2. Interpret this ABG.

The patient has emergency surgery. After a short stay in the high dependency unit (HDU) he returns to the ward. Several days later he complains of further abdominal discomfort after his patient-controlled analgesia (PCA) device is stopped. On examination he is tender in the suprapubic space and this area is dull to percussion. A urinary catheter has been *in situ* since surgery.

His fluid (input/output) chart is observed.

PasTest
HOSPITAL

.... HOSPITAL

AFFIX LABEL HERE OR ENTER

FULL NAME John Dickens

DAILY FLUID CHART

ADDRESS 2 Ford Street, Belfast

24 Hours
Beginning 26/01/2005

D.O.B. 16/04/1951   WD./O.P.D. 5
HOSPITAL NO. 264567

TIME	BY MOUTH Amount ml	Type	INTRAVENOUS OR OTHER ROUTES Amount ml	Type	Add.	Urine ml	Faeces	Vomit ml	Gast. Asp. ml	Drain ml	REMARKS
0800			50			30					
0900			50			34					
1000			50			45					
1100			50			10					
1200			50			10					
1300			50			5					
1400			50			5					
1500			50			0					
1600			50			0					
1700			50			0					
1800			50			0					
1900											
2000											
2100											
2200											
2300											
2400											
0100											
0200											
0300											
0400											
0500											
0600											
0700											

DATE:-   INTAKE   Name ....

TOTAL	By Mouth	Intravenous or Other Routes	Urine	Faeces	Vomit	Gast. Asp.	Drain
Day Total	ML	ML	ML	ML	ML	ML	ML
Night Total	ML	ML	ML	ML	ML	ML	ML
Total for 24 hours	ML	ML	ML	ML	ML	ML	ML

TOTAL INTAKE [   ]   TOTAL OUTPUT [   ]   WCA 225/OS 10290

3. Describe the findings.

Blood and urine are sent for analysis

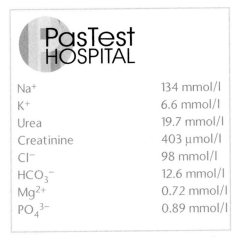

PasTest
HOSPITAL

Na^+	134 mmol/l
K^+	6.6 mmol/l
Urea	19.7 mmol/l
Creatinine	403 µmol/l
Cl^-	98 mmol/l
HCO_3^-	12.6 mmol/l
Mg^{2+}	0.72 mmol/l
PO_4^{3-}	0.89 mmol/l

4. What problem has occurred?

Immediate treatment is given for hyperkalaemia.

5. An ECG was done just before treatment. Describe the findings on the ECG seen below.

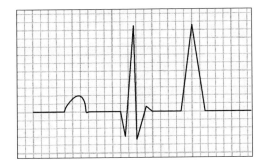

Answer 16.10

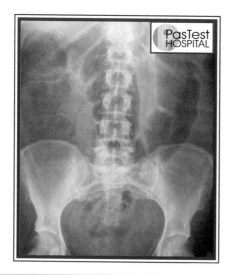 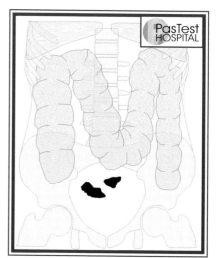

PasTest
HOSPITAL

Abdominal X-ray report

This is a supine abdominal X-ray of Mr D taken on 13 January 2006. The patient is 74 years of age. The technical quality is adequate.

The distribution of gas within the large bowel is abnormal. The luminal diameter is 7 cm at the splenic flexure. Haustral markings can be seen. There is a paucity of gas beyond this point. No extraluminal gas is seen.

Appearances in keeping with large bowel obstruction.

2. Interpretation of the ABG.

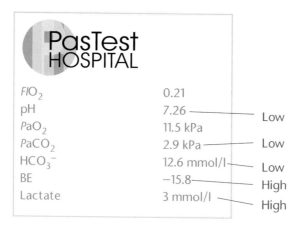

	PasTest HOSPITAL	
FIO_2	0.21	
pH	7.26	Low
PaO_2	11.5 kPa	
$PaCO_2$	2.9 kPa	Low
HCO_3^-	12.6 mmol/l	Low
BE	−15.8	High
Lactate	3 mmol/l	High

The findings on arterial blood analysis are:

- Oxygenation is adequate.

- A low pH. This patient is profoundly acidotic.

- A low $PaCO_2$. Respiratory compensation is occurring.

- A low HCO_3^-. The origin of excess acid is metabolic in nature.

- A high lactate. This is a 'rogue' acid being produced in large quantities. In this case ischaemia of the large bowel is the cause.

The anion gap can be calculated:

$$\text{Anion gap} = (Na^+ + K^+) - (Cl^- + HCO_3^-) = 23.6 \text{ mmol/l}$$

3. This patient has a high anion-gap metabolic acidosis, most likely due to lactic acidosis, secondary to an ischaemic bowel.

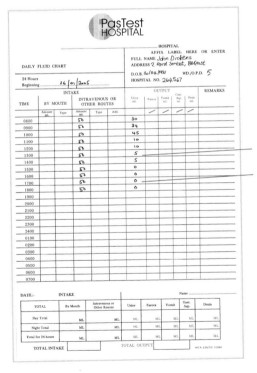

Poor urine output

Anuric

One should infer from the bedside chart that:

- there is a significant positive balance

- the urine output has tailed off in the last 4 hours

- before becoming anuric the urine output was poor.

4. This patient has anuria which was preceded by a period of oliguria. In the first instance the urinary catheter should be checked and flushed to ensure that there is no blockage.

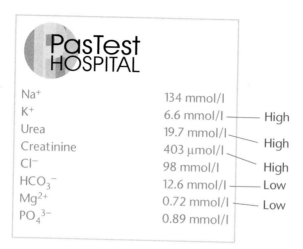

PasTest
HOSPITAL

Na^+	134 mmol/l	
K^+	6.6 mmol/l	High
Urea	19.7 mmol/l	High
Creatinine	403 μmol/l	
Cl^-	98 mmol/l	High
HCO_3^-	12.6 mmol/l	Low
Mg^{2+}	0.72 mmol/l	Low
PO_4^{3-}	0.89 mmol/l	

The blood results show that this patient has developed acute renal failure. From the clinical history it appears that this is due to obstruction of the renal tract.

The patient has life-threatening hyperkalaemia. A potassium of greater than 6.5 mmol/l (in the context of acute renal failure) requires immediate treatment.

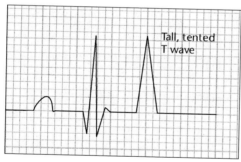

Tall, tented T wave

5. The ECG shows classic changes related to hyperkalaemia. The T waves are tall and peaked.

CASE SUMMARY

Large bowel obstruction
Bowel ischaemia with metabolic acidosis
Acute renal impairment (due to bladder outlet obstruction)
ECG abnormality (due to hyperkalaemia)

Case 16.11

- Biochemistry: urea, electrolytes and CRP
- Haematology: full blood picture (FBP)
- Imaging: chest X-ray
- Respiratory: arterial blood gas
- Pleural fluid analysis
- Microbiology: stool analysis

A 54-year-old pilot is admitted to the local hospital with a complaint of increasing shortness of breath. He has noted this especially while flying recently and he has been seen by his occupational health doctor and prohibited from flying until investigation has been undertaken. He also complains of a cough and intermittent fever.

On examination the trachea is sited centrally. The left lung base is dull to percussion, vocal resonance is decreased and breath sounds are decreased.

Included in your initial investigations are a chest X-ray, FBP, U&Es, CRP and ABG. All are shown below for interpretation.

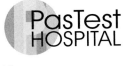

PasTest
HOSPITAL

Hb	14.5 g/dl
MCV	98.7 fl
Plt	293 x 10⁹/l
WCC	14.4 x 10⁹/l
Neutrophils	11.3 x 10⁹/l
Lymphocytes	2.2 x 10⁹/l
Monocytes	0.5 x 10⁹/l
Eosinophils	0.2 x 10⁹/l
Basophils	0.09 x 10⁹/l
Na⁺	137 mmol/l
K⁺	3.8 mmol/l
Urea	8.6 mmol/l
Creatinine	101 µmol/l
Cl⁻	107 mmol/l
CRP	176 mmol/l

1. What abnormalities are seen?

**PasTest
HOSPITAL**

FiO_2	0.21
pH	7.50
PO_2	7.8 kPa
PCO_2	3.1 kPa
HCO_3^-	25.8 mmol/l
BE	+ 6.2 mmol/l

2. Describe the findings on this ABG.

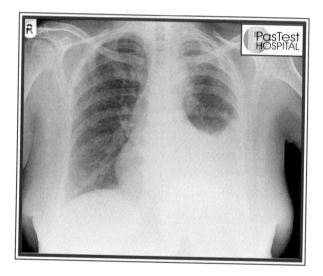

3. Comment on this chest X-ray.

A decision is made to perform a pleural tap for diagnostic purposes based on the findings from the initial investigations. The results are shown.

**PasTest
HOSPITAL**

Total protein	38 g/l
LDH	246 U/l
pH	7.37
Microscopy	Nil seen

4. How would you interpret these results?

He is treated with a cephalosporin antibiotic based on known sensitivities.
Three days into this treatment he develops diarrhoea. Stool samples are sent by
his nurse. The result is shown below.

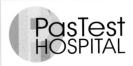

Clostridium difficile toxin positive

5. What is the best course of action based on these findings?

Answer 16.11

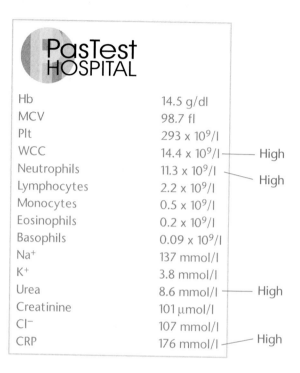

PasTest HOSPITAL		
Hb	14.5 g/dl	
MCV	98.7 fl	
Plt	$293 \times 10^9/l$	
WCC	$14.4 \times 10^9/l$	High
Neutrophils	$11.3 \times 10^9/l$	High
Lymphocytes	$2.2 \times 10^9/l$	
Monocytes	$0.5 \times 10^9/l$	
Eosinophils	$0.2 \times 10^9/l$	
Basophils	$0.09 \times 10^9/l$	
Na^+	137 mmol/l	
K^+	3.8 mmol/l	
Urea	8.6 mmol/l	High
Creatinine	101 μmol/l	
Cl^-	107 mmol/l	
CRP	176 mmol/l	High

1. From the initial investigations one should have identified the following:

   - There is a raised WCC (predominantly comprising neutrophils), along with a raised CRP. The possibility of infection should be entertained.

   - In addition, you will note a mildly raised urea, reflective of a mild degree of dehydration.

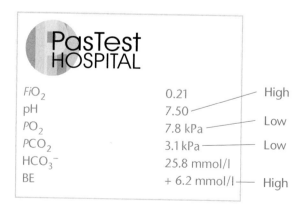

PasTest HOSPITAL		
FiO_2	0.21	High
pH	7.50	
PO_2	7.8 kPa	Low
PCO_2	3.1 kPa	Low
HCO_3^-	25.8 mmol/l	
BE	+ 6.2 mmol/l	High

2. The ABG features two findings:

- A low PaO_2. The patient is hypoxic. He has type 1 respiratory failure.

- A low $PaCO_2$. The patient is short of breath and hyperventilating, causing a low CO_2. This has led to a respiratory alkalosis.

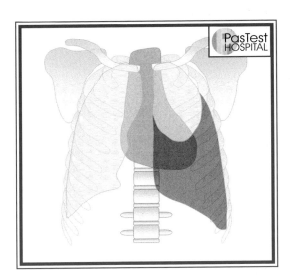

3. The chest X-ray indicates the likely cause for the findings so far.

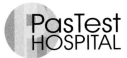

Radiology report

This is a PA chest X-ray of Captain John Boeing taken on 19 December 2005. He is a 54-year-old man. The technical quality of the film is ideal. The most striking finding is an area of radio-opacity on the left side of the chest from the lower zone extending to the midzone. The left hemidiaphragm silhouette and the left costophrenic angle are not seen. A meniscus is noted at the lateral chest wall. No other pathology is noted on the film. These findings are in keeping with a moderate left-sided pleural effusion.

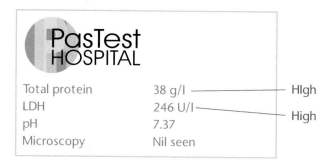

Total protein	38 g/l	High
LDH	246 U/l	High
pH	7.37	
Microscopy	Nil seen	

4. From the pleural fluid analysis one can see:

    -   This is an exudate with an elevated total protein and LDH level.

5. Putting all this information together and correlating it with the patient's clinical features, the likely cause for this pleural effusion is an underlying pneumonia. This is termed a 'parapneumonic pleural effusion'.

    The patient goes on to develop diarrhoea. The most likely cause is simple diarrhoea secondary to the commencement of antibiotics. However, one must be suspicious of *Clostridium difficile* as a causative organism for the diarrhoea, particularly since this patient has received a cephalosporin antibiotic.

    The stool sample indicates the presence of *C. difficile* toxin. Ideally the causative antibiotic should be stopped and a suitable alternative used instead. Oral metronidazole should also be commenced to treat the *C. difficile*.

CASE SUMMARY

Pneumonia
Exudate pleural effusion (parapneumonic)
Type 1 respiratory failure with hyperventilation
Clostridium difficile infection (secondary to antibiotic treatment)

Case 16.12

DATA COVERED IN THIS CLINICAL CASE SCENARIO

- Biochemistry: U&Es
- Endocrine: thyroid function tests
- Endocrine: short Synacthen® test
- Biochemistry: urinary electrolytes and osmolality

A 62-year-old male patient with inoperable lung cancer is admitted on the general medical take-in with acute confusion. Physical examination is unremarkable. Routine blood tests are sent, and the following results are obtained.

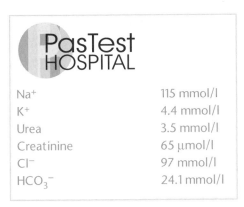

PasTest HOSPITAL

Na^+	115 mmol/l
K^+	4.4 mmol/l
Urea	3.5 mmol/l
Creatinine	65 μmol/l
Cl^-	97 mmol/l
HCO_3^-	24.1 mmol/l

1. His weight is 61 kg. Estimate his glomerular filtration rate.

On the basis of these tests, a host of other investigations are organised. The results of these are shown below.

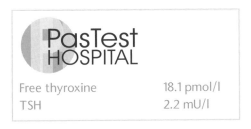

PasTest HOSPITAL

Free thyroxine	18.1 pmol/l
TSH	2.2 mU/l

2. What is his thyroid status?

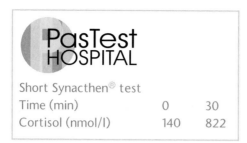

Short Synacthen® test

Time (min)	0	30
Cortisol (nmol/l)	140	822

3. **Interpret this test result.**

4. **His blood glucose is 4.6 mmol/l. Calculate his plasma osmolality.**

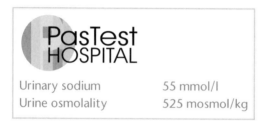

Urinary sodium	55 mmol/l
Urine osmolality	525 mosmol/kg

5. **What is the overall diagnosis?**

Answer 16.12

1. From the information given, the eGFR could be calculated (see page 62 for details). Alternatively, the following formula could be used to give an approximation of the GFR:

$$\text{Creatinine clearance} = \frac{(140 - 62) \times 61}{72 \times 65 \div 88.4} = 89.87 \text{ ml/min}$$

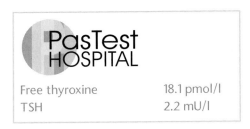

PasTest HOSPITAL

Free thyroxine	18.1 pmol/l
TSH	2.2 mU/l

2. His thyroid status is normal.

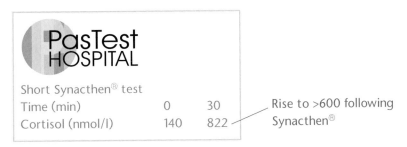

PasTest HOSPITAL

Short Synacthen® test

Time (min)	0	30
Cortisol (nmol/l)	140	822

Rise to >600 following Synacthen®

3. This is a normal short Synacthen® test indicating normal adrenal gland function.

4. Plasma osmolality is calculated as:

Plasma osmolality = 2 x (115 + 4.4) + 3.5 + 4.6 = 246.9 mosmol/kg.

5. This patient fits the diagnostic criteria for SIADH, which is most likely secondary to his lung cancer, most commonly with the small cell subtype. His confusion is probably due to hyponatraemia.

CASE SUMMARY

Hyponatraemia
SIADH

Case 16.13

DATA COVERED IN THIS CLINICAL CASE SCENARIO

- Biochemistry: sweat analysis
- Genetics: mutation analysis
- Miscellaneous: PABA test
- Haematology: D-dimer
- Microbiology: sputum culture
- Miscellaneous: audiogram

A 28-year-old patient is admitted to hospital on account of weight loss. She has an inherited condition. Browsing through old medical notes, the admitting doctor noted the following results.

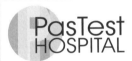

Sweat analysis
112 mg sweat collected
Cl⁻   67 mmol/l
Na⁺   101 mmol/l
Genetics laboratory
ΔF508 mutation on long arm of chromosome 7

1. **What genetic condition does this patient have, and what is the inheritance pattern?**

The medical team are concerned about pancreatic exocrine insufficiency and organise a PABA test. The following result is returned.

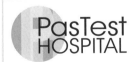

PABA test
45% of oral PABA dose excreted in the urine

2. **Does the patient have pancreatic exocrine insufficiency?**

During the course of her inpatient stay, the patient develops a cough with a degree of haemoptysis. The doctor is concerned about the possibility of a pulmonary embolism, and requests the following test urgently.

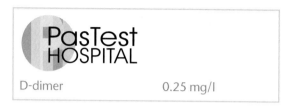

D-dimer	0.25 mg/l

3. How does the D-dimer result help in managing the patient?

The patient then becomes pyrexic, and clinical signs suggest pneumonia. The medical team commence co-amoxiclav. Sputum is sent for culture. Two days later the following result is obtained.

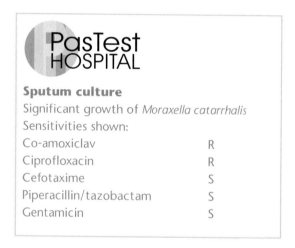

Sputum culture
Significant growth of *Moraxella catarrhalis*
Sensitivities shown:

Co-amoxiclav	R
Ciprofloxacin	R
Cefotaxime	S
Piperacillin/tazobactam	S
Gentamicin	S

On the basis of these sensitivities, and a worsening clinical state, the patient's antibiotics are changed to gentamicin.

A short time later the patient complains of hearing loss. The following audiogram is obtained.

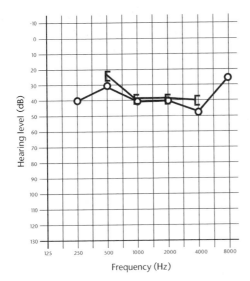

4. **What type of hearing loss has she developed, and how would you explain it?**

Answer 16.13

1. This patient has cystic fibrosis, which is inherited in an autosomal recessive manner.

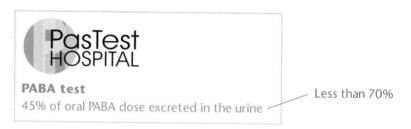

PABA test — Less than 70%
45% of oral PABA dose excreted in the urine

2. Yes. Pancreatic insufficiency is common in cystic fibrosis. More than 70% of the oral PABA should normally be excreted in the urine.

3. The D-dimer is normal. This indicates a very low probability of a thrombo-embolic event such as a pulmonary embolism. Other causes of haemoptysis should be sought. In very rare situations, the D-dimer can be normal in the presence of thrombosis, so clinical judgement is always essential when interpreting this result.

4. The audiogram shows sensorineural deafness. This is a rare but characteristic side effect of aminoglycoside antimicrobials such as gentamicin.

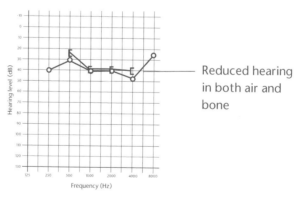

Reduced hearing in both air and bone

CASE SUMMARY

Cystic fibrosis
Pancreatic exocrine insufficiency
Pneumonia
Gentamicin-induced hearing loss

Case 16.14

DATA COVERED IN THIS CLINICAL CASE SCENARIO

- Haematology: full blood picture
- Haematology: haematinics
- Haematology: blood film
- Miscellaneous: CLO test
- Pathology: biopsy result

A 72-year-old man presents with increasing epigastric discomfort. He has been troubled with heartburn for several years. He admits to drinking 'more than he should'. The admitting doctor noted pallor, and requested the following.

PasTest HOSPITAL

Hb	7.7 g/dl
MCV	69.5 fl
Plt	512 x 10^9/l
WCC	8.7 x 10^9/l
Serum iron	5 µmol/l
Ferritin	9 µg/l
TIBC	95 µmol/l
Vitamin B_{12}	265 ng/l
Folate	12.3 µg/l

1. **How would you interpret these results?**

A blood film is examined. The following report is obtained.

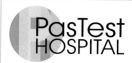

Hypochromic, microcytic cells
Poikilocytosis and anisochromia
Occasional pencil cells seen

2. Is this result in keeping with your answer to question one?

He proceeds to have an oesophagogastroduodenoscopy (OGD). Two abnormalities are noted. First, he is noted to have an abnormal appearance of the lower oesophagus. Second, gastritis is observed. A biopsy is taken from the lower oesophagus and the stomach. A CLO test is performed. You note the following after 24 h.

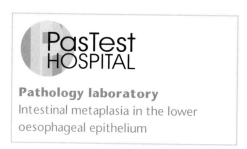

Pink circle

3. What treatment should be commenced on the basis of this CLO result?

One week later, the following result is phoned through from the pathology laboratory:

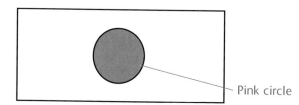

Pathology laboratory
Intestinal metaplasia in the lower
oesophageal epithelium

4. What is the condition affecting the oesophagus?

Answer 16.14

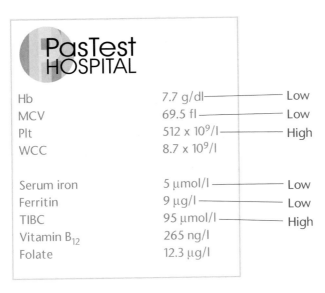

Hb	7.7 g/dl	Low
MCV	69.5 fl	Low
Plt	512 x 10⁹/l	High
WCC	8.7 x 10⁹/l	
Serum iron	5 μmol/l	Low
Ferritin	9 μg/l	Low
TIBC	95 μmol/l	High
Vitamin B₁₂	265 ng/l	
Folate	12.3 μg/l	

1. This patient has a microcytic anaemia. The mild thrombocytosis may be due to active bleeding. The haematinics show iron deficiency.

2. Yes. The abnormal blood cells described can all be found with iron deficiency.

3. The result is CLO positive, indicating gastric infection with *Helicobacter pylori*. The patient should be commenced on a course of antibiotics with a proton pump inhibitor, in an attempt to eradicate the infection.

4. The patient has a Barrett oesophagus, and will require surveillance OGDs for monitoring the disease.

CASE SUMMARY

Iron deficiency anaemia
Helicobacter pylori-positive gastritis
Barrett's oesophagus

Case 16.15

DATA COVERED IN THIS CLINICAL CASE SCENARIO

- Haematology: full blood picture
- Haematology: red cell mass
- Respiratory: arterial blood gas
- Biochemistry: urinary sodium
- Microbiology: urinalysis

An 85-year-old man who is a smoker is admitted complaining of abdominal discomfort. No abnormalities are detected on clinical examination, but some routine blood tests are requested. Your colleague is concerned about the following test result, and asks for your help.

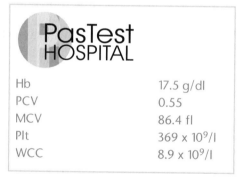

Hb	17.5 g/dl
PCV	0.55
MCV	86.4 fl
Plt	369 x 10⁹/l
WCC	8.9 x 10⁹/l

1. What is this abnormality called, and how would you proceed?

The result is repeated and confirmed. He proceeds to have an estimation of red cell mass.

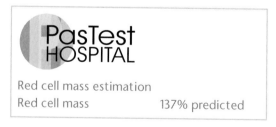

Red cell mass estimation
Red cell mass   137% predicted

2. What does this result indicate?

On the basis of this result, arterial blood gas analysis was performed when the patient was breathing room air.

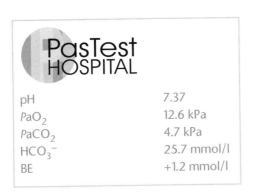

PasTest
HOSPITAL

pH	7.37
PaO_2	12.6 kPa
$PaCO_2$	4.7 kPa
HCO_3^-	25.7 mmol/l
BE	+1.2 mmol/l

3. How would you interpret the blood gas?

An ultrasound scan of the abdomen revealed a mass in keeping with a renal cell carcinoma.

The patient proceeded to surgery, and underwent a nephrectomy. He spent 2 days in the intensive care unit after the operation, but returned to the ward on day 3 after the operation. His urine output deteriorated on day 4, and a urine specimen was sent for analysis.

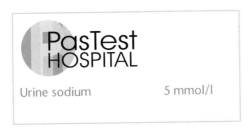

PasTest
HOSPITAL

Urine sodium	5 mmol/l

4. What does this result tell you about the cause of the oliguria, and how would you treat the patient?

The patient's urine output recovers. Several days later he complains of a burning pain on passing urine, and of having to pass urine more often than normal. The following result is obtained on urinalysis.

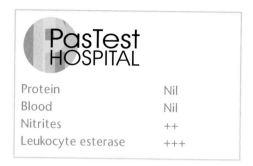

Protein	Nil
Blood	Nil
Nitrites	++
Leukocyte esterase	+++

5. **How would you interpret the urinalysis, and what further urine test would you request?**

Answer 16.15

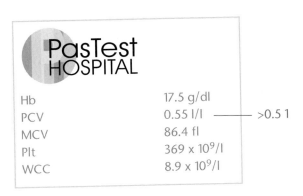

PasTest
HOSPITAL

Hb	17.5 g/dl
PCV	0.55 l/l —— >0.5 1
MCV	86.4 fl
Plt	369 x 10^9/l
WCC	8.9 x 10^9/l

1. The PCV is elevated, indicating polycythaemia. A measurement of the red cell mass is required to distinguish true polycythaemia from apparent polycythaemia.

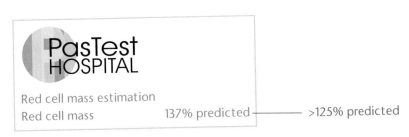

PasTest
HOSPITAL

Red cell mass estimation
Red cell mass   137% predicted —— >125% predicted

2. The red cell mass result indicates true polycythaemia, and a cause should be sought.

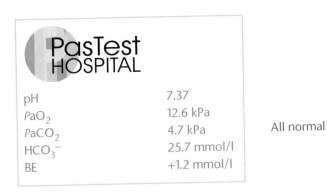

PasTest
HOSPITAL

pH	7.37
PaO$_2$	12.6 kPa
PaCO$_2$	4.7 kPa	All normal
HCO$_3^-$	25.7 mmol/l
BE	+1.2 mmol/l

3. The arterial blood gas analysis is entirely normal.

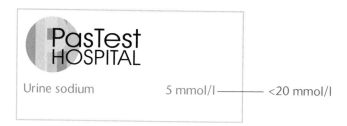

4. The urinary sodium concentration is low, suggesting that the oliguria is due to prerenal causes, ie hypovolaemia. The patient requires intravenous fluid resuscitation.

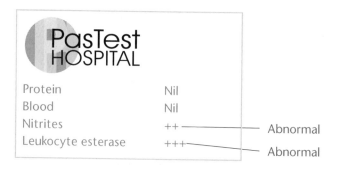

5. The urine contains nitrites and leukocyte esterase. In keeping with the clinical history, these changes are most commonly caused by a urinary tract infection. The most useful next investigation would be a urine culture.

CASE SUMMARY

Renal cell carcinoma
Postoperative prerenal uraemia
Urinary tract infection

INDEX

Page numbers in **bold** refer to the clinical cases.